Early Arrhythmias Resulting from Myocardial Ischaemia

Early Arrhythmias Resulting from Myocardial Ischaemia

Mechanisms and Prevention by Drugs

Edited by

James R. Parratt
MSc, PhD, DSc, FPS

Department of Physiology and Pharmacology, Royal College, University of Strathclyde, Glasgow, Scotland

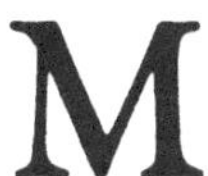

Softcover reprint of the hardcover 1st edition 1982

First published 1982 by
The Scientific and Medical Division of
Macmillan Press Ltd
London and Basingstoke
Companies and representatives throughout the world

Typeset in 10/12pt IBM (Press Roman) by
RDL., 26 Mulgrave Road, Sutton, Surrey

ISBN 978-1-349-06262-1 ISBN 978-1-349-06260-7 (eBook)
DOI 10.1007/978-1-349-06260-7

Contributors

ABRAHMSSON, T. MD	Department of Pharmacology, AB Hässle, S-431 83 Mölndal, Sweden
ALMGREN, O. MD	Department of Pharmacology, AB Hässle, S-431 83 Mölndal, Sweden
BROWNING, R. C. MB, BS, DRCOG	Pfizer Corporation, Africa Middle East Management Centre, International House, PO Box 30340, Nairobi, Kenya
COKER, S. J. PhD	Department of Physiology and Pharmacology, University of Strathclyde, George Street, Glasgow G1 1XW, Scotland
CORR, P. B. MD	Professor, Department of Medicine (Cardiovascular Division), Washington University School of Medicine, 660 South Euclid Avenue, St Louis, Missouri 63110, USA
DENNIS, S. C. PhD	The Lickoff Cardiovascular Institute, Hahnemann Medical College, Philadelphia, Pennsylvania 19102, USA
FITZGERALD, J. D. MD, FRCP	Head of Research Department II, Imperial Chemical Industries PLC Pharmaceuticals Division, Alderley Park, Macclesfield, Cheshire, UK
HEARSE, D. J. PhD	Chief Investigator, Myocardial Metabolism Research Laboratories, The Rayne Institute, St Thomas' Hospital, London SE1, UK
HIRCHE, Hj. MD	Professor and Director, Institute für Angewandte Physiologie, Medizinische

	Einrichtungen der Universität zu Köln, 5 Köln 41, Robert-Koch-Strasse 39, Koln-Lindenthal, West Germany
HOLMGREN, S. MD	Department of Zoophysiology, University of Göteborg, Göteborg, Sweden
JANSE, M. J. MD	Department of Cardiology and Clinical Physiology, University Hospital Wilhelmina Gasthuis, Eerste Halmersstraat 104, 1054 EG, Amsterdam, The Netherlands, and Inter-university Cardiology Institute, Amsterdam, The Netherlands
LAB, M. J. PhD	Department of Physiology, Charing Cross Hospital Medical School, London W6 8RF, UK
MARSHALL, R. J. PhD	Head of Department of Pharmacology, Scientific Development Group, Organon Laboratories Limited, Newhouse, Lanarkshire, Scotland
MEESMANN, W. MD	Professor and Head of Department, Institut für Pathophysiologie, Universitätsklinikum Essen, Hufelandstrasse 55, D4300 Essen, Federal Republic of Germany
OLIVER, M. F. MD, FRCP	Duke of Edinburgh Professor of Cardiology, University Department of Medicine, The Royal Infirmary, Edinburgh EH3 9YW and Cardiovascular Research Unit, Hugh Robson Building, George Square, Edinburgh EH8 9XF, Scotland
PARRATT, J. R. PhD, DSc	Professor, Department of Physiology and Pharmacology, University of Strathclyde, George Street, Glasgow G1 1XW, Scotland
PODZUWEIT, T. MD	Max-Planck-Institute for Physiological and Clinical Research, W.G. Kerckhoff Institut, Parkstrasse 1, D-6350 Bad Nauheim, Federal Republic of Germany

RIEMERSMA, R. A. PhD	University of Edinburgh, Cardiovascular Research Unit, Hugh Robson Building, George Square, Edinburgh EH8 9XF, Scotland
RUSSELL, D. MD, MRCP	Department of Medicine, The Royal Infirmary, Edinburgh EH3 9YW, and Cardiovascular Research Unit, Hugh Robson Building, George Square, Edinburgh EH8 9XF, Scotland
SHANKS, R. G. MD, DSc, MRCP	Whitla Professor of Pharmacology, Department of Therapeutics and Pharmacology, Queen's University, Whitla Medical Building, 97 Lisburn Road, Belfast, BT9 7BL, Northern Ireland
SHERIDAN, D. MD, MRCP	Department of Cardiology, Welsh National School of Medicine, University of Wales, Heath Park, Cardiff CF4 4XN, Wales
SOBEL, B. E. MD	Professor and Head, Department of Medicine (Cardiovascular Division), Washington University School of Medicine, 660 South Euclid Avenue, St Louis, Missouri 63110, USA
SZEKERES, L. MD, DSc	Professor and Head of Institute of Pharmacology, University Medical School of Szeged, Dom ter 12, Szeged, Hungary
WINSLOW, E. PhD	Department of Pharmacology, Scientific Development Group, Organon Laboratories Limited, Newhouse, Lanarkshire, Scotland

Contents

Foreword

This book was based on a meeting of the Cardiac Muscle Research Group organised by Professor Parratt and held in Glasgow in March 1981.

The Cardiac Muscle Research Group was started in 1972 by Keith Gibson and David Hearse. It came into being to provide a forum for scientists in Britain interested in the working of the heart. It has flourished on informality and flexibility. Its proceedings are not published. It has, however, welcomed experiment. This meeting was one such, in that it drew on a more international field of speakers than usual and in that what are in effect its proceedings form the basis for this book.

The meeting well exemplified the Group's purpose in providing for an interdisciplinary approach with basic scientists and clinicians addressing from their different standpoints the focal subjects of, on this occasion, the mechanisms and prevention of early arrhythmias resulting from myocardial ischaemia. The importance of the subject needs no emphasising, 'sudden death' because of just such arrhythmias being perhaps the single biggest medical problem in the developed countries today.

Andrew Henderson MD FRCP,
Professor of Cardiology,
Welsh National School of Medicine;
Former Chairman, Cardiac
Muscle Research Group

Preface

When a coronary artery is occluded in experimental animals ventricular arrhythmias arise within minutes and it is during this early ischaemic period, or during subsequent reperfusion, that ventricular fibrillation is most likely to occur. Later there is an arrhythmia-free period followed, hours later, by further pronounced ventricular ectopic activity. It is the early, life-threatening arrhythmias that are the subject of this book. Their importance lies, as Michael Oliver emphasises in the opening chapter, in their relation to clinical sudden cardiac death.

The present volume has two aims. Firstly, it reviews what is known about how these early arrhythmias arise and especially deals with the relationship between the severity of these arrhythmias, electrophysiological changes and alterations in local myocardial blood flow, metabolism and mechanical 'strain'. It then considers in depth the chemical arrhythmogenic factors (potassium, noradrenaline, cyclic AMP, prostaglandins and lysophosphoglycerides) that might trigger these arrhythmias. Particular emphasis is placed on the role of the sympathetic nervous system in the genesis of these early arrhythmias (chapters 8-10, 16 and 17). The second aim is to review current knowledge about the sensitivity of these arrhythmias to drugs. It is clear that it is possible, at least in the experimental situation, to suppress these life-threatening arrhythmias by appropriate pretreatment with a number of different classes of pharmacological agents (sodium and calcium channel inhibitors, α- and β-adrenoceptor blocking drugs and drugs that inhibit platelet function and thromboxane release). This means that there are now a number of possibilities for the *prophylactic* treatment of individuals at risk from an acute coronary attack. However, we know little about which drugs, if any, are effective in terminating these arrhythmias and in reducing the possibility of ventricular fibrillation occurring, when given *after* the onset of ischaemia.

The majority of the contributions to this volume are based on presentations and review lectures given at a meeting of the Cardiac Muscle Research Group held in the University of Strathclyde (Glasgow) and at Ross Priory (Gartocharn, Loch Lomond) in March 1981. This meeting drew together a number of cardiologists and basic scientists from within the United Kingdom and from the continent of Europe. The presentations have been greatly expanded for the present publication and each contributor was asked to review in depth his or her particular specialised area. I am grateful for the enthusaistic help of all the contributors and especially to those (Michiel Janse, Burton Sobel, Peter Corr and Laszlo Szekeres) who were not present at the original meeting but who so readily agreed to review their own areas of expertise. I am also grateful to those friends in the pharmaceutical industry who provided generous financial support for the original meeting, to the members of my own cardiovascular group for help in proof reading and especially to Liz Marshall who so ably typed the complete edited book and who helped, with Dr Richard Marshall, in the preparation of the index.

My hope for this volume is that it will stimulate, encourage and help those involved in studying the mechanisms and drug treatment of the early arrhythmias arising after myocardial ischaemia. The ultimate purpose of all this research is a deeper understanding and better clinical treatment of these life-threatening arrhythmias.

Glasgow, 1982 J.R.P.

1

Sudden Cardiac Death – An Overview

Michael F. Oliver

1.1 INTRODUCTION AND EPIDEMIOLOGY

Sudden cardiac death was ignored until the last decade because successful reversal of ventricular fibrillation (VF), its most common cause, was a recent medical advance (Zoll *et al.*, 1956), because the brevity of the event pre-empted studies of its causes (and still does) and because it commonly occurs without praecordial tightness or any precise clinical syndrome.

The majority of deaths from coronary heart disease are sudden and, defined as deaths occurring within 1 h of last being seen alive, they represent approximately one-third of the total expression of ischaemic heart disease (IHD) (Armstrong *et al.*, 1972). It can be calculated that there will be about 20-30 deaths per week from sudden cardiac death in most populations of one million (Pisa, 1980).

The Edinburgh Community Study showed that 43 per cent of all deaths occurring within 4 weeks of the onset of a heart attack took place within 1 h and 50 per cent within 2 h (Armstrong *et al.*, 1972). The WHO Myocardial Infarction Register Study (1976) showed that only 8 per cent of patients dying during the first hour were seen by a medical person, and that of 1114 dying within the first half hour only 47 were so attended. It follows that the contribution to the reduction of very early cardiac mortality by coronary care units (where the median time of admission is usually 4 h or more) or even by mobile coronary care units, cannot be expected to be great (Oliver, 1978a).

Removal of the emphasis from coronary care in hospital to the provision in the community of defibrillators for those who suddenly develop lethal ventricular arrhythmias has shown that this is where the maximum yield lies. In Seattle, where the emergency services such as fire brigades have been trained in resuscitation procedures, between 50 and 60 per cent of patients with out-of-hospital VF have been successfully resuscitated and 25-30 per cent were discharged home (Cobb *et al.*, 1980). But this is an unusual community service and it is not widely applicable.

The focus of research should be on how and why VF develops and on the circumstances leading to it - *ante hoc* not *post hoc*.

1.2 PATHOLOGY

The majority of patients dying suddenly have extensive coronary atherosclerosis (Kuller *et al.*, 1975; Perper *et al.*, 1975). Interestingly, predominant involvement of all three main coronary arteries (triple vessel disease) is not the rule and in the Seattle series (Cobb *et al.*, 1975) as many had minimal or one-vessel coronary disease as those with two-vessel, three-vessel or left main vessel disease. A pathological survey (Thomas *et al.*, 1980) has shown that almost as many cases of sudden cardiac death had occlusion of the right coronary artery (39 per cent) as of the left anterior descending coronary artery (43 per cent); in acute myocardial infarction the figures were 28 per cent and 54 per cent respectively.

Acute regional myocardial ischaemia is the basis for the development of the ventricular arrhythmias which lead to sudden cardiac death (figure 1.1). Most sudden cardiac deaths are not associated with identifiable myocardial infarction or coronary thrombosis at autopsy (Lovegrove and Thompson, 1978). Electrocardiographic evidence of myocardial infarction is present in less than 20 per cent of those resuscitated from VF (Cobb *et al.*, 1980). Patients who survive VF without developing myocardial infarction have a worse long term prognosis than those who

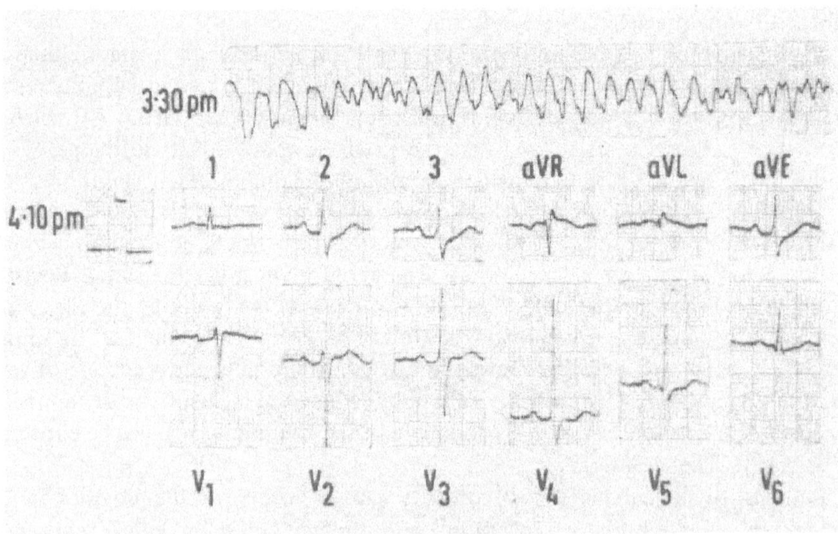

Figure 1.1 This 34 year old man developed ventricular fibrillation when witnessing the birth of his first baby. He had previously been entirely well. The maternity department is equipped with an electrocardiogram and defibrillator and this was immediately applied. Forty minutes later a virtually normal 12-lead electrocardiogram was recorded. The man has been seen annually for the last 7 years and has no symptoms. Coronary arteriography indicated a 70 per cent obstruction of the distal part of the right coronary artery.

survive VF and develop infarction. In the Seattle study (Cobb *et al.*, 1980) 22 per cent of the former category and 2 per cent of the latter category died from sudden death within the next year. Repeated ischaemia could lead to repeated episodes of electrophysiological instability in a regionally vulnerable area of myocardium. In contrast, infarcted and necrotic tissue is not subjected to ischaemia to the same extent since it is no longer viable. The lethal consequences of a wave of regional ischaemia are theoretically and potentially reversible, by treatment of its causes (for example, relief of coronary spasm) or by defibrillation, or both.

1.3 PATHOGENESIS OF VENTRICULAR FIBRILLATION

There has been a tendency in the past to think of myocardial ischaemia as being widespread not regional, uniform not heterogenous and stable not dynamic. This may have arisen in the minds of pathologists because they are accustomed to seeing clearly defined infarcts at post mortem, and in the minds of clinicians because they read electrocardiograms which are not capable of specifying with any accuracy the extent of the ischaemia. The tendency may have arisen in the minds of investigators, because global hypoxia or anoxia is a common experimental model which is often confused with ischaemia. The regionally ischaemic myocardium should be thought of as an area of constantly changing dynamic relationships with regard to blood flow, ionic fluxes and substrate availability.

Primary VF is more likely to be a result of irregular impulse propagation through re-entry circuits in ventricular muscle than of an accelerated impulse from pacemaker fibres (Wit and Bigger, 1975), although the latter may contribute to secondary VF once myocardial infarction has been established. Two basic problems are as follows:

(1) Why does local or regional myocardial ischaemia occur?

(2) Precisely what effects does ischaemia have on myocardial metabolism and on the electrophysiological influences which alter normal propagation of the conducting impulse to produce VF?

The intracellular biochemical response of myocardial tissue to ischaemia has often been reviewed (for example, Opie, 1975; Katz, 1977; Oliver, 1978b), although there are still many aspects requiring clarification. One of the very earliest changes is thought to be the release of myocardial noradrenaline. This was first demonstrated in the isolated blood-perfused dog heart (Shahab *et al.*, 1972). We have, however, been unable to show any overflow of noradrenaline into the venous effluent from either ischaemic or non-ischaemic areas of the dog heart *in vivo* during short coronary artery occlusions (see chapter 8). Loss of fluorescence does take place round nerve endings but, since a net release of noradrenaline does not occur, rapid re-uptake by nerve endings or local catabolism is likely. This question is discussed in detail in chapters 8, 9 and 10. What effects release may have is unclear but local stimulation of adenylate cyclase might be expected during any myocardial redistribution of noradrenaline. An increase in cyclic AMP (cAMP) occurs in the ischaemic region in baboons before the onset of VF (Podzuweit *et al.*, 1978), although more experimental evidence must be accrued before it can be concluded that cAMP really is a precursor stimulus to VF (Lubbe *et al.*, 1976; Podzuweit *et al.*, 1978). Some of the evidence for this hypothesis is outlined by Podzuweit in chapter 11. Another unresolved area is the significance of prostaglandin release from the ischaemic myocardium (chapter 13). Both prostacyclin (as 6-keto $PGF_1\alpha$) and thromboxane (TX) A_2 (as TXB_2) have been identified in the venous effluent from the ischaemic area (Hirsh *et al.*, 1981) and related experimentally to the incidence of ventricular arrhythmias (Coker *et al.*, 1981). Yet another uncertain problem (discussed in chapter 12) is the importance of lysolecithin release (Corr *et al.*, 1979) and whether loss of lysophosphatidylcholine from membranes might lead to arrhythmias or act as a 'carrier' for free fatty acid detergency.

Whatever the significance of catecholamine, cAMP, prostaglandin, phospholipid and substrate changes, an acute and local inhomogeneity of K^+, Na^+ and Ca^{2+} fluxes is likely to be the pathway through which they lead to re-entry arrhythmias. The relative importance of these determinants of re-entry is uncertain, but what has become clear is the probable importance of 'gradients' of difference in local myocardial blood flow (see chapter 3) in ionic equilibria and in substrate availability. The concept has been advanced that non-ischaemic myocardial or Purkinje cells play an essential role in the initial phase of ischaemia by being recipients of premature impulses arising in the ischaemic area and delivering multiple micro re-entry stimuli back to ischaemic tissue (Janse *et al.*, 1980, and discussed in detail by Janse in chapter 4). It has been possible to map some of these 'gradients' immediately before, and at the onset of, VF in dogs with induced myocardial ischaemia, and recently we have constructed three-dimensional diagrams to demonstrate them (reviewed in chapter 3). These and other studies using $NADH_2$ fluorescence photography, K^+ and hydrogen ion concentrations, and ATP content show that multiple patchy areas of ischaemia exist within the affected zone. The ischaemic area is far from uniform and this inhomogeneity may not only cause selective local imbalance of ions and metabolites but modulate energy-dependent electrophysiological effects, such as slow response potential activity.

1.4 CAUSES OF VENTRICULAR FIBRILLATION

There are many local triggers in the coronary circulation and myocardium to the development of regional ischaemia and therefore of VF. Some of these are listed in table 1.1.

Perhaps the most important of all modulating influences for VF is the autonomic nervous system – and especially sympathetic nerve stimulation. This increases the

Table 1.1 Local causes of lethal ventricular arrhythmias

Coronary artery spasm
Reflow after spasm
Platelet thrombosis
Platelet emboli
Ruptured atheromatous plaque with or without emboli
Increased myocardial oxygen demands in the presence of fixed coronary reserve
Local ionic or metabolic disequilibrium
Combination of above

excitability and automaticity of myocardial cells, reduces refractoriness and reduces the threshold at which VF can be induced experimentally (Lown *et al.*, 1973). The influence of psychological stress in angina is well known and there are several well documented examples of VF occurring in otherwise healthy people in association with acute stress. Being 'frightened to death' is not a new concept (figure 1.1) and psychophysiological stimuli, including behavioural stress, can alter cardiac vulnerability and the susceptibility of the myocardium to VF. β-Adrenoceptor blockade prevents stress-induced alterations in cardiac vulnerability, suggesting that the decrease in VF threshold is mediated by the sympathetic limb of the autonomic nervous system (Matta *et al.*, 1976). However, only partial protection can be conferred by removal of the stellate ganglia, suggesting that other adrenergic inputs, probably derived from the adrenal medulla, are important. Enhanced vagal activity has an antiarrhythmic effect and, by decreasing heart rate, improves perfusion of ischaemic tissue and reduces the likelihood of VF. However, if excessive, profound bradycardia could produce hypotension and reduce coronary flow, thus precipitating VF. The role of neural factors has been admirably reviewed recently (Lown *et al.*, 1977).

Distortions of the neural control of the heart may be transient, prolonged or permanent. The former is probably of little importance except where there is co-existing myocardial ischaemia or the potential for its development. In these circumstances, sudden acceleration or slowing of the heart rate, or temporary impairment of atrioventricular conduction, could be critical. More prolonged distortion of neural control can be due to disease involving nerves and ganglia of the heart and this can lead to sudden and unexpected death (James, 1980). This disease may be focal and asymmetrical and may be especially important in causing electrophysiological abnormalities and instability. Inhomogeneous sympathetic neural influences on the ventricular myocardium could lead to serious abnormalities of repolarisation. Neuropathy of this type can occur in collagen disorders, heritable neuromuscular and muscular-skeletal disorders and, quite possibly, inadequate emphasis has been given to it occurring as a consequence of ischaemic degeneration - in other words, another manifestation of ischaemic heart disease with specific involvement of the tissues most likely to lead to ventricular electrical instability. If so, our attention should really be given to the prevention of IHD itself.

1.5 IS PREDICTION OF SUDDEN DEATH POSSIBLE?

The picture of the patient who dies suddenly is really the opposite to that of the patient who is admitted to a coronary care unit with classical symptoms. Studies of the incidence of IHD in communities, and coroner's surveys, have consistently shown that patients who first present with sudden cardiac death are those with the fewest symptoms (Duncan *et al.*, 1976). If the victim of imminent sudden cardiac death actually has no symptoms, or dismisses or denies them sufficiently not to complain, how are we going to predict or institute preventive treatment? Is it possible, at least, to identify individuals with a high risk of sudden cardiac death, that is of VF? It does not seem from the many epidemiological surveys that the usual risk factors for IHD have any greater weighting for sudden cardiac death than for acute myocardial infarction. For example, hypercholesterolaemia, hypertension, diabetes mellitus or obesity are not associated with sudden cardiac death any more than with acute myocardial infarction or angina. There are, however, other possible risk factors to consider (table 1.2).

Table 1.2 Profile of sudden cardiac death

Factors perhaps more associated with sudden death than acute myocardial infarction

Relative youth
Physical inactivity
Excess cigarette smoking
Ventricular premature beats
Sustained tachycardia
Minor QRS conduction defects
Cardiomegaly
Triple vessel disease

Factors equally associated with sudden cardiac death and acute myocardial infarction

Hypercholesterolaemia
Hypertension
Diabetes mellitus
Obesity

Studies on insured persons suggest that sudden cardiac death is more common in young adults than in the elderly (Morgan Jones, 1969). This is not particularly surprising since a major coronary occlusion occurring in a myocardium in which collateral vessels are poorly developed may lead to a larger area of ischaemia than in a heart where there have been a number of small and gradual occlusions over many years with resultant good collateral vessel formation.

A large survey of executive grades of civil servants has concluded that those who regularly undertake really vigorous exercise have less cardiac death than comparable control subjects (Morris *et al.*, 1973); excessive physical activity can also *cause* instantaneous death (Kala *et al.*, 1978).

In a large population survey comprising a 5 year follow-up of 269 755 individuals (Hinkle, 1981) early cycle ventricular premature beats (VPBs), sustained tachycardia and episodes of sinus delay all carried a greater risk of sudden cardiac death. However, the actual risk was small and a large proportion of those who ultimately died had other features of heart disease. In post-infarct patients the occurrence of frequent VPBs is a weak predictor of sudden death.

Atherosclerotic occlusions of all three major coronary arteries is a common autopsy finding in cases of sudden cardiac death. Thus 108 out of 121 patients who died suddenly had triple vessel disease and the remaining 13 had two coronary arteries involved (Lie and Titus, 1972). However, the Seattle experience of angiography in survivors of VF showed single vessel disease in many (Cobb *et al.*, 1975).

What is really required is a prospective community study to determine, after many measurements, the relative importance of each possible risk factor in predicting sudden cardiac death. This would have to be very large, time-consuming and expensive, but until it is done it will not be possible to evaluate the real importance of the above and other risk factors, or to predict with any confidence who is going to die suddenly. This is a real epidemiological and cardiological priority.

More economically, such a study might be conducted in a high risk community (such as patients with unstable angina), although the answers would not necessarily be the same as in an entirely fit population. Two such studies have been made in order to maximise our information about patients likely to die suddenly. In Edinburgh (Duncan *et al.*, 1976) a study was made of 251 ambulant patients with recent onset angina, and in Rotterdam (van der Does and Lusben, 1978) of 252 patients with more severe angina (or the intermediate syndrome of prolonged chest pain) in order to determine their prognosis and whether it might be possible to discriminate those who would develop a heart attack from those who would not and, within the former category, those who would die suddenly. Both studies showed that the 6 month prognosis in patients with recent onset angina is better than often thought, with about 15 per cent developing myocardial infarction, 4 per cent dying and 2.5 per cent dying suddenly. But the level of prediction of any of these events in both studies was poor, although better in the Rotterdam study (as might be expected in view of the greater severity of symptoms in these patients). Multiple regression analyses were made in both studies using a variety of clinical, electrocardiographic (including arrhythmias), haemodynamic and biochemical measurements. None either singly or together provided any firmly useful predictive index. The only consistent adverse prognostic finding was an increased cardiothoracic ratio, radiologically.

In Edinburgh, a second smaller survey of ambulant patients with recent onset angina has shown radionuclide assessment of left ventricular function to be of value in discriminating patients (H. J. Smith, A. L. Muir and M. F. Oliver, unpublished). In most of those patients who subsequently developed myocardial infarction, the left ventricular ejection fraction decreased in response to exercise. In most of the group with a good prognosis, the ejection fraction increased with exercise. While the discrimination between these groups was not absolute, it appears to be a good pointer towards the prediction of immediate outcome.

The combination of exercise electrocardiography and myocardial imaging using thallium-201 to detect the appearance of a defect in myocardial uptake is promising. Together, these techniques are likely to provide more information than either alone. So far neither exercise electrocardiography using multiple leads nor myocardial imaging during exercise have been used prospectively.

But, we are very far from really reliable identification of the characteristics of those likely to develop VF - let alone the individual - and without improved sensitivity and specificity in prediction, prevention of VF is academic.

1.6 PREVENTION OF VENTRICULAR FIBRILLATION

Were we able to predict who is imminently at risk of developing VF, the aim should be to develop an oral treatment which will prevent its onset and protect the potentially vulnerable myocardium before the onset of acute ischaemia. Preventive treatment might have to be given for several weeks or months at a time. One approach in combating the adverse effects of acute myocardial ischaemia is to reduce both the systemic and myocardial catecholamine response. This could be achieved through adrenoceptor blockade. Another approach is to use other antiarrhythmic drugs, but this presupposes that such drugs can be given conveniently, that they are effective and that they are not toxic. The pharmacology of such drugs is considered later in this book. Another and more physiological approach is to 'condition' that myocardium against a wave of ischaemia should an acute occlusion occur.

No prospective studies in healthy or high risk individuals of the effects of β-adrenoceptor blocking drugs, of antiarrhythmic drugs or of interventions to optimise ischaemic myocardial metabolism have been reported - and probably none are in progress. Thus subsequent comments concerning the value of these methods of treatment relate to patients who presumably have IHD.

Several clinical trials in which β-adrenoceptor blocking drugs have been used following myocardial infarction (Multicentre International Study, 1975; Norwegian Multicenter Study Group, 1981; Hjalmarson *et al.*, 1981; BHAT Research Group, 1982) have reported reduction of cardiac deaths (see chapter 16) and most reports distinguish clearly between the effects of these drugs on sudden cardiac death (death occurring within less than 1 h of last being seen alive), later deaths and recurrence of myocardial infarction. As would be expected if the effect of these drugs is primarily antiarrhythmic, the greatest benefit was on sudden cardiac death. Reduction of sudden death rates also occurred in patients with unstable angina given a β-blocker (Yusuf *et al.*, 1980). Experimentally, protection against VF by antagonism of sympathetic influences through β-adrenoceptor blockade is also successful and is also discussed in chapter 16. α-adrenoceptor blockade (see chapter 17) and some coronary dilator drugs (see chapter 18) also reduce susceptibility to VF. This protective effect may be partly due to maintenance of blood flow rather than to any direct myocardial effect.

There has been only one prospective trial (Valentine *et al.*, 1974) of antiarrhythmic therapy in the pre-hospital days of acute myocardial infarction. In a group of 269 patients with suspected or pending myocardial infarction there was a marginal benefit in reduction of sudden death or ventricular fibrillation in those receiving lignocaine compared with those receiving saline. Many trials have been performed with different antiarrhythmic drugs in patients with acute myocardial infarction. Lignocaine is the drug most commonly used and, while there is no doubt that it is a potent suppressor of ventricular arrhythmias, its effectiveness in protecting against primary ventricular fibrillation is not established (see chapters 15 and 20). A review of 13 controlled trials (Noneman and Rogers, 1978) has shown that only two of them suggest a protective effect of lignocaine and only one of the 13 studies was free of major shortcomings and trial design. However, this particular study (Lie *et al.*, 1974) did suggest that lignocaine given during the first 48 h can prevent primary ventricular fibrillation during infarction. A recent report (Chamberlain *et al.*, 1980) has indicated that mexiletine given for 6 months after myocardial infarction has no effect in reducing sudden or non-sudden cardiac death. In chapter 20 of this book Shanks reviews the drug treatment of arrhythmias in the early stages of clinical myocardial infarction. The Anturan re-infarction trial (Anturan Reinfarction Trial Research Group, 1978) suggested that sulphinpyrazone can lead to reduction of sudden cardiac death after myocardial infarction. This trial has been severely and correctly criticised and the results were not confirmed by a recent Italian trial (Anturan Reinfarction Italian Study, 1982). The possibility remains that similar pharmacological approaches to platelet adhesiveness might be associated with reduction of sudden cardiac death, although this has not been shown in trials of aspirin.

The provision of the potentially ischaemic myocardium with a balance of substrates sufficiently optimum to decrease the extent of ischaemia or to reduce inhomogeneity is theoretically attractive. Some experimental approaches have been directed towards improving myocardial blood flow, altering pH, rectifying abnormal electrolyte gradients or improving the availability of substrates for optimum oxidative phosphorylation. Since postulating the free fatty acid (FFA) hypothesis (Kurien and Oliver, 1970), in which we suggested that many episodes of VF might have a metabolic basis, we have been particularly interested in the former approach. Sharp differences in substrate and ion availability could be responsible for local loss of viability and, if these could be ameliorated, the danger of re-entry arrhythmias might be reduced. The aim of metabolic intervention is to decrease excessive peripheral and myocardial lipolysis, to increase available glucose and to conserve lactate production. In dogs, for example, mild ischaemic changes produced in the cardiac muscle action potential as a result of an occlusion of a small branch of a coronary artery can be completely rectified by glucose administration (Russell and Oliver, 1979) and, to some extent, by antilipolytic treatment. In contrast, a higher occlusion with larger areas of ischaemia does not respond in this way and action potential shortening remains unchanged. The analogy in man is that hyperosmolar concentrations of glucose reduce the mortality and morbidity in patients with mild to moderate myocardial infarction but have no beneficial effect in those with severe injury (Rogers *et al.*, 1976). The larger the area of ischaemia, the greater the extent of anaerobic metabolism in the centre and the less likely it is that raising glucose or lowering FFA concentrations in perfusing coronary blood (if it actually penetrates to that area) will make much difference. Inhomogeneities of refractoriness associated with acute myocardial ischaemia can also be rectified by raising the molar concentrations of glucose. Similarly, using an extrastimulus system to induce multiple ventricular premature beats, glucose has been shown to increase the threshold at which they occur and can therefore be regarded as 'protective'.

Antilipolytic treatment, using an analogue of nicotinic acid which reduces elevated serum FFA without any haemodynamic effects, has been shown to reduce the incidence of serious ventricular arrhythmias in patients with acute myocardial infarction, provided that it is given so that FFA concentrations are reduced quickly and consistently during the first few hours after the heart attack (Rowe *et al.*, 1975). ST-segment elevation in patients with acute myocardial ischaemia and infarction has also been reduced by giving antilipolytic treatment. Similarly, the extent of ST depression induced by exercise in patients with angina has been reduced by controlling FFA availability through antilipolytic treatment (Luxton *et al.*, 1976).

An altogether greater effort is needed to test the potential of metabolic intervention in high risk patients with unstable angina. Initial results are encouraging. It is not entirely fanciful to suggest that raising the blood sugar, easily achieved by mouth, could be an otherwise harmless prophylactic for VF during transient episodes of potentially reversible ischaemia.

1.7 CONCLUSION

Perhaps it is too optimistic to continue to search for a unifying cause of VF and sudden cardiac death: it is, after all, no more than a finite endpoint of a very heterogenous set of circumstances in the myocardium. Perhaps we should also recognise that it is not possible to predict who will develop VF: James (1982) has suggested that sudden death might largely be a matter of chance. If so, we may have to re-arrange our thoughts on the subject and accept that preventive treatment of the brief fatal arrhythmia is beyond us and give even more attention to control of the precipitating causes and of IHD.

REFERENCES

Anturan Reinfarction Trial Research Group (1978). Sulfinpyrazone in the prevention of cardiac death after myocardial infarction. *New Engl. J. Med.*, **298**, 289-95

Anturan Reinfarction Italian Study (1982). Sulphinpyrazone in post-myocardial infarction. *Lancet*, *i*, 237-42

Armstrong, A., Duncan, B., Oliver, M. F., Julian, D. G., Donald, K. W., Fulton, M., Lutz, W. and Morrison, S. L. (1972). Natural history of acute coronary heart attacks. A community study. *Br. Heart J.*, **34**, 67-80

Beta-blocker Heart Trial Research Group (1982). A randomized trial of propranolol in patients with acute myocardial infarction. *J. Am. med. Assoc.*, **247**, 1707-14

Chamberlain, D. A., Jewitt, D. E., Julian, D. G., Campbell, R. W. F., Boyle, D. McC. and Shanks, R. G. (1980). Oral mexiletine in high-risk patients after myocardial infarction. *Lancet*, *ii*, 1324-7

Cobb, L. A., Baum, R. S., Alvarez, H. and Schaffer, W. A. (1975). Resuscitation from out-of-hospital ventricular fibrillation: four year follow-up. *Circulation*, **51/52**, Suppl. III, 223-8

Cobb, L. A., Werner, J. A. and Trobaugh, G. B. (1980). Sudden cardiac death. *Mod. Concepts cardiovasc. Dis.*, **49**, 31-42

Coker, S. J., Ledingham, I. McA., Parratt, J. R. and Zeitlin, I. J. (1981). Aspirin inhibits the early myocardial release of thromboxane B_2 and ventricular ectopic activity following acute coronary artery occlusion in dogs. *Br. J. Pharmac.*, **72**, 593-5

Corr, P. B., Cain, M. E., Witkowski, F. X., Price, D. A. and Sobel, B. E. (1979). Potential arrhythmogenic electrophysiological derangements in canine Purkinje fibers induced by lysophosphoglycerides. *Circulation Res.*, **44**, 822-32

Does, E. van der and Lubsen, J. (1978). Acute coronary events in general practice. The Imminent Myocardial Infarction Rotterdam Study. Thesis, Rotterdam.

Duncan, B., Fulton, M., Morrison, S. L., Lutz, W., Donald, K. W., Kerr, F., Kirby, B. J., Julian, D. G. and Oliver, M. F. (1976). Prognosis of new and worsening angina pectoris. *Br. med. J.*, *i*, 981-5

Hinkle, L. E. (1981). The immediate antecedents of sudden death. In *Myocardial Ischaemia* (ed. J. Kjekhus, P. Lund-Johansen and S. Helle Berg), *Acta med. scand.*, Suppl., 207-17

Hirsh, P. D., Hillis, D., Campbell, W. B., Firth, B. G. and Willerson, J. T. (1981). Release of prostaglandins and thromboxane into the coronary circulation in patients with ischaemic heart disease. *New Engl. J. Med.*, **304**, 685-91

Hjalmarson, A., Elmfeldt, D., Herlitz, J., Holmberg, S., Malek, I., Nyberg, G., Ryden, L., Swedberg, K., Vedin, A., Waagstein, F., Waldenstrom, A., Waldenstrom, J., Wedel, H., Wilhelmsen, L. and Wilhelmsson, C. (1981). Effect on mortality of metoprolol in acute myocardial infarction: a double-blind randomised trial. *Lancet*, *ii*, 823-7

James, T. N. (1980). Neural pathology of the heart in sudden death. In *Sudden Death* (ed. H. E. Kulbertus and H. J. J. Wellens), Martinus Nijhoff, The Hague, pp. 49-65

James, T. N. (1981). Chance and sudden death – lessons from nature. *Progr. Cardiol.*, **10**, 101-27

Janse, M. J., Morsink, H., Van Capelle, F. J. L., Klever, A. G., Wilms-Schopman, F. and Durrer, D. (1980). Ventricular arrhythmias in the first 15 minutes of acute regional myocardial ischaemia in the isolated pig heart: possible role of injury currents. In *Sudden Death* (ed. H. E. Kulbertus and H. J. J. Wellens), Martinus Nijhoff, The Hague, pp. 89-103

Kala, R., Romo, M., Siltanen, P. and Halonen, P. I. (1978). Physical activity and sudden cardiac death. *Adv. Cardiol.*, **25**, 28-34

Katz, A. M. (1977). *Physiology of the Heart*, Raven Press, New York

Kuller, L. H., Perper, J. A. and Cooper, M. C. (1975). Sudden and unexpected death due to arteriosclerotic heart diseases. In *Modern Trends in Cardiology*, Vol. 3 (ed. M. F. Oliver), Butterworth, London, pp. 292-332

Kurien, V. A. and Oliver, M. F. (1970). A metabolic cause for arrhythmias during acute myocardial hypoxia. *Lancet*, *i*, 813-5

Lie, J. T. and Titus, J. L. (1972). Early myocardial ischaemia in sudden death from coronary heart disease. *Proc. 5th Asian-Pacific Congr. Cardiol.*, 542-5

Lie, K. I., Wellens, H. J., van Capelle, F. J. and Durrer, D. (1974). Lidocaine in the prevention of primary ventricular fibrillation. *New Engl. J. Med.*, **291**, 1324-6

Lovegrove, T. and Thompson, P. (1978). The role of acute myocardial infarction in sudden cardiac death - a statistician's nightmare. *Am. Heart J.*, **96**, 711-3

Lown, B., Verrier, R. L. and Corbalan, R. (1973). Psychological stress and threshold for repetitive ventricular response. *Science, N.Y.*, **182**, 834-6

Lown, B., Verrier, R. L. and Rabinowitz, S. H. (1977). Neurological and psychological medicine and the problems of sudden cardiac death. *Am. J. Cardiol.*, **39**, 890-902

Lubbe, W. F., Bricknell, O. L., Podzuweit, T. and Opie, L. H. (1976). Cyclic AMP as a determinant of vulnerability to ventricular fibrillation in the isolated rat heart. *Cardiovasc. Res.*, **10**, 697-702

Luxton, M. R., Miller, N. E. and Oliver, M. F. (1976). Antilipolytic treatment in angina pectoris. Reduction of exercise-induced ST segment depression. *Br. Heart J.*, **38**, 1204-8

Matta, R. J., Lawler, J. E. and Lown, B. (1976). Ventricular electrical instability: effects of psychological stress and beta-adrenergic blockade. *Am. J. Cardiol.*, **38**, 594-8

Morgan Jones, A. (1969). Preclinical coronary heart disease. In *Modern Trends in Cardiology*, Vol. 2 (ed. A. Morgan Jones), Butterworth, London, pp. 36-45

Morris, J. N., Chave, S. P. W., Adam, C., Sirey, C., Epstein, L. and Sheehan, D. J. (1973). Vigorous exercise in leisure-time and the incidence of coronary heart disease. *Lancet*, *i*, 333-40

Multicentre International Study (1975). Improvement in prognosis of myocardial infarction by long-term beta adrenoceptor-blockade using practolol. *Br. med. J.*, *iii*, 735-40

Myocardial Infarction Community Registers (1976). *Public Health in Europe No. 5*, World Health Organisation, Geneva

Noneman, J. W. and Rogers, J. F. (1978). Lidocaine prophylaxis in acute myocardial infarction. *Medicine*, **57**, 501-75

Norwegian Multicenter Study Group (1981). Timolol-induced reduction in mortality and reinfarction in patients surviving acute myocardial infarction. *New Engl. J. Med.*, **304**, 801-7

Oliver, M. F. (1978a). Home or hospital for myocardial infarction? *Lancet*, *i*, 1089

Oliver, M. F. (1978b). Metabolism of the normal and ischaemic myocardium. In *Developments in Cardiovascular Medicine* (ed. C. J. Dickinson and J. Marks), Lancaster, Medical and Technical Press, pp. 145-64

Opie, L. H. (1975). Metabolism of FFA, glucose and catecholamines in acute myocardial infarction. *Am J. Cardiol.*, **36**, 938-53

Perper, J. A., Kuller, L. H. and Cooper, M. (1975). Atherosclerosis of coronary arteries in sudden unexpected death. *Circulation*, **51/52**, Suppl. III, 291-3

Pisa, Z. (1980). Sudden death: a worldwide problem. In *Sudden Death* (ed. H. E. Kulbertus and H. J. J. Wellens), Martinus Nijhoff, The Hague, pp. 3-10

Podzuweit, T., Dalby, A. J., Cherry, G. W. and Opie, L. H. (1978). Cyclic AMP levels in ischaemic and non-ischaemic myocardium following coronary artery ligation: relation to ventricular fibrillation. *J. molec. cell. Cardiol.*, **10**, 81-94

Rogers, W. J., Stanley, A. W., Breinig, J. B., Prather, J. W., McDaniel, H. G., Moraski, R. E., Mantle, J. A., Russell, R. O. and Rackley, C. E. (1976). Reduction of hospital mortality rate of acute myocardial infarction with glucose-insulin-potassium infusion. *Am. Heart J.*, **92**, 441-54

Rowe, M. J., Neilson, J. M. M. and Oliver, M. F. (1975). Control of ventricular arrhythmias during myocardial infarction by antilipolytic treatment using a nicotinic-acid analogue. *Lancet*, *i*, 205-300

Russell, D. C. and Oliver, M. F. (1979). The effect of intravenous glucose on ventricular vulnerability following acute coronary artery occlusion in the dog. *J. molec. cell. Cardiol.*, **11**, 31-44

Shahab, L., Wollenberger, A., Krause, E.-G. and Genz, S. (1972). The effect of acute ischaemia on catecholamines and cyclic AMP levels in normal and hypertrophied myocardium. In *Effect of Acute Ischaemia on Myocardial Function* (ed. M. F. Oliver, D. G. Julian and K. W. Donald), Churchill Livingstone, Edinburgh, pp. 97-107

Thomas, A. C., Davies, M. J. and Popple, A. W. (1980). A pathologist's view of sudden cardiac death. In *Sudden Death* (ed. H. E. Kulbertus and H. J. J. Wellens), Martinus Nijhoff, The Hague, pp. 34-48

Valentine, P. A., Frew, J. L., Mashford, M. L. and Sloman, J. G. (1974). Lidocaine in the prevention of sudden death in the prehospital phase of acute infarction. *New Engl. J. Med.*, **291**, 1327-31

Wit, A. L. and Bigger, J. T. (1975). Possible electrophysiological mechanisms for lethal arrhythmias accompanying myocardial ischaemia and infarction. *Circulation*, **51/52**, Suppl. III, 96-115

Yusuf, S., Ramsdale, D., Peto, R., Furse, L., Bennett, D., Bray, C. and Sleight, P. (1980). Early intravenous atenolol treatment in suspected acute myocardial infarction. A preliminary report of a randomised trial. *Lancet*, *i*, 273-6

Zoll, P. M., Linenthal, A. J., Gibson, W., Paul, M. H. and Norman, L. R. (1956). Termination of ventricular fibrillation in man by externally applied electric countershock. *New Engl. J. Med.*, **254**, 727-32

2

Myocardial Ischaemia and Metabolic Changes Associated with the Genesis of Ventricular Arrhythmias

David J. Hearse and Steven C. Dennis

2.1 INTRODUCTION

While a number of pathological conditions may lead to the development of cardiac rhythm disturbances, the one which dominates this book is myocardial ischaemia. The objective of this chapter is to identify the ischaemia-induced changes which may be critical to the genesis of arrhythmias. In order to achieve this it will be necessary to consider the nature and progression of ischaemic injury.

The broad overview presented in this chapter has by necessity been assembled from a multitude of studies using different species and different models. Caution must therefore be exercised in extrapolating many of the findings to the clinical situation. In order to minimise any confusion a number of preliminary points will be made.

The definition of ischaemia

Ischaemia is conveniently defined as a lack of blood in a particular tissue. However, a more broadly based definition (Hearse, 1980) which accounts for the dynamic nature of the condition and for the removal, as well as the supply, of compounds to the myocardium is more appropriate. Essentially ischaemia represents an imbalance between the myocardial demand for, and the vascular supply of, coronary blood. Not only does this create a deficit of oxygen, substrates and energy in the tissue but also, and of considerable importance, it results in an insufficient capacity for the removal of potentially toxic metabolites such as lactate, carbon dioxide and protons. The total cessation of coronary flow is not a prerequisite of myocardial ischaemia. It rarely occurs clinically and, even under experimental conditons with multiple coronary artery ligations, the collateral circulation may provide for substantial perfusion in the ischaemic zone. Indeed, myocardial ischaemia can arise without a reduction in coronary flow under circumstances where there is an inadequate vascular response to an increased energy demand on the heart.

It is most important to distinguish between ischaemia and hypoxia or anoxia, which are totally different (Rovetto *et al.*, 1975) in their origins and their consequences. In anoxia or hypoxia the oxygen delivery to the myocardium is reduced by removing all or some of the oxygen in the coronary flow. Thus, while the P_{O_2} is reduced, coronary flow may be normal or even elevated and substrate delivery and metabolite removal may also be normal. By necessity in later sections some results from hypoxic studies may be included, but the nature of the oxygen deprivation will be stressed.

Evolution of ischaemic injury

In considering ischaemic damage it is important to appreciate that it is not a static condition. Ischaemic tissue evolves through reversible to irreversible damage, cell death and tissue necrosis, the whole process representing myocardial infarction (Jennings and Ganote, 1974, 1976). The rate at which these processes occur and the nature of the processes themselves are influenced by a number of factors including the severity of ischaemia, the age, sex and species of the tissue under investigation, the hormonal, nutritional and metabolic status of the tissue and the co-existence of other disease processes.

The heterogeneity of ischaemia

A striking and important characteristic of ischaemia (and also hypoxia) is its macroscopic and microscopic heterogeneity (Jennings, 1969; Jennings and Ganote, 1974; Steenbergen *et al.*, 1977). Varying conditions of workload, tissue perfusion or ischaemic resistance may create a transient or patchy ischaemia. In the latter instance islands of severely ischaemic tissue may be interspersed with, or lie adjacent to, areas of normal tissue. Within a single ischaemic area, regional differences may exist with concentric zones of decreasing ischaemia radiating outwards from the core of the ischaemic area. Such a situation might create so-called border zones of marginally damaged tissue which separate severely ischaemic from normal tissue (Cox *et al.*, 1968; Opie and Owen, 1976; Hearse *et al.*, 1977b; Hearse and Yellon, 1981). Within these zones gradients of flow, metabolism and electrophysiology will exist. Some investigators (Marcus *et al.*, 1975; Barlow and Chance, 1976; Chance, 1976; Hearse and Yellon, 1981) contend that these gradients are sharp while others (Kloner and Braunwald, 1980) believe them to be less abrupt, with a gradual transition of damage creating quantitatively significant zones of intermediate injury.

Whatever the nature of the interface between normal and ischaemic tissue, the heterogeneity of damage is likely to be a very important factor in the genesis of arrhythmias. The dispersion of refractoriness to conduction between the various zones may predispose to re-entrant arrhythmias (Levites *et al.*, 1975). Further, unidirectional conduction abnormalities between the ischaemic and the non-ischaemic zones may produce premature beats (Schmitt and Erlanger, 1926) and, depending on the sharpness of the border zone (Lubbe *et al.*, 1974), areas of localised fibrillation may occur that can spread to the non-ischaemic tissue (Boineau and Cox, 1973). Since globally ischaemic tissue is relatively stable electrically (Beck, 1958), a number of authors (Harris, 1950, 1966; Brofman *et al.*, 1956; Beck, 1958) have suggested that the border zone is the site of origin of ventricular ectopic impulses.

Models for study

The differences between hypoxia and ischaemia and the heterogeneity of ischaemia make it very difficult to develop an ideal model for the study of arrhythmia development. Species differences compound the problem, as does the debate over the relevance of models involving coronary artery ligation. In this connection it may well transpire that coronary artery thrombosis might not be the initiating event for tissue ischaemia and myocardial infarction (Harris, 1975). Furthermore, the growth of coronary arterial thrombi for at least 72 h after their initial formation in the dog model (Salimi *et al.*, 1977) may well mean that metabolic events defined in models with coronary ligation represent an oversimplification. Finally the possibility that transient coronary artery spasm (Oliva and Breckenridge, 1977) may play a critical role cannot be ignored.

Tissue subtypes and ischaemic injury

A further point to consider when assessing the consequences of ischaemia is the occurrence of tissue subtypes within the myocardium. In the past the consequences of ischaemic damage have been mainly applied to the contractile tissue of the heart. However, the effect of ischaemia upon conducting and vascular tissues warrant equal consideration. There is evidence, for example, for a differential susceptibility to damage between contractile and conducting tissue (Kübler, 1976). Similarly, the susceptibility of myocardial vascular tissue and vascular responses to ischaemia is well known and is critical. Thus, although the contractile tissue of the heart may be quantitatively the most significant component, the responses of the other tissues to ischaemia may be equally important. For instance, Purkinje fibres with a high glycogen content (Opie, 1968-9) have a high capacity for anaerobic glycolysis (Kübler *et al.*, 1972), often survive infarction and become the site of origin of arrhythmias (Lazzara *et al.*, 1973). In this partially depolarised conducting tissue, severe acidosis (pH 6.1) (Davis *et al.*, 1976) and/or hypokalaemic conditions (Cranefield, 1975) can elicit the development of spontaneous phase 4 depolarisation which may be exaggerated by the presence of catecholamines or cyclic AMP (Tsien, 1973).

2.2 METABOLISM AND ISCHAEMIA

Despite the problem of the heterogeneity of ischaemia and the likelihood that at any one time different cells within an ischaemic area will be variably damaged (Jennings and Ganote, 1976), a remarkably detailed picture has emerged of the sequence of events occurring during ischaemia (Braasch *et al.*, 1968; Brachfeld, 1974; Sobel, 1974; Opie, 1976; Hearse, 1980). The following section attempts to give a generalised overview of some of the deleterious changes initiated by myocardial ischaemia. These changes, which affect cellular metabolism, electrical activity, contractile function, vascular responsiveness and tissue ultrastructure are depicted in figure 2.1. This figure is not intended to convey the impression that the events occur in such a strict sequence; indeed many of the changes occur simultaneously. It is, however, likely to represent the situation prevailing following the onset of very severe ischaemia. The dynamic nature of the process and the individual changes should also be appreciated. Thus although figure 2.1 only indicates the *onset* of a change, the individual changes may of course continue for some time. In an attempt to simplify the discussion the changes shown in figure 2.1 have been subdivided into a number of categories, many of which are relevant to the genesis of arrhythmias.

Changes in contractile function

Within a few seconds of the onset of ischaemia there is in the ischaemic zone a precipitous decline of contractile activity (Tennant and Wiggers, 1935; Sonnenblick and Kirk, 1971-2; Jennings, 1969; Katz, 1973). This decline occurs at a time when excitability remains essentially normal (Kardesch *et al.*, 1958). It remains controversial (Tennant and Wiggers, 1935; Katz and Hecht, 1969; Katz, 1973; Hillis and Braunwald, 1977) whether this very rapid conservative response can be attributed to adenosine triphosphate (ATP) depletion (Hearse, 1979) in a small compartment, to a direct ischaemic-induced interference of calcium homeostasis, to an effect of accumulating protons upon calcium binding within the contractile apparatus or to some other as yet unidentified process.

Changes in oxidative metabolism

During the first few seconds in severely ischaemic tissue with little or no collateral

---

Figure 2.1 The progression of myocardial ischaemic injury. Some of the cellular events thought to occur following the onset of severe myocardial ischaemia. This figure, which is highly speculative, is not intended to convey the impression that the events occur in a strict sequence or in the exact order listed; it does, however, indicate that injury becomes more severe with time and eventually leads to cell death. The critical point of transition from reversible to irreversible injury is not known. The progression of change is a dynamic process and only the onset is indicated for some of the changes.

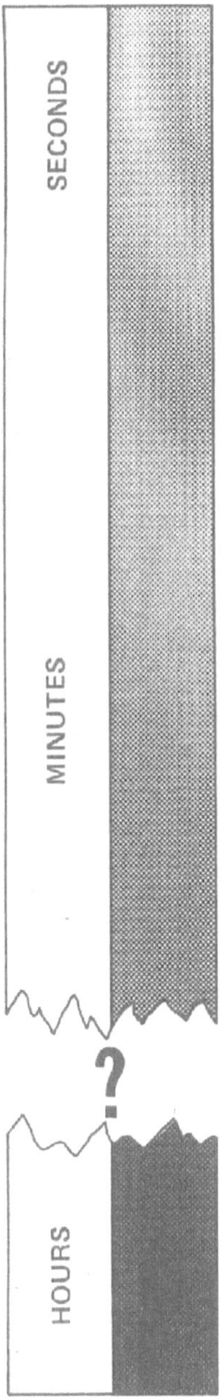

SECONDS

MINUTES

HOURS

ONSET OF SEVERE ISCHAEMIA

Disturbances of transmembrane ionic balance
Utilisation of dissolved oxygen
Reduction of mitochondrial activity and oxidative metabolism
Reduced ATP production
Reduction of creatine phosphate stores
Reduction of amplitude and duration of action potential
Leakage of potassium
ST segment changes
Accumulation of sodium and chloride ions
Catecholamine release
Stimulation of adenyl cyclase
Stimulation of glycogenolysis
Net utilisation of high energy phosphates
Accumulation of protons, carbon dioxide and inorganic phosphate
Stimulation of phosphofructokinase activity
Increase of glycolytic flux
Development of intracellular acidosis
Reduction or blockage of mitochondrial electron transport
Repression of fatty acid oxidation
Utilisation of glycogen
Leakage of inorganic phosphate
Accumulation of NADH
Increased lactate dehydrogenase and α-glycerophosphate dehydrogenase activity
Accumulation and leakage of lactate
Accumulation of fatty acyl CoA derivatives
Depletion of creatine phosphate
Leakage of adenosine, inosine and other metabolites
Vasodilation
Inhibition of adenine nucleotide transferase activity
Possible stimulation of triglyceride synthesis and degradation
Increasing cellular acidosis
Repression of phosphofructokinase and glyceraldehyde-3-phosphate dehydrogenase activity
Slowing of glycolytic flux
Cell swelling
Increase in cytoplasmic ionised calcium content
Leakage of magnesium ions
Possible exhaustion of glycogen reserves
Inhibition of glycolysis
Severe reduction of ATP
Minor ultrastructural changes, for example mitochondrial swelling
Possible onset of contracture

?

ONSET OF IRREVERSIBLE DAMAGE?

Lysosomal changes and activation of hydrolases and lipoprotein lipases
Increasing cellular oedema
Loss of mitochondrial respiratory control
Non-specific electrocardiographic changes
Ultrastructural changes in mitochondria and myofibrils
Complete depletion of energy reserves
Loss of mitochondrial components
Leakage of enzymes to interstitial space and lymph
Severe ultrastructural damage and membrane deterioration
Disruption of mitochondria, myofibrils and cell membranes

CELL DEATH AND TISSUE NECROSIS

coronary flow available oxygen dissolved in the cytoplasm will be utilised and anaerobic conditions will develop within the cell (Kloner *et al.*, 1975; Williamson *et al.*, 1976). Associated with this will be a major reduction (or even a complete abolition) of oxidative metabolism, electron transport and mitochondrial ATP production. Only the much less efficient anaerobic pathways of metabolism will then remain for the production of ATP. In less severely ischaemic tissue with significant collateral flow, there will be a major reduction of oxygen availability and a corresponding reduction of oxidative ATP production; under these conditions ATP will be derived from both aerobic and anaerobic pathways.

In assessing the relative contribution to ATP production made by aerobic and anaerobic pathways, two factors must be considered. First, there is a large difference between the pathways in their efficiency of ATP production. Secondly, substantial collateral flow may exist (Lubbe *et al.*, 1974; Heng *et al.*, 1976; Opie, 1976; Hearse *et al.*, 1977b; Yellon *et al.*, 1981) even in the core of an ischaemic area. Taken together these two factors would suggest (Corabouef *et al.*, 1976; Opie, 1976) that oxidative phosphorylation may often remain the dominant source of ATP despite a severe reduction in oxygen availability.

Changes in carbohydrate metabolism

During the early seconds of ischaemia sensitive cellular control mechanisms trigger major changes in substrate uptake and utilisation patterns (Opie, 1968–9, 1976; Neely and Morgan, 1974; Opie and Stubbs, 1976). Reduced mitochondrial metabolism results in a rapid reduction in glycolytic flux through the β-oxidation pathway for fatty acids (Evans, 1964) - the preferred substrates in well oxygenated hearts (Neely and Morgan, 1974) - and carbohydrate utilisation is stimulated (Rovetto *et al.*, 1973; Opie, 1976). This stimulation of anaerobic glycolysis (the Pasteur effect) represents an attempt to maintain the declining myocardial ATP content through non-oxidative mechanisms of substrate-level phosphorylation. Depending on the degree of coronary flow reduction, increased glycolytic flux is predominantly fuelled by either glucose or glycogen (Opie *et al.*, 1976). In more severe ischaemia, the early release of catecholamines (Wollenberger *et al.*, 1967; Mayer, 1974; Crass *et al.*, 1975) preferentially increases glycogenolysis as a result of cyclic AMP and/or calcium-mediated conversion (Rovetto *et al.*, 1975) of phosphorylase *b* to phosphorylase *a*. In addition, the accumulation of 5′-AMP and inorganic phosphate from the hydrolysis of ATP also stimulates phosphorlyase *b* allosterically (Cox *et al.*, 1968; Neely and Morgan, 1974). Glycolysis is accelerated by the activation of the rate-limiting enzymes phosphofructokinase, glyceraldehyde-3-phosphate dehydrogenase and pyruvate kinase (Rovetto *et al.*, 1973; Hearse, 1977) and, in the first few minutes, regulation of flux oscillates (Patterson, 1971) between these stages. In regional ischaemia control of glycolysis may remain at the level of the phosphofructokinase reaction (Evans, 1964; Opie, 1975) but in global ischaemia glycolytic flux rates are ultimately regulated by glyceraldehyde-3-phosphate dehydrogenase activity (Brachfeld, 1969). The stimulation of glycolysis in the face of reduced mitochondrial activity leads to the accumulation of glycolytic intermediates and reduced nicotinamide adenine dinucleotide phosphate (NADH), which limits flux through glyceraldehyde-3-phosphate dehydrogenase (Neely *et al.*, 1975). In an attempt to regenerate declining and limited reserves of NAD^+ for continued glycolytic activity pyruvate is reduced to lactate, which accumulates in and leaks from the cell (Kübler and Spieckermann, 1970; Opie *et al.*, 1972). Additional regeneration of NAD^+ may be achieved by the activity of α-glycerophosphate dehydrogenase in the conversion of dihydroxyacetone phosphate to α-glycerophosphate (Opie *et al.*, 1973).

Changes in fatty acid metabolism

The conversion of dihydroxyacetone phosphate to a α-glycerophosphate may, through promotion of glyceride synthesis, stimulate the proposed triglyceride fatty acid cycle in ischaemic tissue (Opie, 1975). This paradoxical aspect of fatty acid metabolism involves synthesis of glyceride from the high levels of α-glycerophosphate and the breakdown of glyceride by the cyclic AMP-stimulated lipase. The resulting cycle of lipolysis and resynthesis causes the net utilisation of ATP. Another possible detrimental effect of fatty acid metabolism during early ischaemia is the accumulation of long chain fatty acyl CoA compounds. As stated previously, β-oxidation of fatty acids is reduced during ischaemia but uptake may not be as diminished. As a result of continued fatty acid metabolism (Opie *et al.*, 1973) and possibly of cyclic AMP-stimulated lipolysis (Hough and Gevers, 1975) of endogenous triglycerides (triggered by ischaemia-induced release of catecholamines; Wollenberger and Shahab, 1965; Mayer, 1974; Crass *et al.*, 1975), fatty acyl CoA derivatives accumulate in the cytoplasm and may inhibit adenine nucleotide translocase activity (Shrago *et al.*, 1976). The impaired efflux of ATP produced from residual oxidative phosphorylation in the mitochondria, together with other aspects of fatty acid toxicity (Opie and Stubbs, 1976; Opie *et al.*, 1977), may aggravate the genesis of arrhythmias during the ischaemic period (Kurien and Oliver, 1970; Opie and Lubbe, 1975; Oliver, 1976).

Changes in intracellular pH

As myocardial ischaemia progresses there occurs an accumulation of carbon dioxide from residual oxidative decarboxylation reactions (Khuri *et al.*, 1975) and a build-up of protons from adenine nucleotide degradation and other sources (Opie, 1976; Gevers, 1977). With severe respiratory and metabolic acidosis the earlier activation of glycolysis (by decreased ATP and increased ADP, AMP and inorganic phosphate) may be overridden (Rovetto *et al.*, 1975). In the presence of high concentrations of protons, lactate and NADH, glyceraldehyde-3-phosphate dehydrogenase and phosphofructokinase activity may be inhibited. Glycolytic flux may also be depressed at this stage and this is in part due to severe depletion of available glycogen (Rovetto *et al.*, 1973).

In addition to their inhibitory effect on glycolytic activity and their possible role in early contractile failure, protons may contribute to the development of later stages of ischaemic damage (Opie, 1976). This may result from the activation of lysosomal hydrolases (Brachfeld, 1969; Ricciutti, 1972; Weglicki *et al.*, 1974) and lipoprotein lipase which, together with proton-induced calcium shifts and proton-induced membrane conformational changes, may contribute towards cell leakage.

Changes in high energy phosphate reserves

Despite the conservative effects of contractile failure, the stimulation of anaerobic energy production, the marked vasodilation and the opening of collateral vessels, the myocardium during severe ischaemia is unable to produce sufficient energy for the correct maintenance of basal metabolism and cellular integrity. Thus during the early minutes of ischaemia a progressive fall in myocardial energy reserves occurs (Braasch *et al.*, 1968; Hearse and Chain, 1972; Khuri *et al.*, 1975; Schwartz *et al.*, 1973). This is characterised by a rapid breakdown of creatine phosphate, a less abrupt fall of myocardial ATP and then a transient rise, then fall of ADP, AMP and adenosine. Also associated with net nucleotide degradation is the cellular accumulation and leakage of adenosine, inosine and hypoxanthine.

Changes in coronary vasculature

Changes occur in the coronary vasculature in ischaemia. There is marked coronary vasodilation, perhaps mediated by prostaglandin release (Berger *et al.*, 1977; Hintz and Kaley, 1977) and the efflux of intracellular adenosine (Berne and Rubio, 1974). However, as ischaemia progresses, there is a loss of vascular responsiveness and, although this may in part be compensated for by the development of collateral vessels (Schaper and Pasyk, 1976), there is often a secondary reduction in the remaining coronary perfusion. Two factors may contribute to this secondary reduction of flow (Brachfeld, 1974). First, swelling of capillary endothelial cells may reduce capillary diameter and result in trapping of blood elements. Secondly, the development of contracture may compress the capillary vessels thereby further reducing flow. These combined effects are likely to contribute to the 'no-reflow' phenomenon which is characteristic of more advanced ischaemic damage (Fabiani, 1977).

Changes in mitochondrial function

As the duration of ischaemia increases more severe cellular damage occurs. Mitochondrial malfunction (which may occur despite a continuing limited supply of oxygen) will act to widen the gap between energy demand and energy supply (Hearse, 1977). Studies with mitochondria isolated from ischaemic tissue (Kane *et al.*, 1975; Jennings and Ganote, 1976; Leaf, 1973) reveal that in the early stages of the ischaemic process ADP : O values are near normal but that there is a decreased capacity for oxygen consumption. This suggests an inhibition of phosphorylation rather than an uncoupling. However, as the ischaemic damage progresses inhibition and uncoupling of oxidative phosphorylation are both observed (Patterson, 1971; Leaf, 1973). Dramatic decreases in state 3 and increases in state 4 respiration have been reported (Schwartz *et al.*, 1973; Jennings and Ganote, 1976), as has the loss of electron transport chain components (Jennings *et al.*, 1969). The final result is the total loss of respiratory control and the inhibition of respiration. Mitochondrial calcium depletion probably occurs during the relatively early stages of the ischaemic process (Hearse, 1977). This mitochondrial calcium would contribute to increasing cytoplasmic levels of ionised calcium, the latter arising partly as a result of dechelation of calcium from ATP (as a result of net ATP utilisation) and partly from the reduction of calcium sequestration at various subcellular sites.

Secondary changes in the contractile state

Dependent upon the severity of the ischaemia total contractile failure with diastolic arrest may occur. With increasing durations of ischaemia myocardial contracture (a form of systolic arrest resembling rigour in skeletal muscle) may develop (Cooley *et al.*, 1972). This condition (Katz and Tada, 1972, 1977; Hearse *et al.*, 1977a) is thought to be due to the accumulation of rigour-producing complexes as a direct result of ATP deficiency. The development of contracture or advanced ultrastructural damage (Jennings and Ganote, 1974) is evidenced by the presence of contraction bands, distorted Z bands and myofibrillar disruption. By this stage disruption. By this stage mitochondria are distorted and may appear vesiculated, mitochondria are distorted and may appear vesiculated, glycogen granules are lost and the sarcoplasmic reticulum may be vesiculated. Extensive cellular oedema may have developed and there may be some evidence of distortion or damage to the cell membrane after the first hour or so of ischaemia. The appearance of cytoplasmic proteins and enzymes in the interstitial space and cardiac lymph has been observed at this stage (Spieckermann *et al.*, 1974; Sobel *et al.*, 1976).

Metabolic and ultrastructural disruption

Despite the possibility of a continuing limited supply of oxygen during the later stages of ischaemia, cellular metabolism and ATP production virtually cease, glycogen stores may be depleted and glycolysis and mitochondrial function become totally inhibited. Anabolic and catabolic pathways for proteins, fatty acids, lipids and nucleic acids are no longer functional, cellular autolysis occurs and large quantities of various cellular constituents leak to the extracellular space. A critical process at this stage may be lysosomal activation (Ricciutti, 1972; Weglicki *et al.*, 1974; Fox *et al.*, 1976; Hoffstein *et al.*, 1976; Welman and Peters, 1977). Eventually, electrical activity is lost, extensive ultrastructural damage occurs and (following cell death) fibrous infiltration and tissue necrosis occur.

Although by the time of this advanced ischaemic injury the cell and its metabolism are quiescent, the interface between the injured and normal tissue may still act as an irritable focus for arrhythmogenic activity. Thus autolytic products draining from the infarcted area to the adjacent normal areas may precipitate arrhythmias and lysophospholipid seepage may (Corr *et al.*, 1979) induce electrophysiological changes. This is discussed in detail in chapter 12.

2.3 ELECTROPHYSIOLOGY AND ISCHAEMIA: THE GENESIS OF ARRHYTHMIAS

In the preceding sections emphasis was placed upon the metabolic damages associated with ischaemia and the possibility was alluded to that some of these changes may be involved in the genesis of arrhythmias. In the following sections the electrophysiological changes which occur during ischaemic injury are briefly considered. The changes which may be critical to tissue irritability are summarised in figure 2.2.

Ion movements

Early in ischaemia major ionic and electrophysiological changes occur (Case, 1971-2; Coraboeuf *et al.*, 1976; Hillis and Braunwald, 1977). ST-segment shifts (Pardee, 1920) are detected within 30 s of the onset of ischaemia and usually reach a maximum some 5-10 min later (Hillis and Braunwald, 1977). The electrophysiological basis of ST-segment changes is complex and controversial (Braunwald and Maroko, 1976; Fozzard and DasGupta, 1976; Ross, 1976; Hillis and Braunwald, 1977) but they may result from inadequate polarisation of the ischaemic region during diastole whilst normal tissue is well polarised or from inadequate depolarisation of the ischaemic tissue during excitation (Hillis and Braunwald, 1976).

Disturbances of membrane ion transport appear to be the cause of early ischaemia-induced electrocardiographic changes. With the loss of membrane control (possibly a result of an energy shortage) there is a net cellular accumulation of sodium and chloride and of water (loss of cell volume control; Leaf, 1973) and a net loss of intracellular magnesium (Shen and Jennings, 1972), inorganic phosphate (Opie *et al.*, 1972) and potassium. The resultant increase in extracellular potassium is thought to play a critical role in the genesis of the electrocardiographic changes (Johnson, 1976). Redistribution of potassium and other ions reduces the amplitude and duration of action potential. Although controversial (McDonald *et al.*, 1971; Hyde *et al.*, 1972; Coraboeuf *et al.*, 1976) it is possible that these changes may be related to reduced glycolytic ATP production which may reduce calcium chelation in the subsarcolemma, thus increasing local concentrations of free calcium and reducing the slow inward calcium current.

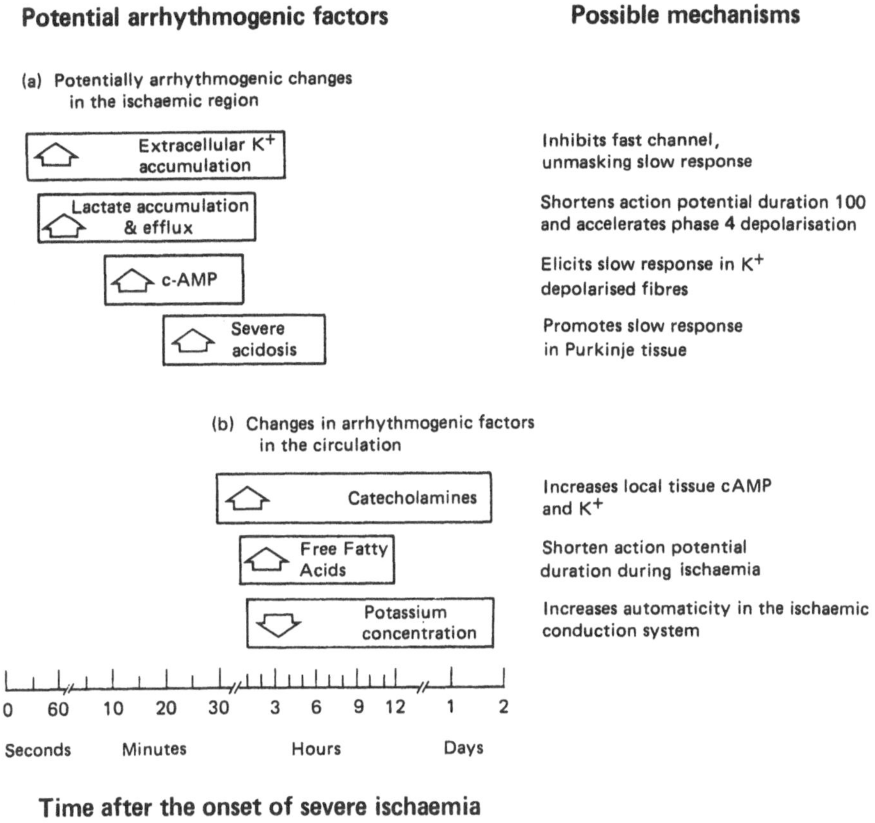

Potential arrhythmogenic factors | **Possible mechanisms**

(a) Potentially arrhythmogenic changes in the ischaemic region

Factor	Mechanism
⇧ Extracellular K^+ accumulation	Inhibits fast channel, unmasking slow response
⇧ Lactate accumulation & efflux	Shortens action potential duration 100 and accelerates phase 4 depolarisation
⇧ c-AMP	Elicits slow response in K^+ depolarised fibres
⇧ Severe acidosis	Promotes slow response in Purkinje tissue

(b) Changes in arrhythmogenic factors in the circulation

Factor	Mechanism
⇧ Catecholamines	Increases local tissue cAMP and K^+
⇧ Free Fatty Acids	Shorten action potential duration during ischaemia
⇩ Potassium concentration	Increases automaticity in the ischaemic conduction system

0 60 10 20 30 3 6 9 12 1 2

Seconds Minutes Hours Days

Time after the onset of severe ischaemia

Figure 2.2 Metabolic effects underlying the genesis of ventricular arrhythmias. Potential arrhythmogenic effects thought to occur following the onset of severe myocardial ischaemia. The time course of events is approximate and serves only to illustrate changes which may explain (1) the maximum ventricular irritability during the first hour of coronary occlusion and (2) the greatest incidence of arrhythmic deaths in the first few hours following infarction.

Extracellular potassium and the inhibition of the fast response

Increased extracellular potassium may also play an important role in the early arrhythmias (Johnson, 1976; Holland and Brooks, 1977), a point discussed in more detail in chapter 7. Within a few minutes (Opie *et al.*, 1979) the coronary venous potassium can rise to levels that are sufficient to depolarise the cells to such an extent (about −50 mV) that the fast response is substantially inhibited (Gettes, 1975), the action potential duration is reduced (Holland and Brooks, 1979) and the threshold for the slow calcium inward current is approached (Gettes, 1975). This favours slow conduction and re-entry (Cranefield *et al.*, 1972); in addition, ectopic activity may also be promoted (Harris *et al.*, 1958).

Inhibition of glycolysis and the shortening of action potential duration

Another early change induced by ischaemia is the increase in tissue lactate. This accelerates phase 4 polarisation in Purkinje fibres (Wissner, 1974) and decreases action potential duration in conducting tissue (Wissner, 1974) and in contractile tissue (Opie *et al.*, 1979). The shortening of the action potential duration (Webb and Hollander, 1956; Prasad and MacLeod, 1969; Wissner, 1974; Coraboeuf *et al.*, 1976; Cowan and Vaughan Williams, 1977; Opie *et al.*, 1979; Russell and Oliver, 1979) by factors which inhibit glycolysis (especially pyruvate), free fatty acids (Newsholme and Randle, 1964), lactate (Rovetto *et al.*, 1975), acidosis (Ui, 1966) and ischaemia (Bruyneel, 1975), and the reversal of these effects by glucose (Prasad and MacLeod, 1969; Cowan and Vaughan Williams, 1977; Opie *et al.*, 1979; Russell and Oliver, 1979), has led to a suggestion that ATP from glycolysis may play some special role in the maintenance of action potential duration in the ischaemic myocardium (Prasad and Macleod, 1969; Bricknell and Opie, 1978). Thus, the accumulation of lactate and protons and the metabolism of fatty acids may, through inhibition of glycolytic flux, combine with the declining energy status further to shorten the action potential duration. As a result of the corresponding reduction of the fast response and the reduced duration of the action potential there is also *et al.*, 1975) the myocardium may become predisposed to arrhythmias.

Catecholamine induction of the slow response

In addition to the loss of the resting membrane potential, the decreased velocity of the fast response and the reduced duration of the action potential there is also initiation of slow responses, for example by increased levels of cyclic AMP (reviewed in chapter 11). Cyclic AMP (cAMP) 'opens' the slow channel (Reuter, 1974) and, in tissues where the fast response is suppressed (partially depolarised) but where sufficient energy remains for inward calcium current activity (Schneider and Sperelakis, 1974), the slow response is stimulated (Sperelakis and Schneider, 1976; Lown *et al.*, 1977) and the ventricular fibrillation threshold is decreased (Lubbe *et al.*, 1976, 1978; Corr *et al.*, 1978). The evidence for a role of cAMP in the generation or arrhythmias is discussed in detail in chapter 11.

As the cAMP produced in response to endogenous catecholamines release starts to decline, further cAMP synthesis may occur as a result of increased circulating catecholamine levels 30 min or so after the onset of ischaemia (Strange *et al.*, 1974). In addition, the associated increased circulating free fatty acids (Vetter *et al.*, 1974) may, as described previously, exaggerate ischaemic damage (Opie, 1972; Opie *et al.*, 1977). Thus, the loss of potassium and the accumulation of lactate, protons, long chain acyl CoA products of fatty acid metabolism and cAMP could explain the maximum ventricular irritability that occurs with the first hour of occlusion.

Circulating catecholamines and enhanced automaticity

In contrast to the early arrhythmias which have been suggested to be associated with slow conduction and re-entry (Wit and Bigger, 1975), later arrhythmias may arise from spontaneous diastolic depolarisations in surviving Purkinje fibres (Lazzara *et al.*, 1973). High circulating catecholamines and related hypokalaemia may enhance automaticity in these fibres (Otsuka, 1958; Cranefield, 1975).

2.4 CONCLUDING COMMENTS

In this chapter we have attempted to describe the sequence of complex changes that are initiated by severe ischaemia. In particular, emphasis has been placed upon metabolic events which may be related to the genesis of arrhythmias and a number of potential factors have been described. However, although each of the events has been shown to be potentially arrhythmogenic, in many cases this was under highly specific conditions. Therefore, it must be stressed that a firm correlation cannot necessarily be made between some of these metabolic changes and the development of arrhythmias following myocardial infarction. It remains to be shown whether many of the proposed interactions underlying the genesis of experimentally induced arrhythmias can be extrapolated to the more complex settings of ischaemic heart disease in man.

ACKNOWLEDGEMENTS

D. J. H. is a British Heart Foundation Senior Lecturer.

REFERENCES

Barlow, C. H. and Chance, B. (1976). Ischemic areas in perfused rat hearts: measurement by NADH fluorescence photography. *Science, N.Y.* **193**, 909-10

Beck, C. S. (1958). Coronary artery disease. *Am. J. Cardiol.*, **1**, 38-45

Berger, H. J., Zaret, B. L., Speroff, L., Cohen, L. S. and Wolfson, S. (1977). Cardiac prostaglandin release during myocardial ischemia induced by atrial pacing in patients with coronary artery disease. *Am. J. Cardiol.*, **39**, 481-6

Berne, R. M. and Rubio, R. (1974). Adenine nucleotide metabolism in the heart. *Circulation Res.*, **34**, Suppl. 3, 109-20

Boineau, J. P. and Cox, J. L. (1973). Slow ventricular activation in acute myocardial infarction. *Circulation*, **48**, 702-13

Braasch, W., Gudbjarnason, S., Puri, P. S., Ravens, K. G. and Bing, R. J. (1968). Early changes in energy metabolism in the myocardium following acute coronary artery occlusion in anaesthetized dogs. *Circulation Res.*, **23**, 429-38

Brachfeld, N. (1969). Maintenance of cell viability. *Circulation*, **39** and **40**, Suppl. 4, 202-19

Brachfeld, N. (1974). Ischemic myocardial metabolism and cell necrosis. *Bull. N.Y. Acad. Med.*, **50**, 261-93

Braunwald, E. and Maroko, P. R. (1976). ST segment mapping, realistic and unrealistic expectations. *Circulation*, **54**, 529-32

Bricknell, O. L. and Opie, L. H. (1978). Effects of substrates on tissue metabolic changes in the isolated rat heart during perfusion and on release of lactate dehydrogenase and arrhythmias during reperfusion. *Circulation Res.*, **43**, 102-15

Brofman, B. L., Leighinger, D. S. and Beck, C. S. (1956). Electric instability of the heart: the concept of the current of oxygen differential in coronary artery disease. *Circulation*, **13**, 161-77

Bruyneel, K. J. J. (1975). Use of moving epicardial electrodes in defining ST-segment changes after acute coronary occlusion in the baboon. Relation to primary ventricular fibrillation. *Am. Heart J.*, **89**, 731-41

Case, R. B. (1971-2). Ion alterations during myocardial ischemia. *Cardiology*, **56**, 245-62

Chance, B. (1976). In discussion of 'The effects of regional ischemia on metabolism of glucose and fatty acids', by L. H. Opie. *Circulation Res.*, **38**, Suppl. 1, 52-74

Cooley, D. A., Reul, J. and Wukasch, D. C. (1972). Ischemic contracture of the heart: stone heart. *Am. J. Cardiol.*, **29**, 575-7

Coraboeuf, E., Deroubais, E. and Hoerter, J. (1976). Control of ionic permeabilities in normal and ischemic heart. *Circulation Res.*, **38**, Suppl. 1, 92-8

Corr, P. B., Witkowski, F. X. and Sobel, B. E. (1978). Mechanisms contributing to malignant dysrhythmias induced by ischemia in the cat. *J. clin. Invest.*, **61**, 109-19

Corr, P. B., Cain, M. E., Witkowski, F. X., Price, D. A. and Sobel, B. E. (1979). Potential arrhythmogenic electrophysiological derangements in canine Purkinje fibres induced by lysophosphoglycerides. *Circulation Res.*, **44**, 822-32

Cowan, J. C. and Vaughan Williams, E. M. (1977). The effects of palmitate on intracellular potentials recorded from Langendorff-perfused guinea-pig hearts in normoxia and hypoxia and during perfusion at reduced rate of flow. *J. molec. cell. Cardiol.*, **9**, 327-42

Cox, J. L., McLaughlin, V. W., Flowers, N. C. and Horan, L. G. (1968). The ischemic zone surrounding acute myocardial infarction. Its morphology as detected by dehydrogenase staining. *Am. Heart J.*, **76**, 650-9

Cranefield, P. (1975). *The Conduction of the Cardiac Impulse: The Slow Response and Cardiac Arrhythmias*, Futura Publishing, Mount Kisco, N.Y., pp. 153-97

Cranefield, P., Wit, A. L. and Hoffman, B. F. (1972). Conduction of the cardiac impulse. III. Characteristics of very slow conduction. *J. gen. Physiol.*, **59**, 227-46

Crass, M. F., Shipp, J. C. and Pieper, G. M. (1975). Effects of catecholamines on myocardial endogenous substrates and contractility. *Am. J. Physiol.*, **228**, 618-27

Davis, L. D., Helmer, P. R. and Ballantyne, F. (1976). Production of slow responses in canine cardiac Purkinje fibres exposed to reduced pH. *J. molec. cell. Cardiol.*, **8**, 61-76

Evans, J. R. (1964). Cellular transport of long chain fatty acids. *Can. J. Biochem.*, **42**, 955-68

Fabiani, J. N. (1977). The no reflow phenomenon following early reperfusion of myocardial infarction and its prevention by various drugs. *Heart Bull., La Haye*, **5**, 134-42

Fisch, C. (1973). Relation of electrolyte disturbances to cardiac arrhythmias. *Circulation*, **47**, 408-19

Fozzard, H. A. and DasGupta, D. S. (1976). ST segment potentials and mapping, theory and experiments. *Circulation*, **54**, 533-7

Fox, A. C., Hoffstein, S. and Weissman, G. (1976). Lysomal mechanisms in production of tissue damage during myocardial ischemia and the effects of treatment with steroids. *Am. Heart J.*, **91**, 394-7

Gettes, L. S. (1975). Electrophysiologic basis of arrhythmias in acute myocardial ischaemia. In *Modern Trends in Cardiology*, Vol. 3 (ed. M. F. Oliver), Butterworth, London, pp. 219-46

Gevers, W. (1977). Generation of protons by metabolic processes in heart cells. *J. molec. cell. Cardiol.*, **9**, 867-74

Harris, A. S. (1950). Delayed development of ventricular ectopic rhythms following experimental coronary artery occlusion. *Circulation*, **1**, 1318-28

Harris, A. S. (1966). Potassium and experimental coronary occlusions. *Am. Heart J.*, **71**, 797-802

Harris, P. (1975). A theory concerning the course of events in angina and myocardial infarction. *Eur. J. Cardiol.*, **3**, 157-63

Harris, A., Toth, L. A. and Hoey, T. E. (1958). Arrhythmic and antiarrhythmic effects of sodium, potassium and calcium salts and of glucose injected into coronary arteries of infarcted and normal hearts. *Circulation Res.*, **6**, 570-9

Hearse, D. J. (1977). Reperfusion of the ischaemic myocardium. *J. molec. cell. Cardiol.*, **9**, 605-16

Hearse, D. J. (1979). Oxygen deprivation and early myocardial contractile failure: a reassessment of the possible role of adenosine triphosphate. *Am. J. Cardiol.*, **44**, 1115-21

Hearse, D. J. (1980). Cellular damage during myocardial ischaemia: metabolic changes leading to enzyme leakage. In *Enzymes in Cardiology: Diagnosis and Research* (ed. D. J. Hearse, and J. de Leiris), John Wiley, Chichester, pp. 1-19

Hearse, D. J. and Chain, E. B. (1972). The role of glucose in the survival and recovery of the anoxic isolated perfused rat heart. *Biochem. J.*, **128**, 1125-33

Hearse, D. J. and Yellon, D. M. (1981). The border zone in evolving myocardial infarction: controversy or confusion? *Am. J. Cardiol.*, **47**, 1321-34

Hearse, D. J., Garlick, P. B. and Humphrey, S. M. (1977a). Ischemic contracture of the myocardium: mechanisms and prevention. *Am. J. Cardiol.*, **39**, 986-93

Hearse, D. J., Opie, L. H., Katzeff, I., Lubbe, W. F., Vander Werff, T. J., Peisach, M. and Boulle, G. (1977b). Characterization of the 'border zone' in acute regional ischemia in the dog. *Am. J. Cardiol.*, **40**, 716-26

Heng, M. K., Singh, B. N., Norris, R. M., John, M. B. and Elliot, R. (1976). Relationship between epicardial ST-segment elevation and myocardial ischemic damage after experimental coronary artery occlusion in dogs. *J. clin. Invest.*, **58**, 1317-26

Hillis, L. D. and Braunwald, E. (1977). Myocardial ischemia. *New Engl. J. Med.*, **296**, 971-8

Hintz, T. H. and Kaley, G. (1977). Prostaglandins and the control of blood flow in the canine myocardium. *Circulation Res.*, **40**, 313-20

Hoffstein, S., Weissmann, G. and Fox, A. C. (1976). Lysomes in myocardial infarction: studies by means of cytochemistry and subcellular fractionation, with observations on the effects of methyl prednisolone. *Circulation*, **53**, Suppl. 1, 34-40

Holland, R. P. and Brooks, H. (1977). TQ-ST segment mapping: critical review and analysis of current concepts. *Am. J. Cardiol.*, **40**, 110-29

Hough, F. S. and Gevers, W. (1975). Catecholamine release as a mediator of intracellular enzyme activation in ischaemic perfused rat hearts. *S. Afr. med. J.*, **49**, 538-43

Hyde, A., Chevnal, J. P., Blondel, B. and Cirardier, L. (1972). Electrophysiological correlates of energy metabolism in cultured rat heart cells. *J. Physiol., Paris*, **64**, 269-92

Jennings, R. B. (1969). Early phase of myocardial ischemic injury and infarction. *Am. J. Cardiol.*, **24**, 753-65

Jennings, R. B. and Ganote, C. E. (1974). Structural changes in myocardium during acute ischemia. *Circulation Res.*, **34** and **35**, Suppl. III, 156-68

Jennings, R. B. and Ganote, C. E. (1976). Mitochondrial structure and function in acute myocardial ischemic injury. *Circulation Res.*, Suppl. 1, 82-4

Jennings, R. B., Herdson, P. B. and Sommers, H. M. (1969). Structural and functional abnormalities in mitochondria isolated from ischemic dog myocardium. *Lab. Invest.*, **20**, 548-57

Johnson, E. A. (1976). First electrocardiographic sign of myocardial ischemia: an electrophysiological conjecture. *Circulation*, **53**, Suppl. 1, 82-4

Kane, J. J., Murphy, M. L., Bisset, J. K., de Soyza, N., Doherly, J. E. and Straub, K. D. (1975). Mitochondrial function, oxygen extraction, epicardial ST segment changes and tritiated digoxin distribution after reperfusion of ischemic myocardium. *Am. J. Cardiol.*, **36**, 218-24

Kardesch, M., Hogancamp, C. E. and Bing, R. J. (1958). The effect of complete ischaemia on the intracellular electrical activity of the whole mammalian heart. *Circulation Res.*, **6**, 715-20

Katz, A. M. (1973). Effects of ischemia on the contractile processes of heart muscle. *Am. J. Cardiol.*, **32**, 456-80

Katz, A. M. and Hecht, H. H. (1969). The early pump failure of the ischemic heart. *Am. J. Med.*, **47**, 497-502

Katz, A. M. and Tada, M. (1972). The stone heart, a challenge to the biochemist. *Am. J. Cardiol.*, **39**, 1073-7

Katz, A. M. and Tada, M. (1977). The stone heart and other challenges to the biochemist. *Am. J. Cardiol.*, **39**, 1073-7

Khuri, S., Flaherty, J. T., O'Riordan, J. B., Pitt, B., Brawley, R. K., Donahoo, J. S. and Gott, V. L. (1975). Changes in intramyocardial ST segment voltage and gas tensions with regional myocardial ischemia. *Circulation Res.*, **37**, 455-63

Kloner, R. A. and Braunwald, E. (1980). Observations on experimental myocardial ischaemia. *Cardiovascular Res.*, **14**, 371-95

Kloner, R. A., Ganote, C. E., Reimer, K. A. and Jennings, R. B. (1975). Distribution of coronary arterial flow in acute myocardial ischemia. *Archs Path.*, **99**, 86-94

Kübler, W. (1976). Comparative metabolism of contractile and conductive tissue. *Proc. 7th Eur. Congr. Cardiol.*, **2**, 127

Kübler, W. and Spieckermann, P. G. (1970). Regulation of glycolysis in the ischaemic and the anoxic myocardium. *J. molec. cell. Cardiol.*, **1**, 351-77

Kübler, W., Moll, W., Roggendorf, H. and von Smekal, P. (1972). Comparative studies of the energy metabolism of the conducting tissue and of the myocardium. In *Les Surcharges Cardiaques* (ed. P. Y. Hatt), Editions INSERM, Paris, pp. 139-49

Kurien, V. A. and Oliver, M. F. (1970). A metabolic cause for arrhythmias during acute myocardial hypoxia. *Lancet*, *i*, 813-5

Lazzara, R., El-Sherif, N. and Scherlag, B. J. (1973). Electrophysiological properties of canine Purkinje cells in one day-old myocardial infarction. *Circulation Res.*, **33**, 722-34

Leaf, A. (1973). Cell swelling, a factor in ischemic injury. *Circulation*, **48**, 455-6

Levites, R., Banka, V. S. and Helfant, R. H. (1975). Electrophysiological effects of coronary occlusion and reperfusion. Observations of dispersion of refractoriness and ventricular automaticity. *Circulation*, **52**, 760-5

Lown, B., Verrier, R. L. and Rabinowitz, S. H. (1977). Neural and physiologic mechanisms and the problem of sudden cardiac death. *Am. J. Cardiol.*, **39**, 890-902

Lubbe, W. F., Peisach, M., Pretorius, R., Brunneel, K. J. J. and Opie, L. H. (1974). Distribution of myocardial blood flow before and after coronary artery ligation in the baboon; relation to early ventricular fibrillation. *Cardiovasc. Res.*, **8**, 478-87

Lubbe, W. F., Bricknell, O. L., Podzuweit, T. and Opie, L. H. (1976). Cyclic AMP as a determinant of vulnerability to ventricular fibrillation in the isolated rat heart. *Cardiovasc. Res.*, **10**, 697-702

Lubbe, W. F., Podzuweit, T., Daries, P. S. and Opie, L. H. (1978). The role of cyclic adenosine monophosphate in adrenergic effects of ventricular vulnerability to fibrillation in the isolated perfused rat heart. *J. clin. Invest.*, **61**, 1260-9

McDonald, T. F., Hunter, E. G. and McLeod, D. P. (1971). Adenosine triphosphate partition in cardiac muscle with respect to transmembrane electrical activity. *Pflügers Arch. ges. Physiol.*, **322**, 95-108

Marcus, M. L., Kerber, R. E., Ehrhardt, J. and Abboud, F. M. (1975). Three dimensional geometry of acutely ischemic myocardium. *Circulation*, **52**, 254-63

Mayer, S. E. (1974). Effect of catecholamines on cardiac metabolism. *Circulation Res.*, **34/35**, Suppl., 129-35

Neely, J. R. and Morgan, H. E. (1974). Relationship between carbohydrate and lipid metabolism and the energy balance of the heart muscle. *A. Rev. Physiol.*, **36**, 413-59

Neely, J. R., Whitmer, J. T. and Rovetto, M. J. (1975). Effect of coronary blood flow on glycolytic flux and intracellular pH in isolated rat hearts. *Circulation Res.*, **37**, 733-41

Newsholme, E. A. and Randle, P. J. (1964). Regulation of glucose uptake by muscle. 7. Effects of fatty acids, ketone bodies, and pyruvate, and of alloxan-diabetes, starvation, hypophysectomy and adrenalectomy on the concentrations of hexose phosphates, nucleotides and inorganic phosphate in perfused rat heart. *Biochem. J.*, **93**, 641-51

Oliva, P. B. and Breckenridge, J. C. (1977). Arteriographic evidence of coronary arterial spasm in acute myocardial infarction. *Circulation*, **56**, 366-74

Oliver, M. F. (1976). The influence of myocardial metabolism on ischemic damage. *Circulation*, **53**, Suppl. 1, 168-70

Opie, L. H. (1968-9). Metabolism of the heart in health and disease. *Am. Heart J.*, **76**, 658-98; **77**, 101-22; **77**, 383-410

Opie, L. H. (1972). The general and local response to acute myocardial infarction. *Acta biol. med. germ.*, **28**, 873-92

Opie, L. H. (1975). Metabolism of free fatty acids, glucose and catecholamines in acute myocardial infarction. *Am. J. Cardiol.*, **36**, 938-53

Opie, L. H. (1976). Effects of regional ischaemia on metabolism of glucose and fatty acids. *Circulation Res.*, **38**, Suppl. 1, 52-74

Opie, L. H. and Lubbe, W. F. (1975). Are free fatty acids arrhythmogenic? *J. molec. cell. Cardiol.*, **7**, 155-9

Opie, L. H. and Owen, P. (1976). The effect of glucose-insulin-potassium infusions on arteriovenous differences of glucose and of free fatty acids on tissue metabolic changes in dogs with developing myocardial infarction. *Am. Heart J.*, **38**, 310-21

Opie, L. H. and Stubbs, W. A. (1976). Carbohydrate metabolism in cardiovascular disease. *Clinics Endocr. Metab.*, **5**, 703-29

Opie, L. H., Thomas, M., Owen, P. and Shulman, G. (1972). Increased coronary venous inorganic phosphate concentrations during experimental myocardial ischemia. *Am. J. Cardiol.*, **30**, 503-13

Opie, L. H., Owen, P., Thomas, M. and Samson, R. (1973). Coronary sinus lactate measurements in assessment of myocardial ischemia. *Am. J. Cardiol.*, **32**, 295-305

Opie, L. H., Owen, P. and Lubbe, W. (1976). Estimated glycolytic flux in infarcting heart. In *Recent Advances in Studies on Cardiac Structure and Metabolism* (ed. P. Harris, R. J. Bing and A. Fleckenstein), University Park Press, Baltimore, pp. 249-55

Opie, L. H., Tansey, M. and Kennelly, B. M. (1977). Proposed metabolic vicious circle mechanism in patients with large myocardial infarcts and high plasma free fatty acid concentrations. *Lancet*, *ii*, 890-2

Opie, L. H., Nathan, D. and Lubbe, W. F. (1979). Biochemical aspects of arrhythmogenesis and ventricular fibrillation. *Am. J. Cardiol.*, **43**, 131-48

Otsuka, M. (1958). Die Wirkung von Adrenalin auf Purkinje-Fasern von Saugetierherzen. *Pflügers Arch. ges. Physiol.*, **266**, 512-7

Pardee, H. E. B. (1920). An electrocardiographic sign of coronary artery obstruction. *Archs int. Med.*, **26**, 244-57

Patterson, R. A. (1971). Metabolic control of rat heart glycolysis after acute ischaemia. *J. molec. cell. Cardiol.*, **2**, 193-210

Prasad, K. and MacLeod, D. P. (1969). Influence of glucose on the transmembrane action potential of guinea-pig papillary muscle. Metabolic inhibitors, ouabain, calcium chloride, and their interaction with glucose, sympathomimetic amines, and aminophylline. *Circulation Res.*, **24**, 939-50

Reuter, H. (1974). Localisation of beta-adrenergic receptors, and effects of noradrenaline and cyclic nucleotides on action potentials, ionic currents and tension in mammalian cardiac muscle. *J. Physiol., Lond.*, **242**, 429-51

Ricciutti, M. A. (1972). Lysomes and myocardial cellular injury. *Am. J. Cardiol.*, **30**, 498-502

Ross, J. (1976). Electrocardiographic ST-segment analysis in the characterization of myocardial ischemia and infarction. *Circulation*, **53**, Suppl. 1, 73-81

Rovetto, M. J., Whitmer, J. T. and Neely, J. R. (1973). Comparison of the effects of anoxia and whole heart ischemia on carbohydrate utilization in isolated working rat hearts. *Circulation Res.*, **32**, 699-711

Rovetto, M. J., Lamberton, W. F. and Neely, J. R. (1975). Mechanisms of glycolytic inhibition of ischemic rat heart. *Circulation Res.*, **37**, 742-51

Russell, D. C. and Oliver, M. F. (1979). The effects of intravenous glucose on ventricular vulnerability following acute coronary artery occlusion in the dog. *J. molec. cell. Cardiol.*, **11**, 31-44

Salimi, A., Oliver, G. C., Lee, J. and Sherman, L. A. (1977). Continued incorporation of circulating radiolabeled fibrinogen into preformed coronary artery thrombi. *Circulation*, **56**, 213-7

Schaper, W. and Pasyk, S. (1976). Influence of collateral flow on the ischemic tolerance of the heart following acute and sub-acute coronary occlusion. *Circulation*, **53**, Suppl. 1, 57-65

Schmitt, F. O. and Erlanger, J. (1926). Directional differences in the conduction of the impulse through heart muscle and their possible relation to extrasystoles and fibrillary contractions. *Am. J. Physiol.*, **87**, 326-47

Schneider, J. A. and Sperelakis, N. (1974). Valinomycin blockade of slow channels in guinea-pig hearts perfused with elevated K^+ and isoproterenol. *Eur. J. Pharmac.*, **27**, 349-54

Schwartz, A., Wood, J. M., Allen, J. C., Bornet, E. P., Entman, M. L., Goldstein, M. A., Sordahl, L. A. and Suzuki, M. (1973). Biochemical and morphological correlates of cardiac ischemia. *Am. J. Cardiol.*, **32**, 46-61

Shen, A. C. and Jennings, R. B. (1972). Myocardial calcium and magnesium in acute ischemic injury. *Am. J. Path.*, **67**, 417-40

Shrago, E., Shug, A. L., Sul, H., Bittar, N. and Folts, J. D. (1976). Control of energy production of myocardial ischemia. *Circulation Res.*, **38**, Suppl. 1, 75-9

Sobel, B. E. (1974). Salient biochemical features in ischemic myocardium. *Circulation Res.*, **34/35**, Suppl. III, 173-80

Sobel, B. E., Roberts, R. and Larson, K. B. (1976). Considerations in the use of biochemical markers of ischemic injury. *Circulation Res.*, **38**, Suppl. 1, 99-106

Sonnenblick, E. H. and Kirk, E. S. (1971-2). Effects of hypoxia and ischemia on myocardial contraction. *Cardiology*, **56**, 302-13

Sperelakis, N. and Schneider, J. A. (1976). A metabolic control mechanism for calcium ion influx that may protect the ventricular myocardial cell. *Am. J. Cardiol.*, **37**, 1079-85

Spieckermann, P. G., Nordbeck, H., Knoll, D., Kohl, F. V., Sakai, K. and Bretschneider, H. J. (1974). The role of cardiac lymph in the transport of cardiac enzymes into the blood stream after myocardial infarct. *Dt. med. Wschr.*, **99**, 1143-4

Steenbergen, C., Peleeuw, G., Barlow, C. H., Chance, B. and Williamson, J. R. (1977). Heterogeneity of the hypoxic state in perfused rat heart. *Circulation Res.*, **41**, 606-15

Strange, R. C., Vetter, N., Rowe, M. J. and Oliver, M. F. (1974). Plasma cyclic AMP and total catecholamines during acute myocardial infarction in man. *Eur. J. clin. Invest.*, **4**, 115-9

Tennant, R. and Wiggers, C. J. (1935). The effect of coronary occlusion on myocardial contraction. *Am. J. Physiol.*, **123**, 351-61

Tsien, R. W. (1973). Adrenaline-like effects of intracellular iontophoresis of cyclic AMP in cardiac Purkinje fibres. *Nature new Biol.*, **245**, 120-2

Ui, M. (1966). A role of phosphofructokinase in pH-dependent regulation of glycolysis. *Biochim. biophys. Acta*, **124**, 310-22

Vetter, N. J., Strange, R. C., Adams, W. and Oliver, M. F. (1974). Initial metabolic and hormonal response to acute myocardial infarction. *Lancet*, *i*, 284-8

Webb, J. L. and Hollander, P. B. (1956). Metabolic aspects of the relationships between the contractility and membrane potentials of the rat atrium. *Circulation Res.*, **4**, 618-26

Weglicki, W. B., Owens, K., Ruth, R. C. and Sonnenblick, E. H. (1974). Activity of endogenous myocardial lipases during incubation at acid pH. *Cardiovasc. Res.*, 8, 237-42

Welman, E. and Peters, T. J. (1977). Enhanced lysosomal fragility in the anoxic perfused guinea-pig heart: effects of glucose and mannitol. *J. molec. cell. Cardiol.*, **9**, 101-20

Williamson, J. R., Schaffer, S. W., Ford, C. and Safer, B. (1976). Contribution of tissue acidosis to ischemic injury in the perfused rat heart. *Circulation*, **53**, Suppl. 1, 3-14

Wissner, S. B. (1974). The effect of excess lactate upon the excitability of the sheep Purkinje fibre. *J. Electrocardiol.*, 7, 17-26

Wit, A. L. and Bigger, J. T. (1975). Possible electrophysiological mechanisms for lethal arrhythmias accompanying myocardial ischemia and infarction. *Circulation*, **52**, Suppl. III, 96-115

Wollenberger, A. and Shahab, L. (1965). Anoxia-induced release of noradrenaline from isolated perfused heart. *Nature, Lond.*, **207**, 88-9

Wollenberger, A., Krause, E. G. and Shahab, L. (1967). Endogenous catecholamine mobilisation and the shift to anaerobic energy production in acutely ischaemic myocardium. In *International Symposium on the Coronary Circulation and Energetics of the Myocardium, Milan*, Karger, Basel, pp. 200-19

Yellon, D. M., Hearse, D. J., Crome, R., Grannell, J. and Wyse, R. K. H. (1981). Characterization of the lateral interface between normal and ischemic tissue in the canine heart lining involving myocardial infarction. *Am. J. Cardiol.*, **47**, 1233-9

3

Early Ventricular Arrhythmias: Relationship of Electrophysiology to Blood Flow and Metabolism

Douglas C. Russell

3.1 INTRODUCTION

An early phase of malignant ventricular arrhythmias occurs in the experimental animal within the first 15-30 min of acute coronary arterial ligation and ventricular fibrillation may result. The period of maximum vulnerability to fibrillation is between 5 and 10 min after the onset of occlusion, although a further burst of arrhythmias has been observed in some instances between 15 and 30 min of ischaemia (for references see chapter 6). Thereafter, despite continuing ischaemia, an arrhythmia-free period ensues for several hours.

The importance of these early arrhythmias and their mechanisms of pathogenesis lies in their possible relationship to mechanisms of sudden cardiac death in man in association with coronary heart disease. A large proportion of these deaths occur within the first 1-2 h of the acute heart attack and are due to ventricular fibrillation. This is during the phase of acute and potentially reversible myocardial ischaemia and is often prior to the onset of actual infarction. Indeed, of 239 patients resuscitated from out-of-hospital ventricular fibrillation, 200 had no evidence of myocardial infarction (Cobb *et al.*, 1975). Conversely, ventricular fibrillation is rare in patients with established myocardial infarction 6 h or more after the onset of the acute heart attack. Furthermore, the incidence of recurrent ventricular fibrillation in patients resuscitated from out-of-hospital early ventricular fibrillation is three times greater in patients who did not sustain myocardial infarction.

Profound alterations occur during this first few minutes of ischaemia, not only in the electrophysiological properties of the myocardium but also in regional blood flow distribution and cellular metabolism. Evidence would suggest that the early ventricular arrhythmias generated at this time result from re-entrant excitation or electrical circus movement within the myocardium. These are reviewed by Janse in chapter 4. The possibility arises therefore that underlying abnormal patterns of regional blood flow distribution or metabolism might predetermine or predispose to exact patterns of re-entrant excitation which may ultimately lead to ventricular arrhythmias or fibrillation. Furthermore, it has been suggested that modulation of the cellular metabolic response to acute ischaemia by alterations in substrate availability may influence the electrophysiological changes and hence exert an anti-arrhythmic effect.

To understand the mechanisms of genesis of these early ventricular arrhythmias, therefore, it is necessary to consider the nature of the early electrophysiological response and of associated alterations in cardiac metabolism and regional blood flow distribution during the acute phase of ischaemia.

3.2 ELECTROPHYSIOLOGICAL RESPONSES TO ISCHAEMIA

The phasic nature of ventricular arrhythmias during this early period of acute myocardial ischaemia is illustrated in figure 3.1. Data are taken from an experiment involving acute ligation of the left anterior descending coronary artery in an anaesthetised dog preparation. A burst of ventricular premature beats occurs within the first 10 min of coronary occlusion and is maximal in frequency after 5 min of ischaemia. Despite continuing occlusion and ischaemia these so-called Harris phase 1 arrhythmias subsided. These very early arrhythmias have been designated phase 1a arrhythmias as a second wave of arrhythmias (phase 1b) may follow more pro-

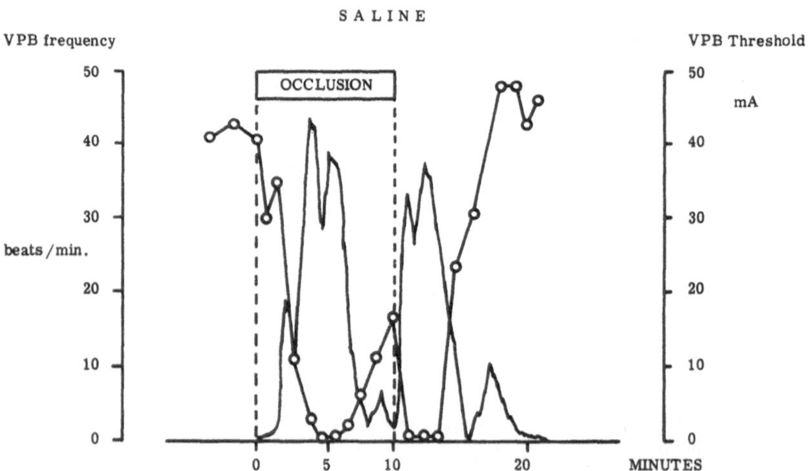

Figure 3.1 Frequency of ventricular premature beats during and following a 10 min period of occlusion of the left anterior descending coronary artery in a dog. Note the bursts of ventricular arrhythmias after 5 min of ischaemia and also on reperfusion. These phases of arrhythmias are mirrored by depressions in the ventricular premature beat threshold curve (open circles) of the current strength required to induce additional ventricular premature beats by extrastimulus testing.

longed periods of coronary occlusion of between 15 and 30 min of ischaemia. This figure also illustrates the appearance of reperfusion arrhythmias immediately on release of the coronary occlusion clip and which persist for only 2-3 min. Both early and late reperfusion arrhythmias have been described in the dog (Kaplinsky *et al.*, 1980).

Ventricular fibrillation may arise in association with both phases of early ischaemic arrhythmias and also on reperfusion. The electrophysiological mechanisms involved in the genesis of these various categories of arrhythmia are likely, however, to differ. Two major mechanisms are possible: first, enhancement or induction of automatic or spontaneous pacemaker activity; secondly, formation of continuous electrical circus movements of so-called re-entrant activation within the myocardium. Evidence, both indirect and direct, suggests that the dominant mechanism of genesis, at least of the first phase (1a) of early arrhythmias is that of re-entry. Both macro and micro re-entry circuits have been demonstrated with continuous electrical activity during the course of ventricular tachycardias resulting in fibrillation in the pig and the dog (Janse *et al.*, 1980). However, the additional possibility exists that excessive flow of current of injury between normal and ischaemic tissue may be sufficient to trigger a re-entrant impulse (Kleber *et al.*, 1978). Different mechanisms may operate during the second wave of early arrhythmias (phase 1b). In contrast to findings during phase 1a arrhythmias, low voltage continuous electrical bridging activity linking normal to ectopic beats and suggestive of re-entry is not demonstrable. Dominant mechanisms of genesis of reperfusion arrhythmias would seem to be that of enhanced, automatic activity (Penkoske *et al.*, 1978), although very early reperfusion arrhythmias immediately following release of experimental coronary occlusion may be re-entrant in origin (Kaplinsky *et al.*, 1980).

During ventricular fibrillation patterns of impulse propagation are fragmented and disorganised. Exact spatial patterns of conduction vary from moment to moment and it is believed that multiple asynchronous electrical circus movements are generated within the myocardium. The exact patterns of impulse propagation, however, must depend upon the patterns of distribution of electrophysiological abnormalities within individual myocardial cells. Abnormalities which could predispose to re-entrant activity include (1) marked slowing of conduction, (2) unidirectional conduction block and (3) inhomogeneities or regional variability in refractoriness. Each of these effects has indeed been observed during the first few minutes of experimental ischaemia.

During this time electrophysiological events occur extremely rapidly within the ischaemic zone. Surface recordings show ST-segment elevation within 20 s and surface bipolar electrograms demonstrate rapid loss of potential amplitude and marked slowing and fragmentation of surface activation at the time of genesis of early ventricular arrhythmias (Scherlag *et al.*, 1970; Boineau and Cox, 1973; Corr *et al.*, 1978). Strong evidence for re-entry is the finding of continuous electrical activity in surface recordings linking normally propagated impulses to ectopic beats in early (Janse *et al.*, 1980, and discussed in detail in chapter 4) and also in later (El-Sherif *et al.*, 1977) stages of ischaemia as a result of markedly delayed conduction.

More detailed information may be obtained from *in vivo* recordings of intracellular cardiac action potentials using a floating micro-electrode technique (Downar *et al.*, 1977; Russell *et al.*, 1977). An initial transient prolongation of action potential duration is followed by progressive shortening associated with loss of action potential amplitude, reduction in resting membrane potential and a marked reduction of initial upstroke velocity. This latter change coincides with a progressive delay and fractionation of epicardial activation. An example of the time course of these changes is given in figure 3.2, the data being taken from a dog developing ventricular fibrillation 4.5 min after coronary occlusion. Fibrillation can be seen to occur at a time of maximum endocardial-epicardial conduction

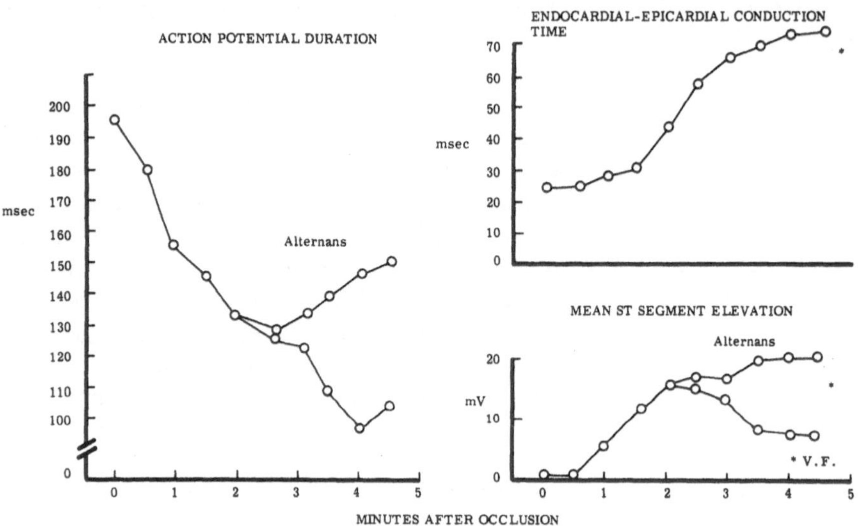

Figure 3.2 Changes in action potential duration, endocardial and epicardial conduction delay and mean ST-segment elevation preceding ventricular fibrillation in a dog following acute ligation of the left anterior descending coronary artery.

delay in the central ischaemic area and is preceded by maximal shortening in action potential duration. Potentials recorded at this time demonstrate electrical alternans of duration and amplitude and have markedly depressed initial upstroke velocities. This may represent either true electrical alternans or alternatively electrotonic interaction between areas of normal activation and intermittent conduction block. In one series of animals, ventricular fibrillation was preceded by recordings of electrical alternans in over 90 per cent of cases and by regional conduction block in over 60 per cent. This intermittency and regional inhomogeneity of distribution of conduction within the ischaemic myocardium may be critical for formation of re-entrant circuits. Furthermore, the morphology of potentials recorded immediately preceding fibrillation is very similar to that of the slowly conducting slow response potentials recorded *in vitro* under conditions of partial depolarisation (Cranefield, 1975). A reduction of membrane potential to below –60 mV inactivates the fast sodium current responsible for initial rapid depolarisation and unmasks a much slower inward current carried largely by calcium ions. Such potentials have the exact conduction properties necessary for re-entry and are also prone to alternating activity and conduction block. In addition, the conditions during the first few minutes of ischaemia of increased concentrations of extracellular potassium together with intracellular and extracellular acidosis should predispose to slow response depolarisation. It is possible, however, that recorded depressed depolarisations *in vivo* may represent fast response action potentials resulting from depressed inward sodium current rather than true slow response activity.

The likelihood of re-entry is further enhanced by findings of regional variability in excitability thresholds and refractoriness immediately preceding early ventricular arrhythmias and fibrillation (Russell and Oliver, 1978). Dispersion of refractoriness is known to be increased during ischaemia and to be related to a decrease in fibrillation threshold (Han and Moe, 1964). Indeed, disparities in refractoriness of as little as 11 ms in adjacent areas are sufficient to generate local re-entrant activity. During mild ischaemia refractory periods shorten in parallel with changes in action potential

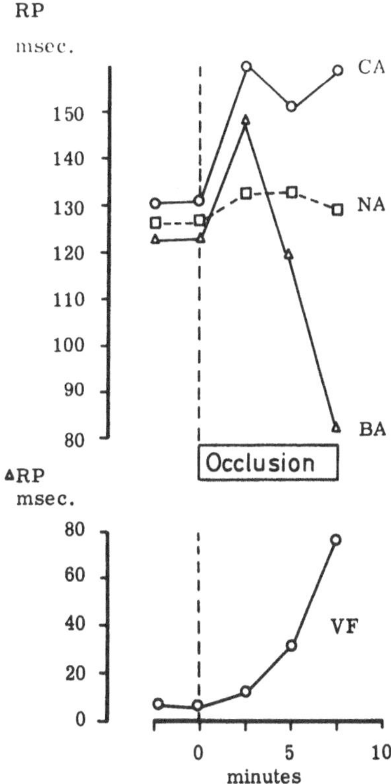

Figure 3.3 Changes in ventricular refractory period (RP) in non-ischaemic (NA), central (CA) and border ischaemic (BA) zones preceding early ventricular fibrillation in a dog. Little change in refractoriness is seen in the normal area but marked divergence in refractoriness occurs between central and border ischaemic zones preceding fibrillation.

duration. However, during more severe ischaemia associated with arrhythmias a wide variety of divergent patterns of change of refractoriness occur with prolongation of refractoriness despite further shortening of action potential duration (Downar *et al.*, 1977; Russell and Oliver, 1978). Figure 3.3 demonstrates changes in refractory period determined in central ischaemic, border ischaemic and non-ischaemic myocardium immediately preceding fibrillation in a dog. Marked divergence of refractoriness occurs between central and border areas with few or no changes in the normal zone. Inhomogeneity of recovery of excitability is therefore generated across the ischaemic zone which is of an order to permit asynchrony of ventricular activation necessary for fibrillation. Infusion of catecholamines or sympathetic stimulation further increases these inhomogeneities (Han and Moe, 1964). Underlying metabolic factors may also be of importance. Additional electrophysiological inhomogeneity of conduction may result from abnormal electrical coupling between cells which may induce localised conduction blocks and abnormal flow of current or injury.

3.3 INTRACELLULAR RESPONSES TO ISCHAEMIA

The early and rapid electrophysiological changes associated with arrhythmogenesis occur in association with profound metabolic changes within the first few minutes of myocardial ischaemia. These have been discussed in detail in chapter 2. The distribution of these metabolic changes within the myocardium is by no means uniform. An immediate reduction of coronary blood flow and hence of oxygen supply to the ischaemic zone follows acute coronary occlusion. The regional severity of induced ischaemia is dependent upon multiple factors including the degree of collateral perfusion and regional metabolic demands. Cyanosis and regional contractile abnormalities are apparent within 5 s. Creatine phosphate levels fall within 30 s and ATP levels within 1 min accompanied by a rapid decline in intracellular pH (Braasch *et al.*, 1968). At the same time an outpouring of potassium, lactate, adenosine and inosine into the extracellular space may be detected together with a fall in extracellular pH. Glycogen stores are diminished within 30 s and anaerobic glycolysis is stimulated. In addition either transient or sustained increases in tissue cyclic AMP have been reported which may relate to sympathetic stimulation, local noradrenaline release from post-ganglionic nerve terminals or elevations in plasma concentration of catecholamines. This is discussed in chapter 11.

In addition to these gross effects a major shift occurs in cardiac metabolism away from the normal oxidation of free fatty acids towards aerobic and anaerobic glucose metabolism. These effects could be of relevance to arrhythmogenesis as *in vitro* studies have shown a dependence of likely activity of the so-called slow channels in the cell membrane (and hence slowly conducting 'slow response' potentials) on intracellular ATP derived from the anaerobic phase of glycolysis (McDonald *et al.*, 1971). Slowly conducting potentials of this type could generate the slow circus movements of activation of re-entry. Stimulation of glycolysis, however, is transient and inhibition finally results from excessive lactate or hydrogen ion accumulation. At the same time as glycolysis is enhanced the normal β-oxidation of fatty acids is inhibited. Tissue levels of long chain acyl CoA are increased and by inhibiting adenine nucleotide translocases may reduce ATP transport from mitochondria to the cytosol (Shug *et al.*, 1975). This in turn could limit ATP availability for electrophysiological processes. These processes may be accelerated by increases in plasma concentrations of free fatty acids and indeed it has been suggested that under certain circumstances this may be arrhythmogenic. This may be so particularly if concentrations of fatty acids in plasma exceed the binding capacity of albumin. In the presence of accumulation of unoxidised intracellular fatty acids or long chain acyl CoA with inhibition of oxidative ATP production, the major source of energy for the ischaemic cell would be that derived from anaerobic glycolysis. The possibility arises, therefore, that low levels of residual high energy phosphate synthesis from glycolysis might have important electrophysiological effects.

3.4 REGIONAL METABOLIC ABNORMALITIES AND ARRHYTHMIAS

Many observed electrophysiological effects of myocardial ischaemia may be explained on the basis of the biochemical and metabolic response to ischaemia. The major possible factors of importance are outlined in table 3.1 and are believed to be as discussed below.

Table 3.1 Possible metabolic influences of ischaemia on arrhythmogenesis

(1) Ionic shifts
Increased extracellular potassium
Acidosis
(2) Toxic metabolites
Free fatty acids
Lactate
Lysophosphatides
Fatty acyl carnitine
(3) Adrenergic activation
cAMP
(4) Cellular energy status
ATP, ADP, AMP, creatine phosphate

Accumulation of intracellular (H^+) or extracellular (H^+, K^+) ions

Elevation of extracellular potassium is known to reduce conduction velocity and shorten duration of the cardiac action potential (see chapter 7). It may also cause partial membrane depolarisation sufficient to inactivate the rapid inward sodium current and generate slowly conducting slow response potentials, this effect being facilitated by catecholamines. In the dog and pig the ventricular fibrillation of early ischaemia occurs at levels of around 14 mM extracellular potassium but regional inhomogeneity of potassium distribution has been observed at this time (Hill and Gettes, 1980). Regional acidosis has a depressant effect on excitability and may modulate conduction of slow potentials or induce conduction block.

Accumulation of toxic metabolites

The rapidity of onset of electrophysiological changes during myocardial ischaemia and the rapid reversibility of changes on reperfusion even with persistence of hypoxia suggest a possible effect of accumulating metabolites. Certainly not all observed phenomena can be accounted for by potassium and hydrogen ion accumulation. Accumulation of excess unoxidised free fatty acids and fatty acyl CoA derivatives have been implicated in arrhythmogenesis on the basis of a clinical association between elevated free fatty acids and arrythmias in man in the early stages of acute myocardial infarction (Kurien and Oliver, 1970). More recently, a possible toxic effect of lysophosphoglyceride has been suggested (Corr *et al.*, 1979) and this hypothesis is discussed in detail in chapter 12. These substances are elevated in ischaemic tissue and also in ischaemic venous effluent due to the action of phospholipase on membrane phospholipid and have produced *in vitro* depressant effects similar to effects observed *in vivo* during ischaemia, particularly under conditions of acidosis. Similar effects which are additive to those of lysophosphatides are obtained with fatty acyl carnitine, which also accumulates in the cytosol during ischaemia.

Adrenergic influences

Catecholamines are arrhythmogenic and their role during early ischaemia is discussed elsewhere in this volume (chapters 8–10 and 16). Cellular effects include shortening of action potential duration and refractory period, hyperpolarisation of partially depolarised fibres and stimulation of slow response activity in depressed tissue. Regional dispersion of refractoriness is enhanced and this may promote re-entry and stimulate automatic activity. An additional hypothesis is that a sudden increase in intracellular cyclic AMP may be arrhythmogenic (chapter 11). It is of interest that slowly conducting slow response potentials are sensitive to alterations in cyclic AMP, probably by modulation of calcium influx through slow channels in the cell membrane.

Cellular ATP production

Cellular high-energy phosphate production is necessary for maintenance of ionic active transport mechanisms and for the maintenance of normal resting levels of transmembrane potential. Of more importance, however, may be an energy dependency of the slow inward current mediated largely by ATP derived from the anaerobic phase of glycolysis (McDonald and MacLeod, 1973). The beneficial effects of exogenous creatine phosphate in the early stages of acute myocardial ischaemia, which include suppression of ventricular ectopic activity (Marshall and Parratt, 1974; Fagbemi *et al.*, 1982), have also been explained by the provision of energy to activate the slow (ATP-dependent) cation (Na^+ and Ca^{2+}) channels.

3.5 METABOLIC MAPPING AND ARRHYTHMIAS

A major factor in the genesis of early re-entrant arrhythmias would appear to be inhomogeneity of electrophysiological responses in the ischaemic myocardium with particular respect to regional abnormalities in conduction and refractoriness. Furthermore, it is likely that this electrophysiological non-uniformity may relate to the known heterogeneity of biochemical responses to ischaemia. The specific changes which may have electrophysiological effects have been outlined above. However, the degree to which any individual metabolic effect contributes to the overall electrophysiological response to ischaemia remains ill-defined. The possibility arises therefore that specific patterns of conduction in the ischaemic myocardium may relate to specific patterns of biochemical abnormality which in turn could relate to patterns of collateral perfusion of the ischaemic zone.

A further possibility is that critical modulations of local electrophysiological effects induced by ionic shifts, accumulation of metabolites or adrenergic influence may result from regional variations in cellular energy production. For example, active ionic pumping may maintain the resting membrane potential against an adverse transmembrane gradient of potassium ions. Slowly conducting slow response potentials are highly sensitive to small fluctuations in ATP at the inner cell membrane (McDonald *et al.*, 1971). Marked slowing and fractionation of conduction has been observed in the central ischaemic zone at exactly the time when glycolysis might be expected to be stimulated or depressed but not completely inhibited (Boineau and Cox, 1973; Russell *et al.*, 1979). It is possible, therefore, that regional variations in glycolytic ATP production within the central ischaemic area might control patterns of slow conduction in depressed tissue and hence patterns of impulse propagation and re-entry. Furthermore, this might enhance regional electrophysiological gradients and hence inhomogeneity. It might also account for certain rapid beat-to-beat modulation of electrophysiological properties such as electrical alternans and intermittent conduction block.

For these reasons a series of detailed mapping studies have been performed at the time of onset of early ventricular arrhythmias following experimental myocardial ischaemia in order to attempt to interrelate patterns of regional flow, metabolism and conduction in the ischaemic zone.

Studies were performed in open chest dogs under pentobarbitone anaesthesia. The left anterior descending coronary artery was occluded proximally (but distal to the septal branch) to induce a large area of myocardial ischaemia. This resulted in ventricular arrhythmias or fibrillation within 3-5 min of onset of ischaemia. A

50 mm × 40 mm area of left ventricle was selected for analysis, encompassing the major part of the ischaemic border, some non-ischaemic tissue and the 'border area' between the two. At the time of onset of arrhythmias simultaneous or near simultaneous maps were derived within this area of epicardial activation patterns, regional myocardial blood flow, tissue lactate and indices of glycolytic activity. Each map was derived from 80 data points and for tissue analysis separate maps were made for endocardial and epicardial patterns. Visualisation of the complex changes occurring was aided greatly by use of a three-dimensional computer plotting program.

Epicardial activation patterns were derived by analysis of individual epicardial activation delays from multiplexed electrograms recorded from an 80-point flexible multi-electrode grid sutured to the anterior surface of the left ventricle in the area of distribution of the left anterior descending coronary artery. Inter-electrode separation was 5 mm. Signals were recorded on tape and subsequently demultiplexed. Only data from normally propagated non-ectopic beats were analysed. Simultaneous determination of regional myocardial blood flow was made by the tracer microsphere technique after left atrial injection of large numbers (25×10^6) of 9 μm microspheres. Such large numbers were chosen to permit adequate resolution of flow at the low flow levels of ischaemia. After collection of a reference arterial blood sample for calibration of blood flow data, the heart was rapidly excised and immersed in liquid nitrogen. Tissue samples were then taken from endocardium and epicardium respectively at 80 sites corresponding to the overlying electrode positions at the termination of the study. Regional flow was assessed from microsphere radioactivity in each sample. Analysis was also performed on each sample of lactate concentration and ^3H_2O content, animals previously having been infused over a 90 min period with [2-^{3}H] glucose. This latter measurement may be taken as a rough index of on-going glycolytic breakdown of [2-^{3}H] glucose. Corrections were not made, however, for regional variations resulting from differential regional washout. By this means a series of three-dimensional maps could be constructed in each animal for regional flow, regional lactate and regional ^3H_2O distribution from endocardium and from epicardium in the 50 mm × 40 mm area of interest for comparison with simultaneous maps of patterns of epicardial activation. This was all carried out within a minute of the onset of early ventricular arrhythmias.

An example of one such series of maps is shown in figures 3.4–3.7. This animal developed ventricular arrhythmias within 3.5 min of coronary occlusion and the maps refer to data at 5 min of ischaemia. Horizontal axes of the maps refer to the section taken of the anterior wall of the left ventricle underlying the attached electrode grid. Vertical axes refer respectively to epicardial activation delays and epicardial and endocardial regional blood flow, lactate and ^3H_2O distribution.

Examination of the epicardial activation maps (figure 3.4) reveals considerable delays in surface activation within the central ischaemic area during an abnormally propagated impulse. In addition fragmentation of activation delays are seen in areas of depressed conduction. Maps from other studies (not shown) show quite variable patterns and in some animals discrete zones of conduction block occur.

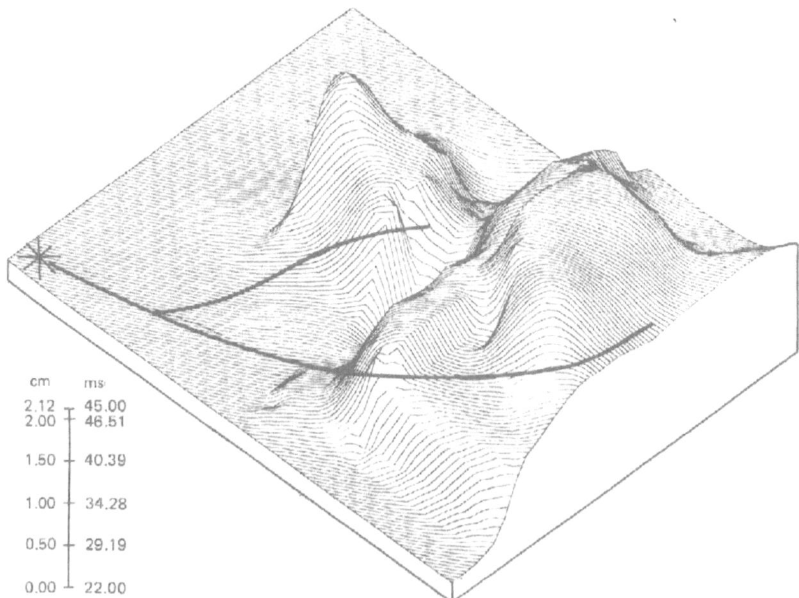

Figure 3.4 Three-dimensional computer map of epicardial activation delay at the time of onset of early ventricular arrhythmias. Horizontal axes refer to a selected 40 mm x 50 mm area of epicardium in the region of distribution of the left anterior descending coronary artery. Vertical axis refers to epicardial activation delay (in milliseconds). For discussion see text.

These findings are consistent with subsequent or associated formation of re-entrant circuits as a mechanism of arrhythmogenesis. Comparison with simultaneous flow maps (figure 3.5) reveals a number of important features. First, the area of conduction delays and fractionation of conduction is found to lie within a zone of markedly depressed flow to levels of 25 per cent or less of that in the non-ischaemic area. In addition, within this central ischaemic area considerable heterogeneities of flow values are observed, in some studies ranging from 5 to 25 per cent of non-ischaemic values. This spatial heterogeneity of flow occurred in the same areas as the inhomogeneities of epicardial activation (see figures 3.4 and 3.5), although values did not correlate directly. This relation between epicardial activation delay and regional flow in one experiment is shown in figure 3.8. Little or no delay in activation is observed at intermediate flow values above 25 per cent of normal. At least in these experiments, therefore, the properties of the so-called border region would not appear to influence the genesis of re-entrant circuits. Preliminary studies suggest that in some animals steep profiles of flow reduction across the border may be the site of intermittent conduction block. It is of interest, therefore, that variability in profiles of flow is observed across this border area in some animals (figure 3.9). These profiles of flow are sharp in some areas but more progressive (over three or four tissue samples) in other areas. These variable gradients would seem likely to reflect true areas of intermediate flow rather than tissue sampling artefacts across a sharp border region.

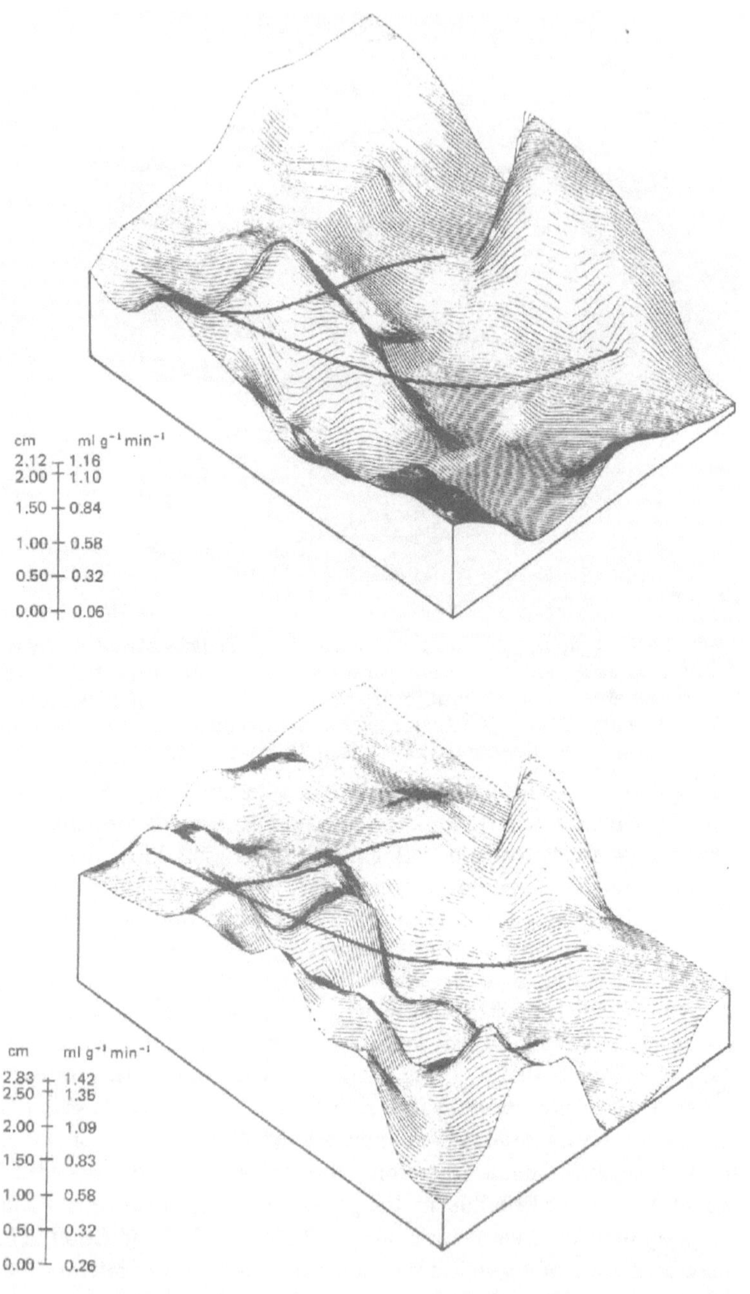

Figure 3.5 Three-dimensional computer map of (above) epicardial and (below) endocardial blood flow in a selected 40 mm × 50 mm area of myocardium at the time of onset of early ventricular arrhythmias. The vertical axis refers to blood flow in millilitres per gram per minute. For full discussion see text.

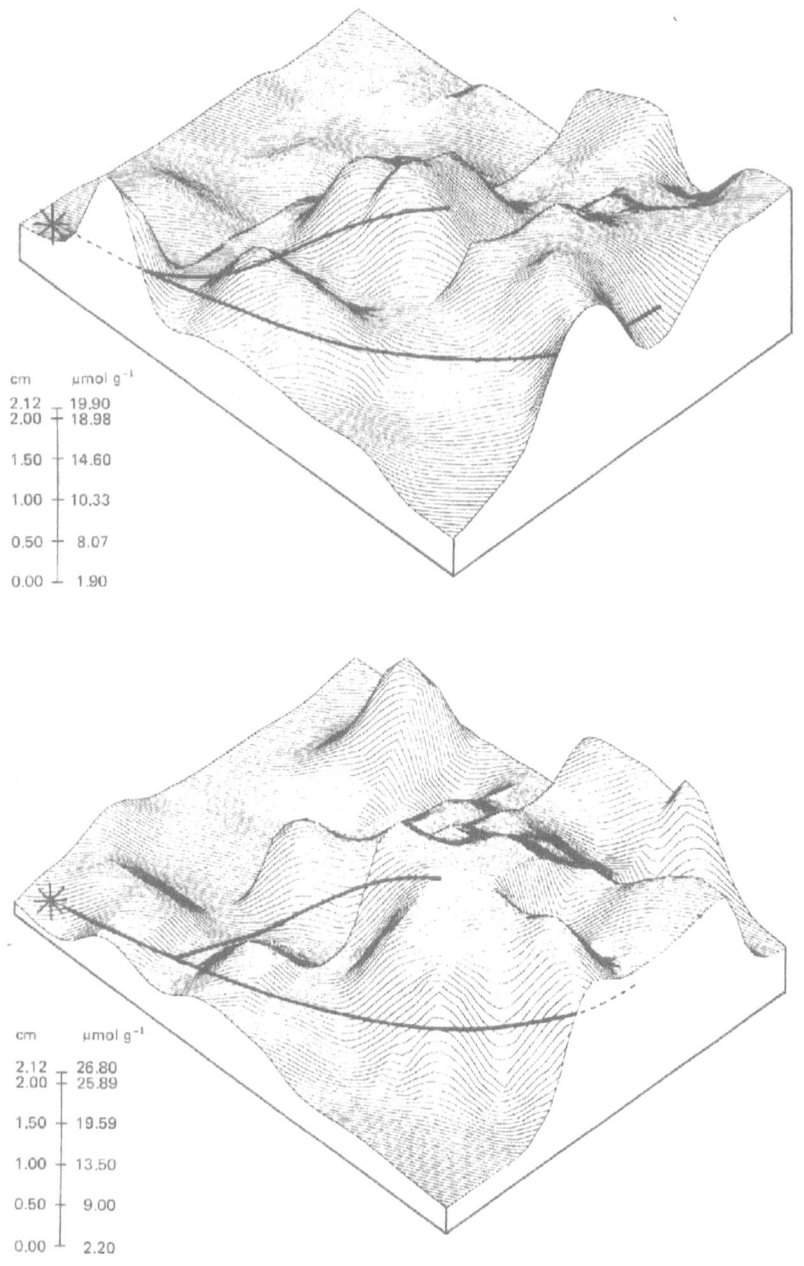

Figure 3.6 Three-dimensional computer maps of (above) epicardial and (below) endocardial tissue lactate content (in micromoles per gram) in a selected 40 mm × 50 mm area of myocardium (the same as in figure 3.5) at the time of onset of early ventricular arrhythmias. For full discussion see text.

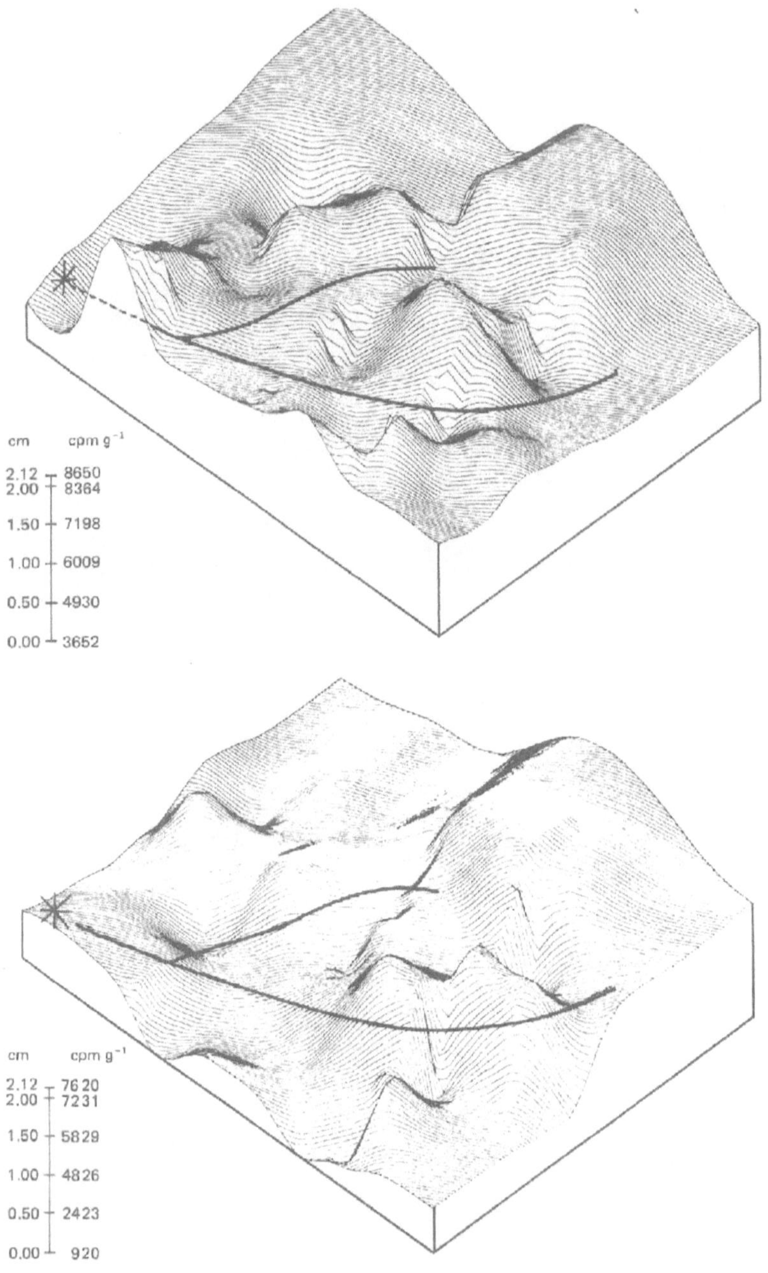

Figure 3.7 Three-dimensional computer maps of (above) epicardial and (below) endocardial tissue ^3H_2O content (in counts per minute per gram) in a selected 40 mm × 50 mm area of myocardium (corresponding to those in figures 3.5 and 3.6) at the time of onset of early ventricular arrhythmias. For full discussion see text.

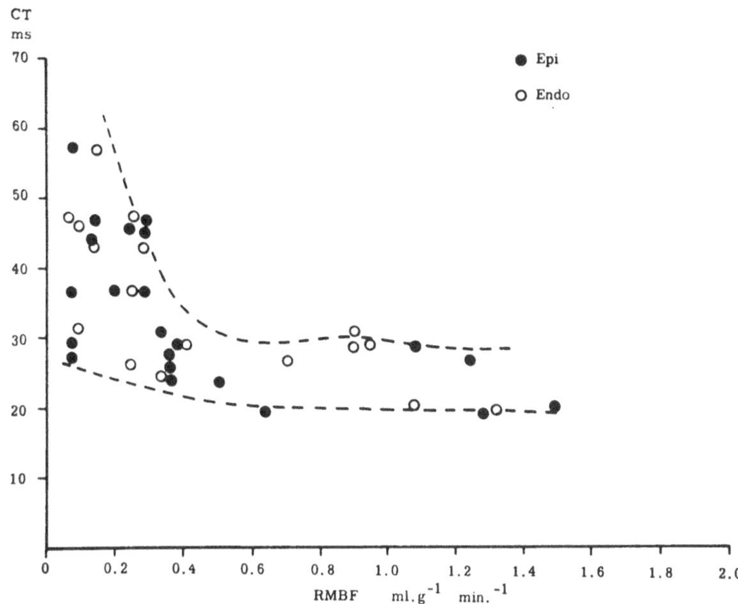

Figure 3.8 Relation between epicardial activation delay (CT) and regional myocardial blood flow (RMBF) in one animal at the time of onset of early ischaemic arrhythmias. Flow values are taken from endocardium and epicardium. Conduction is little impaired until flow is reduced to below 0.3 ml g^{-1} min^{-1}.

Similar inhomogeneities are revealed in the three-dimensional plots of tissue lactate (figure 3.6) and ^3H_2O distribution (figure 3.7). Tissue lactate levels are increased within the ischaemic zone (more so in endocardium than epicardium) reflecting anaerobic glycolysis. This is not, however, uniform. A highly significant correlation was found between regional flow and lactate in individual 5 mm^2 samples of tissue ($P < 0.001$), highest lactate levels being found in areas of lowest flow and vice versa (see figures 3.5 and 3.6). One possibility is that the extent of aerobic glycolysis and hence oxidation of lactate may vary within the ischaemic zone. Examination of the ^3H_2O maps (figure 3.7) reveals some similarities with the lactate maps (figure 3.6) but also some important differences. Similar inhomogeneity of distribution is found within the central ischaemic area of conduction abnormality. In the so-called border region at the edge of the ischaemic zone, however, a ridge of enhanced ^3H_2O content is observed in an area where conduction is little impaired (figure 3.7). An interpretation of these observations is that an area of enhanced glycolytic activity is present near the edge of the ischaemic zone and that variable patterns of glycolysis, and hence glycolytic energy production, co-exist in the central ischaemic area. The spatial relation of these changes to the border area are shown more clearly in figure 3.9. Profiles of lactate and ^3H_2O are shown in tangential sections at several points across the edge of the ischaemic area in one animal and contrasted with profiles of flow and activation delay. The dotted line

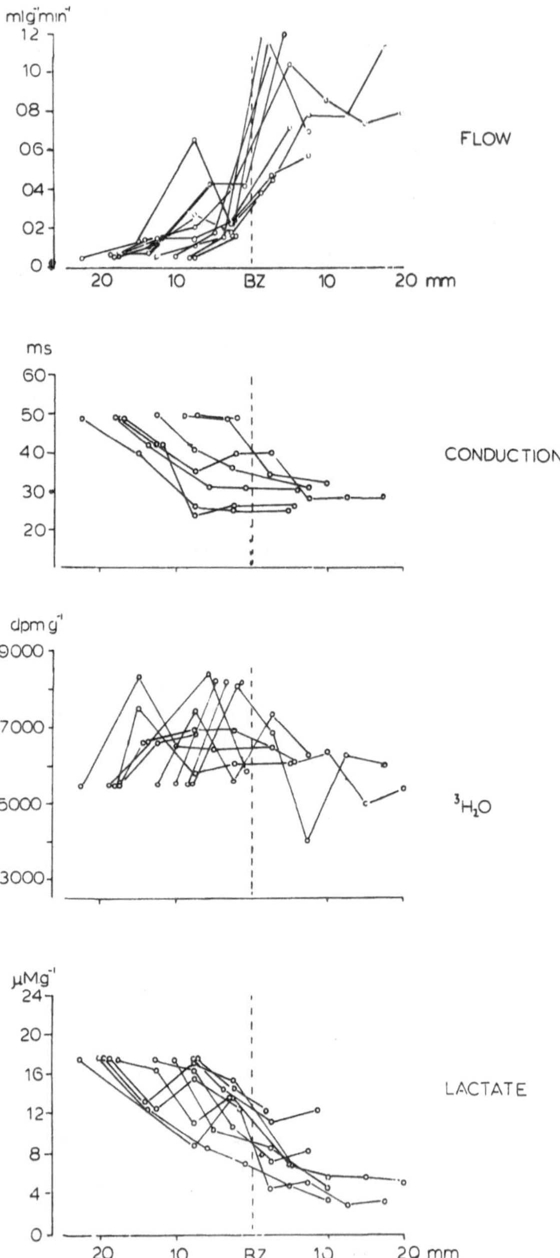

Figure 3.9 Profiles of flow, conduction delay, lactate and ^3H_2O (as an index of glycolytic activity) between non-ischaemic and ischaemic myocardium in one animal at the time of onset of early arrhythmias. The dotted line refers to the position of 50 per cent reduction in regional flow. Continuous lines refer to radial sections across the edge of the ischaemic area at different sites (see text).

arbitrarily refers to a line of 50 per cent reduction in regional flow and the ischaemic area is to the left of the diagram. The spatial heterogeneity of flow, conduction and metabolic activity with respect to the edge of the ischaemic area is clearly seen.

It is suggested on the basis of these studies that inhomogeneities of glycolytic activity within the central ischaemic area may be of critical importance in determining exact pathways of re-entrant excitation by virtue of effects on energy-dependent slow conduction, possibly mediated by slow response activity.

3.6 METABOLIC INTERVENTIONS

Should such a mechanism be operative a basis is provided for understanding potential antiarrhythmic effects resulting from manipulation of the efficiency of cellular energy production by alteration in myocardial substrate availability. Studies in our laboratory have shown that an approximate doubling of arterial glucose levels is effective in reducing the arrhythmia threshold (Russell and Oliver, 1979) and also in reversing abnormalities in conduction and refractoriness. This is accompanied by an increase in glucose extraction by the ischaemic zone. This is true, however, only for a mild degree of ischaemia such as that which follows a distal branch occlusion and does not hold for more severe ischaemia resulting in early ventricular fibrillation (Russell, 1979). Similar disparities in antiarrhythmic effectiveness of glucose-insulin-potassium regimes have been borne out in clinical studies. Although the initial studies of Sodi-Pallares *et al.* (1963) in patients with acute myocardial infarction appeared to show an antiarrhythmic effect of glucose-insulin-potassium, other large scale studies have been inconclusive. Findings of many of these studies may be dismissed as therapy was commenced well after the early hours of ischaemia when arrhythmias are most severe (Opie, 1980). The findings of Rogers *et al.* (1976) are of particular interest. Hospital mortality rate was approximately halved by administering glucose-insulin-potassium in 70 patients commencing within the first few hours after onset of symptoms of myocardial infarction. The greatest reduction in mortality was in patients with least complications - those without previous myocardial infarction and those with single vessel coronary arterial disease. A possible explanation of this differential effect of glucose might lie in its effects on the spatial heterogeneity of glycolysis under differing degrees of severity of ischaemia. During mild ischaemia a stimulation of glycolysis might influence preferentially areas of depressed metabolic activity and so diminish electrophysiological inhomogeneities in the ischaemic zone. By contrast, in more severe ischaemia stimulation of glycolysis might affect multiple small areas within depressed tissue and so enhance, rather than diminish, electrophysiological inhomogeneity. Furthermore, transient stimulation of anaerobic glycolysis during severe ischaemia might either enhance or depress glycolytic ATP production in adjacent areas of tissue with consequent effects on conduction, refractoriness and arrhythmogenicity.

Similar mechanisms could play a role in the antiarrhythmic action of antilipolytic therapy. An analogue of nicotinic acid has been shown to reduce the incidence of ventricular arrhythmias within the first 6 h of onset of myocardial infarction, but only in a subgroup of patients showing a large fall in serum-free fatty acid concentrations (Rowe *et al.*, 1975). This same agent is effective in reducing ST segment in patients with acute myocardial ischaemia and infarction and in decreasing ST-segment depression during exercise-induced myocardial ischaemia with stable angina (Luxton *et al.*, 1976). Animal studies have shown less striking effects than with glucose with amelioration of abnormalities in refractoriness, although not in conduction (Russell, 1979). Antilipolytic therapy markedly reduces myocardial oxygen consumption, particularly during adrenergic stimulation, and might be expected to influence the distribution of metabolically dependent electrophysiological processes during myocardial ischaemia.

Inroads have thus been made into the potential management of malignant arrhythmias by metabolic rather than pharmacological means. The ultimate goal of metabolic intervention might be to reduce the inhomogeneities of tissue metabolism which could set the scene for re-entry, rather than manipulate the absolute severity of ischaemic injury. This might be achieved by improvement of collateral flow, reduction of the adrenergic response to ischaemia or by increased supply of glucose or decreased intracellular accumulation of free fatty acids.

REFERENCES

Boineau, J. P. and Cox, J. L. (1973). Slow ventricular activation in acute myocardial infarction. A source of re-entrant premature ventricular contraction. *Circulation*, **48**, 702–13

Braasch, W., Gudbjarnason, S., Pari, P. S., Ravens, R. G. and Bing, R. J. (1968). Early changes in energy metabolism in the myocardium following acute coronary occlusion in anesthetized dogs. *Circulation Res.*, **23**, 429–38

Cobb, L. A., Baum, R. S., Alvarez, H. and Schaffer, W. A. (1975). Resuscitation from out-of-hospital ventricular fibrillation. 4 years follow-up. *Circulation*, **52**, Suppl. III, 223-9

Corr, P. B., Witkowski, F. X. and Sobel, B. E. (1978). Mechanisms contributing to malignant dysrrhythmias induced by ischemia in the cat. *J. clin. Invest.*, **61**, 109–19

Corr, P. B., Cain, M. E., Witkowski, F. X., Price, D. A. and Sobel, B. E. (1979). Potential arrhythmogenic electrophysiological derangements in canine Purkinje fibres induced by lysophosphoglycerides. *Circulation Res.*, **44**, 822-32

Cranefield, P. F. (1975). *The Conduction of the Cardiac Impulse: The Slow Response and Cardiac Arrhythmias*, Futura Press, Mount Kisco, N.Y.

Downar, E., Janse, M. J. and Durrer, D. (1977). The effect of coronary artery occlusion on subepicardial transmembrane potentials in the intact porcine heart. *Circulation*, **56**, 217-24

El-Sherif, N., Scherlag, B. J., Lazzara, R. and Hope, R. R. (1977). Re-entrant ventricular arrhythmias in the late myocardial infarction, period 1. Conduction characteristics in the infarction zone. *Circulation*, **55**, 686-702

Fagbemi, O., Kane, K. A. and Parratt, J. R. (1982). Creatine phosphate suppresses ventricular arrhythmias resulting from coronary artery ligation. *J. cardiovasc. Pharmac.*, **4**, 53-8

Han, J. and Moe, G. K. (1964). Non-uniform recovery of excitability in ventricular muscle. *Circulation Res.*, **14**, 44-60

Hill, J. L. and Gettes, L. S. (1980). Effect of acute coronary artery occlusion on local myocardial extracellular K^+ activity in swine. *Circulation*, **61**, 768-78

Janse, M. J., Capelle, F. J. L. van, Morsink, H., Kleber, A. G., Wilms-Schopman, F., Cardinal, R., Naumann D'Alnoncourt, C. and Durrer, D. (1980). Flow of 'injury' current and patterns of excitation during early ventricular arrhythmias in acute regional myocardial ischemia in isolated porcine and canine hearts. *Circulation Res.*, **47**, 151-65

Kaplinsky, E., Ogawa, S., Michelson, E. L. and Dreifus, L. S. (1980). Spontaneous and delayed ventricular arrhythmias after reperfusion of acutely ischemic myocardium: evidence for multiple mechanisms. *Circulation*, **63**, 333-40

Kleber, A. G., Janse, M. J., Capelle, F. J. L. van and Durrer, D. (1978). Mechanism and time course of ST and T-Q segment changes during acute regional myocardial ischaemia in the pig's heart determined by extracellular and intracellular recordings. *Circulation Res.*, **42**, 603-13

Kurien, V. A. and Oliver, M. F. (1970). A metabolic cause of arrhythmias during experimental myocardial infarction. *Lancet*, *ii*, 185-7

Luxton, M. R., Miller, N. E. and Oliver, M. F. (1976). Antilipolytic therapy in angina pectoris: reduction of exercise-induced ST-segment depression. *Br. Heart J.*, **38**, 1204-8

McDonald T. F. and MacLeod, D. P. (1973). Metabolism and electrical activity of anoxic ventricular muscle. *J. Physiol., Lond.*, **229**, 559-82

McDonald, T. F., Hunter, E. G. and MacLeod, D. P. (1971). Adenosine triphosphate partition in cardiac muscle with respect to transmembrane electrical activity. *Pflügers Arch. ges. Physiol.*, **322**, 95-108

Marshall, R. J. and Parratt, J. R. (1974). Reduction in ventricular arrhythmias following acute coronary artery ligation in the dog after the administration of creatine phosphate. *Naunyn-Schmiedebergs Arch. Pharmac.*, **281**, 437-41

Opie, L. H. (1980). Myocardial infarct size. Comparison of anti-infarct effects of beta-blockade, glucose-insulin-potassium, nitrates and hyaluronidase. *Am. Heart J.*, **100**, 531-52

Penkoske, P. A., Sobel, B. E. and Corr, P. B. (1978). Disparate electrophysiological alterations accompanying dysrhythmias due to coronary occlusion and reperfusion in the cat. *Circulation*, **58**, 1023-35

Rogers, W. J., Stanley, A. W., Breinig, J. B., Prather, J. W., McDaniel, H. E., Moraski, R. E., Mantue, J. A., Russell, R. O. and Rackley, C. E. (1976). Reduction of hospital mortality rate of acute myocardial infarction with glucose-insulin-potassium infusion. *Am. Heart J.*, **92**, 441-54

Rowe, M. J., Neilson, J. M. M. and Oliver, M. F. (1975). Control of ventricular arrhythmias during myocardial infarction by antilipolytic treatment using a nicotinic acid analogue. *Lancet*, *i*, 295-300

Russell, D. C. (1979). Electrophysiological effects of substrate manipulation during acute myocardial ischaemia. PhD thesis, University of Edinburgh

Russell, D. C. and Oliver, M. F. (1978). Ventricular refractoriness during acute myocardial ischaemia and its relationship to ventricular fibrillation. *Cardiovasc. Res.*, **12**, 221-7

Russell, D. C. and Oliver, M. F. (1979). The effect of intravenous glucose on ventricular vulnerability following acute coronary artery occlusion in the dog. *J. molec. cell. Cardiol.*, **11**, 31-44

Russell, D. C., Oliver, M. F. and Wojtczak, J. (1977). Combined electrophysiological techniques for assessment of the cellular basis of ventricular arrhythmias. Experiments in dogs. *Lancet*, *ii*, 686-8

Russell, D. C., Smith, H. J. and Oliver, M. F. (1979). Transmembrane potential changes and ventricular fibrillation during repetitive myocardial ischaemia in the dog. *Br. Heart J.*, **42**, 88

Scherlag, B. J., Helfant, R. H., Haft, J. I. and Damato, A. N. (1970). Electrophysiological changes underlying ventricular arrhythmias due to coronary ligation. *Am. J. Physiol.*, **219**, 1665-71

Shug, A. L., Shrago, E., Bittar, N., Folts, J. D. and Koke, J. R. (1975). Acyl-CoA inhibition of adenine nucleotide translocation in ischemic myocardium. *Am. J. Physiol.*, **228**, 689-92

Sodi-Pallares, D., Bisteni, A., Medrano, G. A., Testelli, M. R. and Micheli, A. de (1963). The polarizing treatment of acute myocardial infarction - possibility of its use in other cardiovascular conditions. *Dis. Chest*, **43**, 424-32

4

Electrophysiological Changes in the Acute Phase of Myocardial Ischaemia and Mechanisms of Ventricular Arrhythmias

Michael J. Janse

4.1 INTRODUCTION

It has been known for a long time that occlusion of a coronary artery in dogs results in the frequent occurrence of ventricular arrhythmias and that these occur in different phases (Harris, 1950). In the first 15-30 min ventricular arrhythmias are particularly malignant, frequently leading to ventricular fibrillation. Then follows a period during which arrhythmias are rare, until the second phase of arrhythmias begins after 4-8 h. These can continue for several days. Although it is not known whether such a bimodal distribution occurs in all animals, including man, the early phase of arrhythmias may be related to the 'pre-hospital' phase of arrhythmias in humans with coronary artery disease. It is by no means certain that all ventricular arrhythmias, particularly fibrillation, occurring in the setting of coronary artery disease are caused by the electrophysiological alterations due to the cessation of blood flow to part of the ventricular myocardium. It is well known that, in the experimental animal, release of a coronary artery occlusion induces ventricular fibrillation much more frequently than does the occlusion itself, provided that the occlusion is released abruptly and not too long after the vessel was occluded (Tennant and Wiggers, 1935; Stephenson *et al.*, 1960). It is also known that the majority of patients resuscitated from out-of-hospital fibrillation subsequently show no signs of myocardial necrosis (Baum *et al.*, 1974). One may therefore speculate whether in some cases spasm of coronary artery could occur, the release of which after a few minutes, and the subsequent reperfusion of the ischaemic region, induces ventricular fibrillation.

The purpose of this chapter is to describe the electrophysiological changes occurring in the very first minutes after coronary artery occlusion and also upon re-perfusion after short-lasting occlusions. Mapping experiments will be described both during coronary occlusion and following reperfusion, which allowed the analysis of patterns of activation during the spontaneously occurring ventricular arrhythmias in both conditions. From these experiments it emerged that two different mechanisms play a role in the genesis of the arrhythmias; re-entry and a 'focal' mechanism, the exact nature of which remains to be determined.

4.2 CHANGES IN TRANSMEMBRANE POTENTIAL AND DC EXTRACELLULAR POTENTIALS DURING ACUTE ISCHAEMIA

Most experiments were performed in intact, isolated, Langendorff-perfused hearts of dogs and pigs, although the results were verified in experiments on hearts *in situ* (Downar *et al.*, 1977; Kléber *et al.*, 1978; Janse *et al.*, 1979; Cinca *et al.*, 1980). The hearts were perfused with a 1 : 1 mixture of blood and modified Tyrode solution. Transmembrane potentials were recorded from the subepicardium by using pairs of so-called floating micro-electrodes. The tip of one micro-electrode was placed intracellularly; the other micro-electrode was located as close as possible in the extracellular space; the potential difference between the two electrodes is the transmembrane potential. At the same location, local DC extracellular electrograms were recorded, using cotton- or silk-wick electrodes soaked in isotonic saline, which recorded the DC potential of the extracellular space with respect to the DC potential of the aortic root, obtained via another wick electrode.

Figure 4.1 shows results obtained from an isolated pig heart. Transmembrane potentials are shown in the upper rows, where the horizontal line indicates the zero potential obtained when both micro-electrodes were in the extracellular space. The lower signals are the DC extracellular electrograms in which the horizontal line represents the DC potential of the aortic root. In the control situation, before occlusion of the anterior descending branch of the left coronary artery (LAD), the transmembrane potential has a rapid upstroke corresponding to a fast intrinsic deflection in the extracellular complex. There is a marked plateau and in the extracellular complexes the TQ and ST segments are isoelectric. Following occlusion of the left anterior descending coronary artery the resting membrane potential decreases (see the recordings made $3\frac{1}{2}$, 8 and 30 min after occlusion) and action potential amplitude, upstroke velocity and duration decrease. In the extracellular potential the decrease in resting membrane potential is reflected by the depression of the TQ segment; the reduced action potential amplitude is expressed in the elevation of the ST segment. The smaller, slower, intrinsic deflection is a consequence of the low upstroke velocity and reduced amplitude of the rising phase of the action potential.

It is remarkable that electrical activity within the ischaemic zone is improved after 30 min of occlusion, compared to the situation after 8 min. Resting membrane potential has increased and the action potential is faster and longer than in earlier phases of ischaemia. In the extracellular potential, the magnitude of TQ

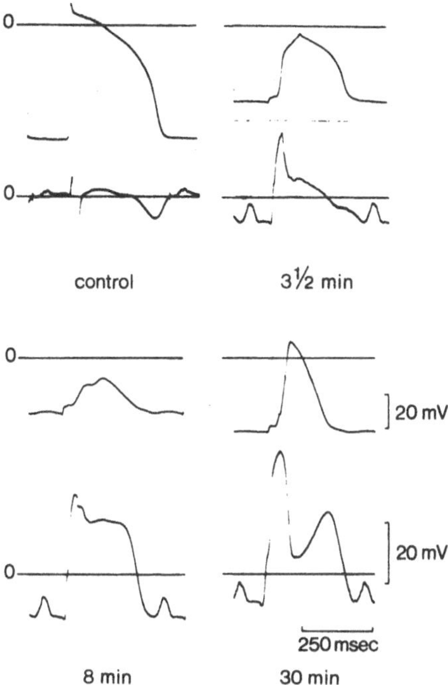

Figure 4.1 Ventricular transmembrane potentials (upper tracings) and local DC extracellular electrograms (lower tracings) before and after occlusion of the left anterior descending coronary artery of an isolated, Langendorff-perfused pig heart. Note the reduction in resting membrane potential, the decrease in action potential amplitude leading to depression of the TQ segment, and the elevation of the ST segment in the extracellular potentials. The increase in action potential amplitude and upstroke velocity after 30 min of ischaemia, as compared to the situation 8 min after coronary artery occlusion, is reflected in the large, fast intrinsic deflection of the extracellular complex and a reduction in magnitude of ST and TQ potential changes. (Reproduced with permission from Cinca *et al.*, *Chest*, 77, 499–505, 1980.)

depression and ST elevation has diminished and the intrinsic deflection has become faster and longer. This improvement of electrical activity is temporal because, after 40–60 min, ischaemic cells lose their excitability and no longer exhibit action potentials. Such temporal improvement, which has been noted by others as a decrease in the delay of epicardial activation (Scherlag *et al.*, 1974; Lazzara *et al.*, 1978), is as yet unexplained.

4.3 CHANGES IN EXCITABILITY

It is generally assumed that since action potential duration shortens in acute ischaemia, refractory periods shorten as well. Although this may be true when the definition of refractory period is confined to the shortest interval between two electrical stimuli delivered to the heart at which the second stimulus elicits a response, it is not quite true when the nature of the premature response is taken into account (Lazzara *et al.*, 1978). Gettes and Reuter (1974) have shown that, in the partially depolarised myocardium, recovery from inactivation of both fast and slow inward currents is markedly delayed and that complete recovery of excitability occurs well after repolarisation is completed. Schütz (1936) noted that under certain circumstances, such as an elevated extracellular K^+ concentration, monophasic potentials elicited after repolarisation was complete were graded. Such a discrepancy between action potential duration and full recovery of excitability has been reported in isolated fibres of the His–Purkinje system excised several hours after coronary artery occlusion. The term post-repolarisation refractoriness has been used to describe this phenomenon (Lazzara *et al.*, 1975, 1978).

As shown in figure 4.2, post-repolarisation refractoriness occurs also in the very early phase of myocardial ischaemia. In the example shown, cathodal test stimuli were delivered at a distance of less than 1 mm from the recording micro-electrode. In the control situation the refractory period was strictly related to the duration of the transmembrane action potential and the earliest successful test stimulus S_2, having an intensity of four times diastolic threshold, could be given 280 ms after the basic stimulus S_1. Twelve minutes after the left anterior descending coronary

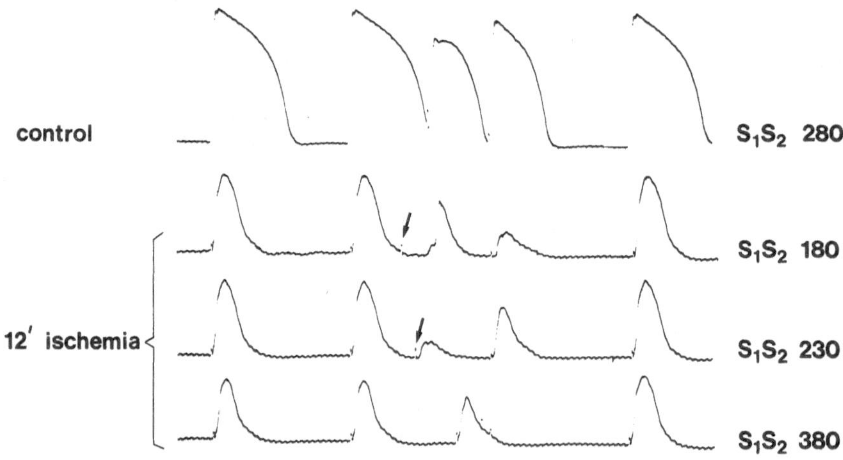

Figure 4.2 Transmembrane potentials recorded from an isolated pig heart. Stimuli were delivered within 1 mm of the cell from which the recordings were taken. In the control situation, recovery of excitability follows the time course of repolarisation. After 12 min of ischaemia, the heart responds to a test stimulus S_2 given 100 ms earlier than in the control situation. However, the latency between stimulus and response is more than 100 ms. Action potentials of fairly large amplitude without any latency were only obtained when the coupling interval was increased to 380 ms, well after completion or repolarisation. (Reproduced with permission from Downar *et al.*, *Circulation*, **56**, 217–24, 1977.)

artery was occluded a test pulse delivered 100 ms earlier was successful. In one sense, therefore, the refractory period had shortened. However, the latency between test stimulus (arrow) and response was longer than 100 ms, and the premature action potential, as well as the response elicited by the next basic stimulus, had smaller amplitudes than the basic action potentials. Only when the test stimulus was applied 230 ms after the basic stimulus did a very small response occur with minimal latency. Sizeable action potentials were obtained only when the test stimulus was given much later, even though after 380 ms the action potential amplitude was still lower than that of the basic beats.

The fact that recovery of excitability is a function of resting membrane potential (and that in partially depolarised tissue graded responses can be elicited long after repolarisation has been completed) is one of the most important determinants for the occurrence of slow conduction and conduction block. Adjacent cell groups having differences in resting membrane potential of only a few millivolts in the critical range can have widely disparate refractory periods. Whereas at relatively slow heart rates the action potentials in such adjacent areas may be very similar, premature impulses, or basic impulses when heart rate is suddenly increased, may elicit graded responses which will propagate slowly in the least depolarised cells but find slightly more depolarised cells unresponsive so that conduction in those areas will fail.

Figure 4.3 shows four simultaneously recorded action potentials several minutes

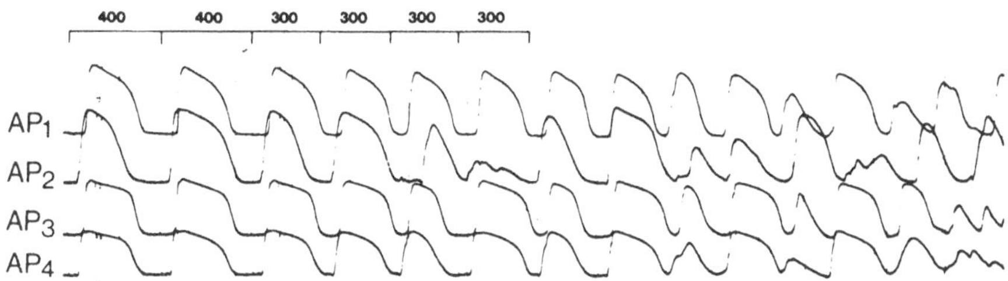

Figure 4.3 Four simultaneously recorded action potentials from an isolated porcine heart. The atrium was paced, initially at a cycle length of 400 ms. Activation of all four cells was fairly synchronous. When the cycle length was suddenly shortened to 300 ms this synchronicity is lost, cell 2 becomes activated later and in the sixth beat conduction block occurs. At the end of this recording the chaotic activity of ventricular fibrillation is seen. (Reproduced with permission from Janse *et al.*, *Annls Cardiol. Angéiol.*, **26**, 551–4, 1977.)

after coronary artery occlusion. The atria were stimulated initially at basic cycle lengths of 400 ms. The four cells are activated fairly synchronously and the action potentials have a similar configuration. When cycle length is decreased to 300 ms an alternation in action potential duration first results and then the activation pattern changes. In the second cell, the fifth action potential is markedly delayed, and the sixth response is a very low amplitude potential indicating local conduction block. Finally the chaotic activity of ventricular fibrillation is seen.

4.4 CHANGES FOLLOWING REPERFUSION

Provided that a period of ischaemia does not last too long, that is, not longer than about 40 min, the electrophysiological changes are completely reversible following reperfusion. Cells which were inexcitable during the occlusion exhibit within seconds following reperfusion near normal action potentials. However, the recovery of electrical activity following reperfusion does not occur at the same rate in all cells within the previously ischaemic zone.

Figure 4.4 shows four action potentials simultaneously recorded when, following

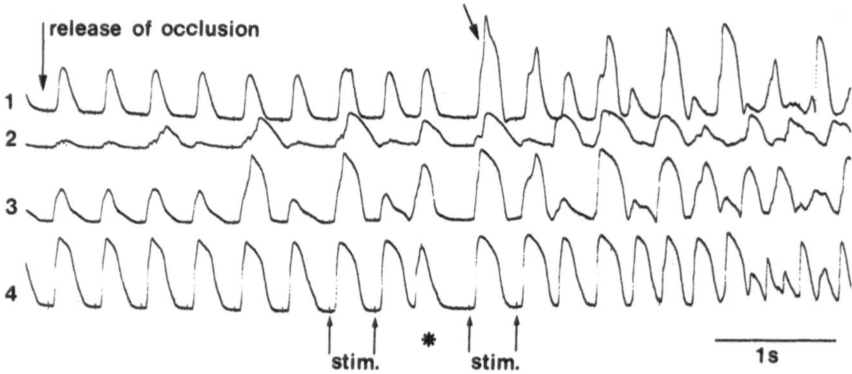

Figure 4.4 Release of a coronary artery occlusion 6 min after occlusion, resulting in ventricular fibrillation. Within beats following re-perfusion cell 2 shows 2 : 1 responses and cell 3 shows alternation between large and small action potentials. After the pause following the ventricular premature beat (asterisk) the alternation in cells 2 and 3 gets out of phase. (Reproduced with permission from Downar *et al.*, *Circulation*, **56**, 217–24, 1977.)

6 min of LAD occlusion, the clamp on the artery was released. The heart was paced from a location on the non-ischaemic myocardium. Within a few beats following release of the occlusion, 2 : 1 responses occur in cell 2 and large and small action potentials alternate in cell 3. A premature beat occurs (asterisk) and is followed by synchronised responses to the first post-extrasystolic stimulus. Thereafter the alternation in the responses of cell 2 and cell 3 is out of phase, the loss of synchrony increases and a chaotic arrhythmia follows.

4.5 PATTERNS OF ACTIVATION DURING VENTRICULAR ARRHYTHMIAS

To analyse the patterns of excitation during the spontaneously occurring arrhythmias, both during occlusion and following release, we simultaneously recorded the DC extracellular electrogram from 60 epicardial or intramural sites. By using an

A/D converter and a computer, signals recorded during a 2 s period could be stored and analysed later (van Capelle *et al.*, 1980; Janse *et al.*, 1980). Figure 4.5 shows the 60 extracellular potentials recorded from the anterior aspect at the left ventricle of an isolated pig heart. The right atrium was paced at a cycle length of 400 ms. At this time scale differences in shape and timing of the intrinsic deflection between the individual complexes are hardly noticeable. The short horizontal lines at the left are the zero potentials for each signal, corresponding to the DC potential of the active root. TQ- and ST-segment potentials of all signals are isoelectric. The general impression conveyed in this figure is one of striking synchrony in the electrical activity of this part of the heart. Figure 4.6 shows the signals recorded from the same electrodes, 3 min after occlusion of the LAD. In many signals TQ depression, ST elevation, delayed intrinsic deflection and alternation of the ST–T segments are visible, whereas other signals have retained their original configuration. At the end of the recording spontaneous premature beats occurred, which in this case led to ventricular tachycardia (depicted in figure 4.7) which finally degenerated into ventricular fibrillation (figure 4.8). Note that in figures 4.7 and 4.8 several signals still show some degree of synchrony, indicating that part of the heart was activated in some organised manner, whereas other signals have a more disorganised, chaotic appearance.

By measuring the moments of activation of each of these signals isochrone maps could be constructed. These show in a simplified manner the activation patterns during such arrhythmias. The accuracy of such activation maps depends of course on the accuracy with which the extracellular potential can be interpreted. In particular, it is necessary to recognise the intrinsic deflections (indicating local regenerative inward currents) or their absence (indicating local inexcitability). Even in transmembrane recordings it cannot always be determined with certainty whether a low amplitude, slowly rising response truly represents an active response or is merely an electronic potential reflecting activity elsewhere. In extracellular potentials it is even more difficult to distinguish between deflections which indicate local activity and those which are electrotonic deflections due to active responses in adjacent cells. Thus there is some degree of inaccuracy in the reconstruction of activation maps. Also, since simultaneous recordings were made of only 60 sites, some uncertainties exist as to whether, for example, the earliest activated site found is truly the earliest activated part of the heart. Likewise, since only a part of the heart was mapped we do not know how the rest of the heart is activated during the arrhythmias. These restrictions must be borne in mind when discussing the activation patterns presented below.

4.6 VENTRICULAR FIBRILLATION DURING OCCLUSION AND FOLLOWING REPERFUSION

In figures 4.9, 4.10 and 4.11 activation patterns are depicted during the spontaneous occurrence of ventricular fibrillation 3 min after occlusion and when, after success-

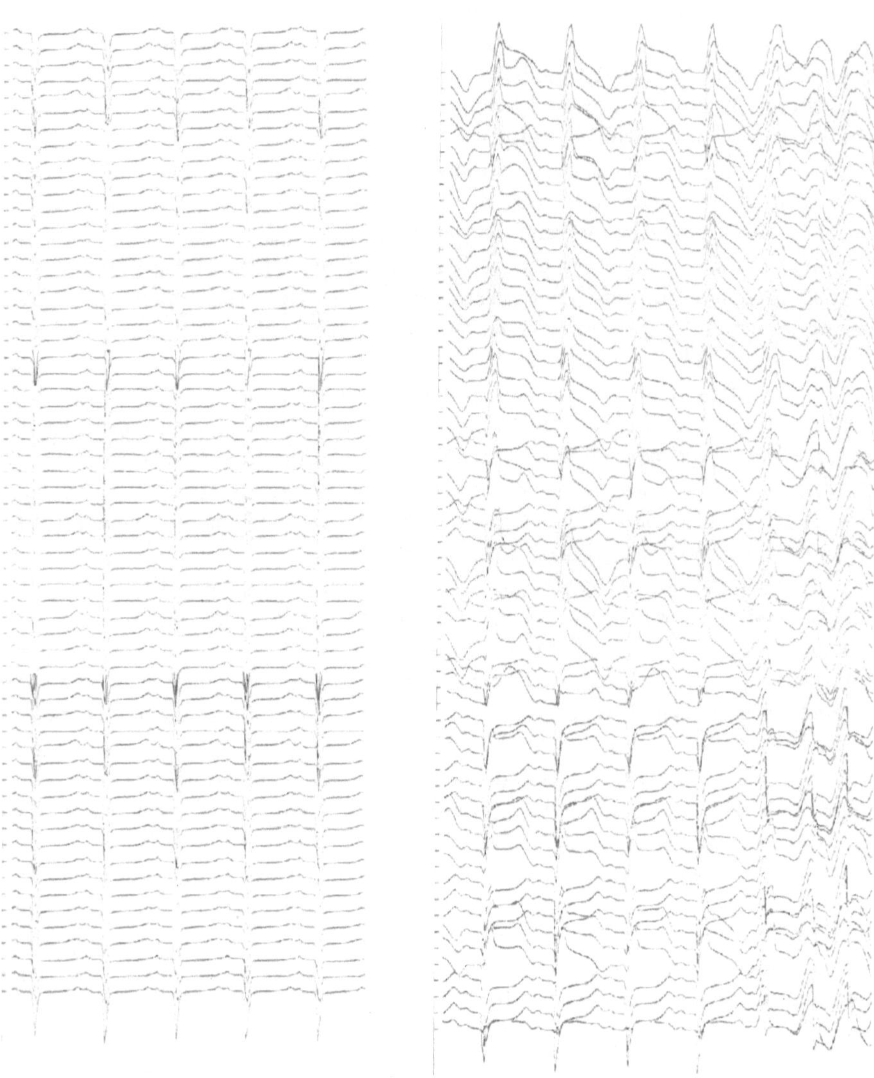

Figure 4.5 Sixty DC extracellular electrograms simultaneously recorded from the anterior surface of the left ventricle of an isolated pig heart before a coronary occlusion. Note the isoelectric TQ and ST segments and the nearly synchronous activation of this area of the heart.

Figure 4.6 Recordings from the same 60 sites as in figure 4.5, 3 min after occlusion of the left anterior descending coronary artery. Note TQ depression and ST elevation and alternation of T waves in many signals; in these signals the intrinsic deflection occurs late.

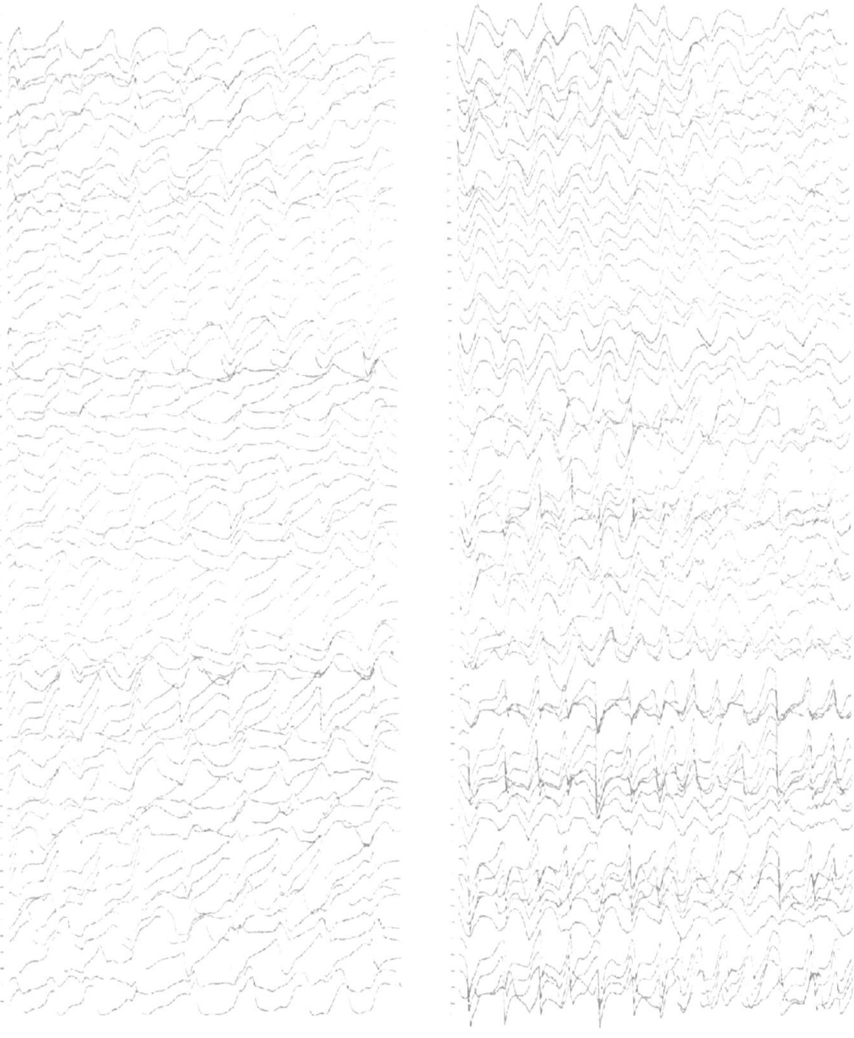

Figure 4.7

Figure 4.8

Figure 4.7 and 4.8 Recordings from the same 60 sites as in figure 4.5, 4 min after occlusion of the left anterior descending coronary artery. At the end of the recordings of figure 4.6 spontaneous ventricular beats occur which initiate a long run of ectopic activations (ventricular tachycardia, figure 4.7) and finally degenerate into ventricular fibrillation (figure 4.8)

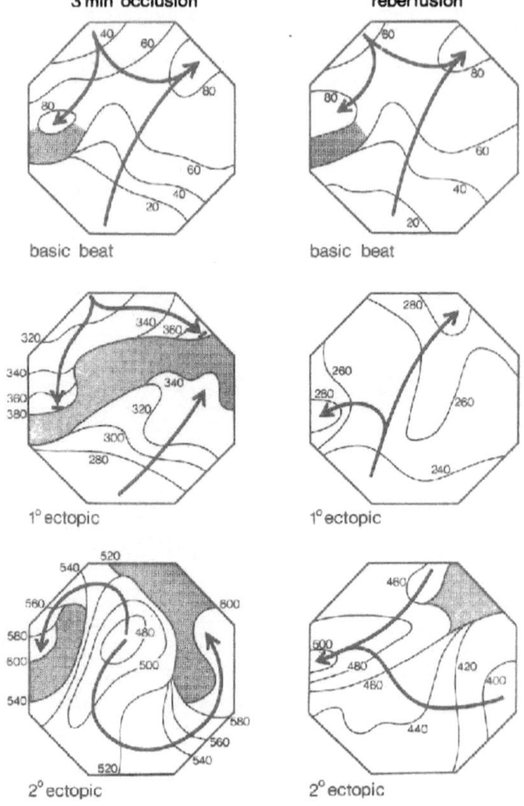

Figure 4.9

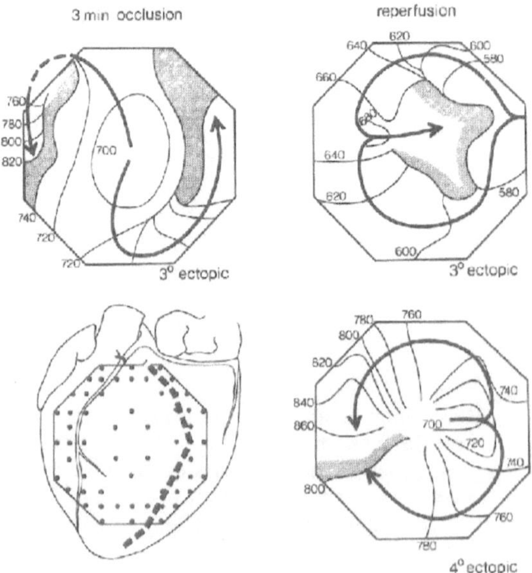

Figure 4.10

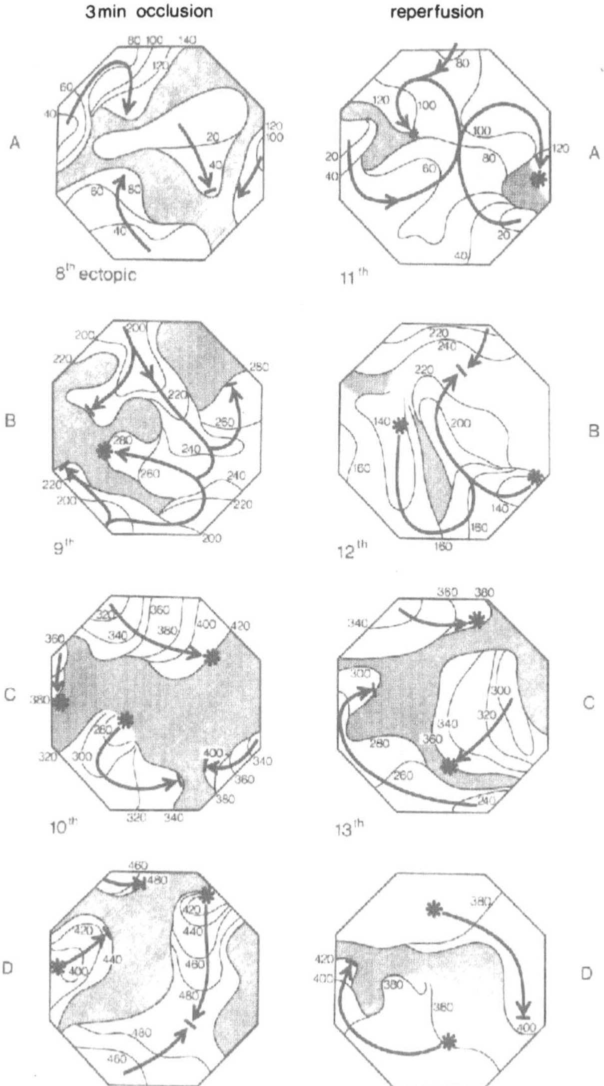

Figure 4.11

Figures 4.9, 4.10 and 4.11 Pattern of activation in an area of the left ventricle covered by a multiple electrode, schematically depicted in lower left panel of figure 4.10. Each dot is an individual electrode terminal; the heavy dotted line is the electrophysiological border zone. In figure 4.9 are shown the pattern of activation of the last basic beat (paced from the atrium) and the first two ectopic beats of an arrhythmia which developed into ventricular fibrillation. In the left panels the arrhythmia occurring 3 min after occlusion is depicted; in the right panels is shown the arrhythmia which followed reperfusion after 6 min of occlusion when successful defibrillation had occurred. In figure 4.10, ectopic beats no. 3 (occlusion arrhythmia) and nos 3 and 4 (reperfusion arrhythmia) are shown which marked the end of the first recordings in both arrhythmias. New recordings were made about 1 s later, when the heart was fibrillating, and activation patterns at those stages are shown in figure 4.11. Shaded areas are zones of conduction block. Isochrones separate areas activated within the same 20 ms interval (time zero was arbitrarily chosen) and thick arrows indicate general spread of activation. See text for further discussion.

ful defibrillation, the occlusion was released 6 min after coronary ligation. In each case two recordings were made, one of the initial phase and one about 1 s later. In the arrhythmia occurring during occlusion the activation pattern of the first three ectopic beats could be analysed; in the reperfusion arrhythmia that of the first four ectopic beats. In the lower left panel of figure 4.10 the position of each terminal on the anterior surface of the isolated pig heart is indicated by a dot. Because DC recordings were made the position of the electrophysiological border zone (indicated by a heavy dotted line in the lower left panel of the figure) could be determined by making an isopotential map during the TQ segment of a normally propagated beat from the atrium and delineating the area where TQ potentials became negative. During the last basic beat, propagated from the atrium, the activation patterns during occlusion and also following reperfusion are very similar (upper panels of figure 4.9). An arbitrary zero time was chosen and isochrone separate areas activated within the same 20 ms interval. The ischaemic zone is invaded from two sides, the two wavefronts merge and latest activation occurs 80 ms after the earliest activity was recorded in the area covered by the electrode. A small zone of conduction block is present on the left side of the electrode (areas of block are shaded). Although the activation pattern of the first spontaneous premature beat, which initiates ventricular fibrillation, was not identical in both instances, the following common features may be noted: (1) there is a considerable gap between latest activity during the basic beat and the earliest ectopic activity and (2) the earliest ectopic activity is recorded from the non-ischaemic myocardium close to the border zone. In the second and third ectopic beats during occlusion (figures 4.9 and 4.10) the earliest activated site is found within the ischaemic zone and epicardial activation patterns show attempted circus movements, activity turning around two different areas of conduction block which are not, however, completed. In the reperfusion arrhythmia complete circus movement can be demonstrated on the epicardial surface between the third and fourth ectopic beats. In the third beat earliest activity is recorded on the non-ischaemic side of the border, as was the case during first and second ectopic beats. This wavefront is blocked and the excitatory wave bypasses the inexcitable area on two sides. At the opposite end the two wavefronts fuse and retrogradely invade the area of unidirectional block to re-excite the site of origin after 700 – 600 ms (that is, 100 ms). In the fourth beat two semicircular wavefronts are again set up which seem to collide between 800 and 860 ms. Since the recording ended at this moment we do not know the subsequent activation patterns. In figure 4.11 activation patterns are shown from recordings made less than 1 s later when in both instances the heart was fibrillating. For each arrhythmia four consecutive 'beats' are shown (zero times were arbitrarily chosen). The characteristic features of the excitation pattern of fibrillation are clearly visible: (1) multiple wavelets are simultaneously present; (2) re-excitation frequently occurs, and is indicated by asterisks; (3) circus movements are seldom completed.

The general pattern can best be described as multiple wavelets travelling slowly along tortuous routes among multiple islets of conduction block which change position and magnitude from moment to moment. This pattern bears a striking resemblance to the pattern of fibrillation in the computer model of Moe (1962).

Although the arrhythmias during occlusion and following reperfusion show many similarities, there are also differences. In the first place, conduction during the reperfusion arrhythmia seems faster than during occlusion; the difference between earliest and latest activity during the four beats shown are during ischaemia 460 ms and during the reperfusion arrhythmia 400 ms. Secondly, refractory periods seem shorter during the reperfusion period since re-excitation occurs at shorter coupling intervals than during ischaemia. For example in a beat during ischaemia (in the upper left part) a circus movement is attempted but the wavefront at 140 ms fails to re-excite the region in which block had occurred after 20 ms (coupling interval 120 ms). In beat during a reperfusion successful re-entry occurs in the same area at a coupling interval of 140 – 80 = 60 ms.

4.7 RE-ENTRY AND FOCUS

Our mapping experiments showed that circus movement re-entry plays the dominant role in ventricular tachycardia and ventricular fibrillation. In ventricular tachycardia (defined as a series of more than five consecutive ectopic impulses), which could either terminate spontaneously or degenerate into ventricular fibrillation, there was basically one large circus movement present with a diameter of 10-20 mm. The centre around which activity circles consisted of ischaemic myocardium, which at that moment was inexcitable. Thus, as has already been described, ischaemic cells often show 2 : 1 alternation and may exhibit sizeable action potentials at long cycle lengths; the tissue in the centre of such a circus movement was not completely inexcitable and had a longer time to recover than the cells which formed part of the circulating excitation front. Therefore, in the next activation, conduction could occur in cells which showed no response in the previous activation, and cells which were excited in that cycle could be unresponsive in the next. The position, dimension and revolution time of circus movement in ventricular tachycardia changes from beat to beat and the centrifugal wavefronts emerging from the circus movement to excite the rest of the ventricles changed direction and frequency. It is therefore not surprising that the rate of ventricular tachycardia in acute ischaemia is not constant. Also local electrograms could have a very irregular, chaotic appearance and be interpretated as 'local fibrillation' since in one beat they could show a fast, large intrinsic deflection indicating local activity whilst in another beat they could show slow, multiphasic, low amplitude potentials indicating local block and electrotonic depolarisation due to activity in adjacent tissue. By looking at some of the signals displayed in figures 4.7 and 4.8, it is impossible to decide whether one deals with a tachycardia or fibrillation, and the distinction could only be made when activation patterns were analysed, or when the arrhythmia ended spontaneously. In the last instance, circus movement re-entry was not completed when the advancing wavefront found the tissue ahead in a state of too low excitability. In fibrillation, where multiple re-entrant wavelets are present, the extinction of one wavefront or the collision of two wavefronts does not lead to termination of the arrhythmia since the many other wavelets will simply continue their chaotic routes.

Thus for tachycardia and fibrillation re-entry within the ischaemic myocardium is the underlying mechanism. This implies that the electrical activity of the ischaemic cells must be depressed, since both slow conduction and the occurrence of areas of unidirectional block are required, but that the activity must not cease altogether. It is no coincidence that at the time the majority of the ischaemic cells become totally inexcitable (at resting membrane potentials in the order of −60 to −65 mV; Kléber *et al.*, 1978) tachycardia and fibrillation are no longer seen. The fact that re-entry becomes impossible when ischaemic cells are inexcitable has implications for drug therapy, as will be discussed later. The reason that ventricular fibrillation occurs so frequently upon reperfusion is related to the fact that electrical activity returns quickly to previously inexcitable cells. Probably the inhomogeneity in the first seconds after blood flow is restored is greater than during occlusion, although this is difficult to quantify. Not all areas within the ischaemic zone will be equally perfused when a coronary occlusion is suddenly released, and therefore the return of electrical activity does not occur at the same speed at all sites. The changes, which during ischaemia take several minutes to develop, occur in the reverse order in a matter of seconds during reperfusion; re-entry will be facilitated by both the return of electrical activity and the greater degree of inhomogeneity.

One of the surprising findings of our mapping experiments was that no evidence was found that re-entry was also responsible for the occurrence of single ventricular premature beats or for the initial ectopic activations of a tachycardia, whether ending spontaneously or continuing as fibrillation (Janse *et al.*, 1980). The experimental findings, in porcine and in canine hearts, can be summarised as follows:

(1) Earliest activity during single premature beats (or initial beats of a series of ectopic activations) was found in the normal myocardium adjacent to the electrophysiological border, that is, the zone in which TQ potentials of normally propagated beats became negative.

(2) During either epicardial or intramural recording no evidence was found for re-entrant activity bridging the gap between the latest activity during the last basic beat and the earliest activity in the first ectopic beat.

(3) Whenever Purkinje activity was recorded in subendocardial leads (dog hearts) or from both intramural and endocardial recordings (pig hearts) it preceded myocardial activity in the ectopic activations.

(4) Epicardial activation patterns were similar during spontaneous ectopic beats and during stimulation of subendocardial sites where Purkinje activity was recorded.

(5) Very frequently, just before the occurrence of ectopic activity on the non-ischaemic side of the border zone, large 'injury' currents were flowing across the ischaemic border.

The possibility that injury current may play an arrhythmogenic role has been considered by many authors (for example, Harris, 1950; Hoffman, 1966) and some of the mechanisms by which injury currents could induce local ectopic activity are discussed below.

4.8 ROLE OF INJURY CURRENTS

Current will flow between adjacent areas in the heart whenever there are at any one moment potential differences between the intracellular compartments of both cell groups so long as the cells are well coupled. It has long been known that when heart cells are mechanically injured, the injured part will be 'sealed off' from the healthy part (Adrian, 1921; Délèze, 1970). This 'healing over' process includes the formation of high resistance connections between healthy and injured cells and prevents current flow between these cells. It is known that in hypoxia an increase in longitudinal resistance eventually occurs so that hypoxic cells gradually become uncoupled (Wojtczak, 1979). It is more than likely that in ischaemia such an uncoupling will eventually seal off the ischaemic part of the heart from the normal part so that current flow between these two parts will be impeded. However, it is equally likely that in the very early phase (that is, the first 10-15 min) ischaemic and normal cells remain well coupled via low resistance intercellular connections. In the rat heart ultrastructural changes in the nexus, which is the anatomical site of the low resistance pathway, are found only after 24 min of ischaemia (McCallister *et al.*, 1979).

In acute ischaemia the so-called injury current changes magnitude and direction. In figure 4.12 the flow of current in diastole and systole is schematically depicted. In the left part of the figure transmembrane potentials (upper row) and local DC electrograms (lower row) at ischaemic and normal sites are superimposed. The signals recorded from the normal myocardium are indicated by dotted lines and those from ischaemic myocardium by solid lines. In the right part of the figure current flow between ischaemic (I), border (B) and normal (N) cells is schematically depicted. Two different moments (indicated by the dotted vertical line in the recordings) were selected, one during diastole and one during systole. The numbers in the diagrams indicate transmembrane potentials and the intra- and extracellular potentials (in millivolts) at those moments. In diastole, 4 min after occlusion, the resting membrane potential of the ischaemic cell has markedly decreased. Consequently the intracellular compartment of the ischaemic cells is positive with respect to that of normal cells and an intracellular current flows towards the normal cells across the ischaemic border. This current will cross the cell membranes, leading to the establishment of current sources in the normal extracellular space, and the current then sinks in the ischaemic extracellular space; current flow in the extracellular space has an opposite direction to that of intracellular current flow. It is this local current circuit which is responsible for the depression of the TQ segment in the local DC extracellular electrogram recorded from the ischaemic myocardium.

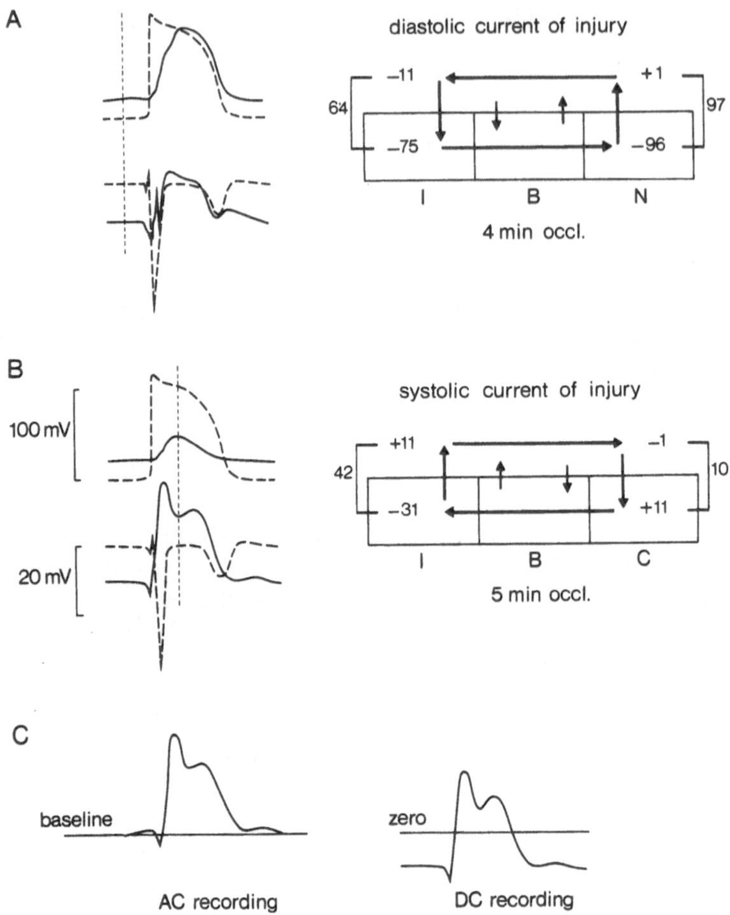

Figure 4.12 Intra- and extracellular potentials of normal myocardium (dotted lines) are superimposed over potentials recorded after 4 and 5 min of ischaemia (solid lines). In the diagrams, the local current circuits in systole and diastole are depicted; the moments in the cardiac cycle are indicated by a vertical dotted line in the re-drawn potentials. Transmembrane potentials and intra- and extracellular potential levels are given in millivolts. I = ischaemic area, B = border zone, N = normal myocardium, each represented in one cell. In C, extracellular potentials are shown, recorded in the ischaemic area 5 min after coronary occlusion with both AC and DC amplifiers. (Reproduced with permission from Janse and Durrer, in *Myocardial Ischaemia* (ed. W. Schaper), Marcel Dekker, New York, in press.)

When 5 min after occlusion action potential amplitude of the ischaemic cell is considerably reduced a large systolic current of injury of opposite direction is set up, and this now results in elevation of the ST segment in extracellular DC recordings. In the bottom row of figure 4.12 the extracellular complexes recorded at this moment from the ischaemic area are shown, when they are recorded via metal electrodes and AC amplifiers and also when wick electrodes and DC amplifiers are used. In AC recordings no distinction, of course, can be made between TQ-segment depression and true ST-segment elevation, and the 'ST elevation' recorded via conventional electrocardiographs is in fact a combination of TQ depression and ST elevation.

We have estimated the strength of the injury current in the different phases of the cardiac cycle by recording DC potentials at 60 terminals, placed in a regular grid across the ischaemic border (Kléber *et al.*, 1978; Janse *et al.*, 1980). At each moment of the cycle, an isopotential map of the extracellular space could be made and from such maps the distribution of current sources and sinks could be calculated. To determine the source or sink current at a particular site C we used the potential values of the eight surrounding sites:

$$\begin{array}{ccc} B_1 & A_1 & B_2 \\ A_2 & C & A_3 \\ B_3 & A_4 & B_4 \end{array}$$

The source current is then given by

$$i = -\frac{4 \sum_{k=1}^{4} V(A_k) + \sum_{k=1}^{4} V(B_k) - 20\, V(C)}{6 \rho L^2}$$

in amps per cubic metre, in which V is the DC potential at each site, ρ the specific resistance of the tissue (we used a value of 4 Ω m based on measurements of van Oosterom *et al.* (1979), L is the distance between sampling points and the number 6 is a geometrical factor.

We found that the strongest currents were flowing across the ischaemic border in one particular situation, namely at that point in the cycle when normal cells had repolarised and ischaemic cells were still in their 'plateau' phase. At that moment current sources on the normal side of the border were of the order of $2 \mu A\ mm^{-3}$ tissue. Since at that moment normal cells had recovered their excitability and the injury current has a depolarising effect on normal cells, this current might be strong enough to re-excite the normal cells. We measured the current sources which are set up by a broad wavefront propagating through normal myocardium in the same way; current sources in tissue which is about to be excited by such a wavefront were of the order of $5 \mu A\ mm^{-3}$, which gives some idea as to the strength of the injury current flowing across the ischaemic border.

There are several other mechanisms by which injury currents could induce ectopic activity. Katzung *et al.* (1975) observed in isolated papillary muscle preparations (in which one part was normally superfused and another part depolarised by a solution containing 145 mM K^+) that, due to current flow between the two parts, abnormal automaticity was induced in the normally superfused part provided that catecholamines were present and that the extracellular K^+ concentration was not higher than 3.5 mM.

Current flow could induce some form of triggered automaticity by inducing either early or delayed after-depolarisations (Cranefield, 1975). When Purkinje fibres are in electrotonic contact with ischaemic myocardium via Purkinje-muscle junctions in, or close to, the ischaemic border then those fibres could be the site of abnormal impulse formation under the influence of current.

Electrotonic currents flowing through small segments of inexcitable cells in the ischaemic border zone can influence normal automaticity in Purkinje fibres located close by (Jalife and Moe, 1976). Thus when electrotonic depolarisation falls late in the spontaneous cycle of such automatic Purkinje fibres the spontaneous discharge may be speeded up and an extrasystole will occur.

Finally, micro re-entry and reflection may occur within the border zone, in which the dimensions of the tissue involved could be of the order of several millimetres (Wit *et al.*, 1972; Antzelevitch *et al.*, 1980).

It will be clear that the exact nature of the 'focal' mechanism responsible for the genesis of premature beats will be very difficult to demonstrate in the intact heart. Because the nature of this mechanism is as yet unknown, no speculation will be made concerning which antiarrhythmic drugs could suppress these premature beats. Since these premature beats form the 'trigger' for re-entrant mechanisms, their suppression may be of great importance. At present only the ways in which re-entry may be suppressed will be discussed.

4.9 THE PREVENTION OF RE-ENTRY

In principle there are two ways in which re-entry may be abolished. The key to the prevention of re-entrant arrhythmias is the prevention of the occurrence of areas of unidirectional block. This can be done either by converting an area of unidirectional block into an area of total (bidirectional) block or to change it into tissue where conduction is possible in all directions. A relatively simple way to achieve this last condition is to keep heart rate within normal limits. As already discussed, an increase in heart rate may, due to post-repolarisation refractoriness, unmask slight differences in recovery properties in adjacent areas within the ischaemic tissue. This would lead to unidirectional block in one area and slow conduction in the next. At slower rates more or less synchronous activation is still possible. It is in this respect noteworthy that of the patients with acute myocardial infarction seen within 30 min after the onset of chest pain (when the incidence of ventricular fibrillation is highest) 24 per cent had sinus tachycardia (Pantridge *et al.*, 1981). The relationship between fast heart rates and the occurrence of re-entrant arrhythmias in acute ischaemia in the experimental animal has been emphasised by Scherlag *et al.* (1970).

The idea that measures which improve the action potential upstroke characteristics (and thus conduction) have an antiarrhythmic effect in all instances is not, however, quite correct. For one thing, reperfusion, which quickly leads to an improvement in conduction, is one of the most effective ways to induce ventricular fibrillation. Preliminary experiments in our laboratory indicate that stimulation of the left stellate ganglion during regional ischaemia of the heart improves conduction through the ischaemic myocardium. At the same time, however, the incidence of ventricular arrhythmias, including fibrillation, was greatly increased.

We have recently studied the effect of lignocaine on the electrophysiological changes induced by ischaemia (Cardinal *et al.*, 1981). Figure 4.13 shows transmembrane potentials and DC electrograms recorded from the same site on the left ventricle during two successive coronary artery occlusions, separated by a long reperfusion period during which lignocaine was administered. Lignocaine exaggerated and accelerated the changes in transmembrane potential; after 7 min only small local responses were present, whereas in the absence of drug sizeable action potentials could still be recorded after 12 min of ischaemia. Mapping studies revealed that at comparable times after coronary artery occlusion the inexcitable area within the ischaemic region was much larger in the presence of lignocaine than in its absence. Spontaneous ventricular arrhythmias still occurred when lignocaine was given prior to the occlusion but the incidence of ventricular fibrillation was greatly reduced. In 13 hearts ventricular tachycardia occurred 11 times during an occlusion without lignocaine, and nine times when the drug was present. Ventricular fibrillation occurred eight times during 13 control occlusions but only once in 13 occlusions when lignocaine was present in high dosage (5 μg ml^{-1}). Lignocaine did not influence the occurrence of fibrillation when the occlusion was released.

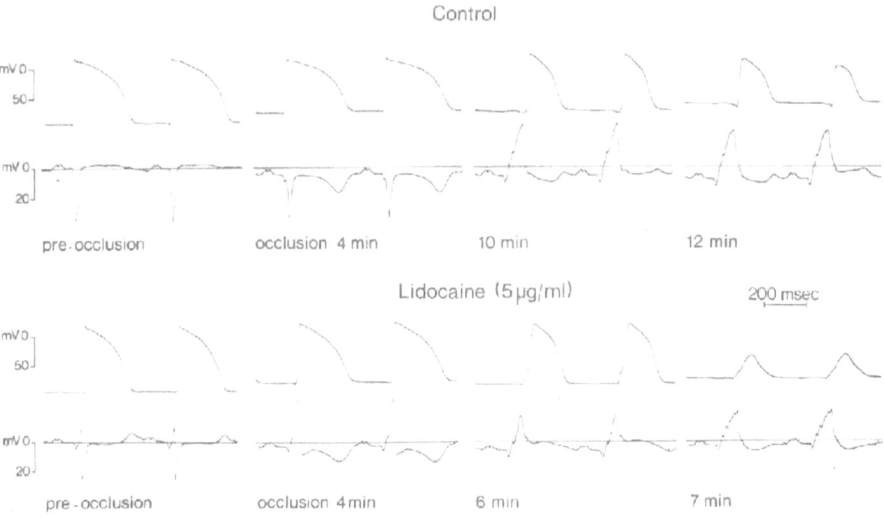

Figure 4.13 Effects of 5 μg ml^{-1} lignocaine (lidocaine) on intra- and extracellular potentials prior to and during coronary artery occlusion. Note that lignocaine accelerates the time course of ischaemic changes. (Reproduced with permission from Cardinal *et al.*, *Circulation Res.*, **49**, 792–806, 1981.)

In figure 4.14 activation patterns are depicted during spontaneous arrhythmias during coronary occlusions in the absence of lignocaine. In figure 4.14A, in the first ectopic beat two premature wavefronts invaded the ischaemic region. In the upper right panel the electrode position is shown together with isopotential lines during the TQ segment of a normally propagated beat. The border zone corresponds to the 0 mV line and earliest ectopic activity originated on the normal side of this border. During the next beats of the tachycardia activation patterns were similar but islands of conduction block were appearing; eventually a large circus movement was set up in which the activation wave travelled around a central area of conduction block. This had a diameter of 10–20 mm. This pattern (not shown) continued for about 15 beats and then the circulating wave fragmented into multiple wavelets and the activation pattern of fibrillation, shown in the two middle panels, appeared. There is one complete circus movement around an area of conduction block with a diameter less than 10 mm and other wavelets sketching out incomplete circus movements of even smaller dimensions. About 10 s later a DC shock was applied.

In Figure 4.14B, the activation pattern during a tachycardia in the same heart is shown in the presence of lignocaine. In the first ectopic beat premature wavefronts again propagated from the periphery of the electrode over border regions and collided in the centre of the ischaemic zone. In the following beats activation patterns were similar; sometimes complete, large circus movements could be demonstrated. Two middle panels represent activity during the 35th and 36th ectopic beat. A wavefront propagating from the apical part of the heart was blocked on its way into the ischaemic zone and was conducted in the border zone and the non-ischaemic myocardium in a counter-clockwise fashion. This wavefront completed a full revolution, re-excited tissue proximal to the initial block and then was blocked after almost another half-revolution. This circus movement was similar to the one in the middle diagram of figure 4.14A, except that no multiple wavelets were present. In the last beat of this tachycardia (the 54th successive ectopic beat) an attempt at large circus movements was made, but the wavefront travelling around the zone of block was itself blocked after only one half-revolution. The tachycardia ended and sinus rhythm was restored. Lignocaine thus converted an area of unidirectional block into one of total block. In this way lignocaine is effective against re-entry and is particularly able to prevent the fragmentation of one large circus movement into multiple re-entrant wavelets. Because lignocaine increases the number of sites where excitation fails, and because it accelerates the transition from areas of depressed conduction to failure of activation in the ischaemic zone, it is effective against fibrillation. However, since the activation delay in ischaemic areas where conduction still persisted was greater in the presence of lignocaine than in control occlusions, large circus movements could still occur. Furthermore, lignocaine has no effect on the 'focal' mechanism responsible for the occurrence of premature beats. It is therefore not surprising that in animal experiments and also in the coronary care unit lignocaine does not abolish 'warning arrhythmias' and ventricular tachycardia, although it does prevent ventricular fibrillation (Lie *et al.*, 1974). In the out-of-hospital situation lignocaine may not be as effective. Adgey

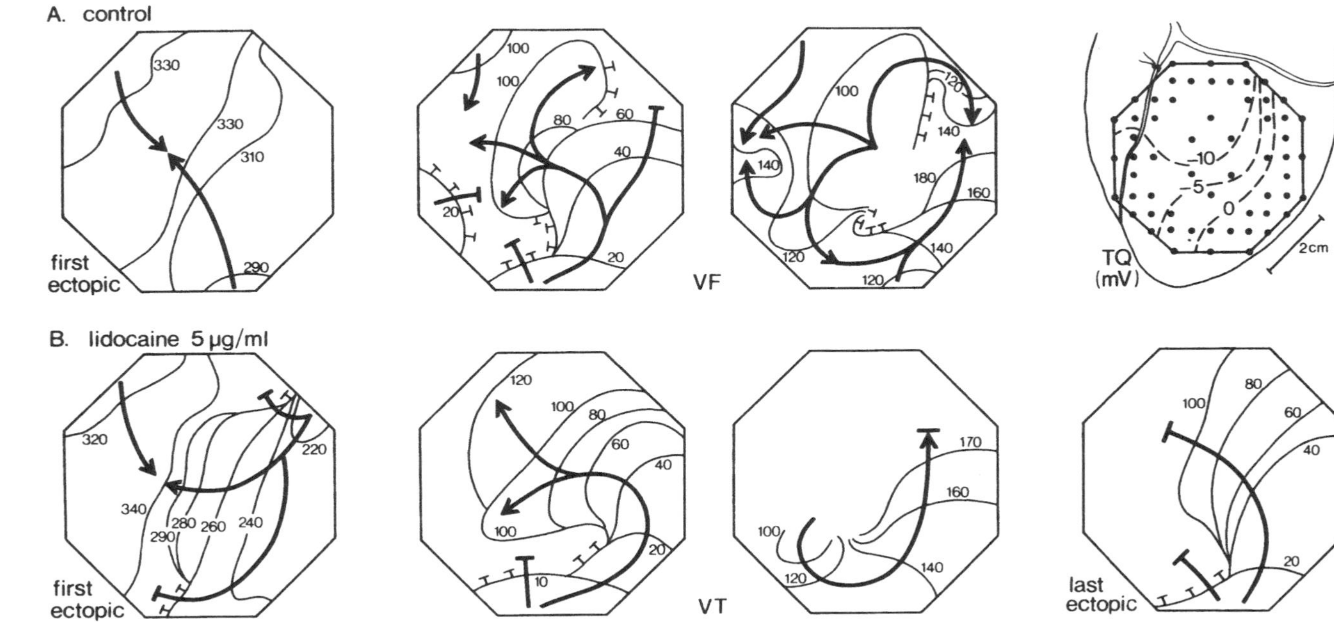

Figure 4.14 Effects of lignocaine (lidocaine) on patterns of activation during spontaneous arrhythmias. In the control occlusion a spontaneous ventricular beat (left panel) triggered a tachycardia which eventually changed into ventricular fibrillation (middle panels). In the presence of lignocaine premature beats and tachycardias still occurred (lower panels) and circus movement re-entry was occasionally observed but no fragmentation into multiple wavelets re-entry occurred. See text. (Reproduced with permission from Cardinal *et al.*, *Circulation Res.*, **49**, 792–806, 1981.)

and Webb (1979) have indicated that in the very early phase of myocardial infarction the deleterious effects of over-activity of the sympathetic nervous system may override the beneficial effects of lignocaine and that this drug is less effective in the presence of sinus tachycardia. In our experiments the only instance of ventricular fibrillation in the presence of lignocaine occurred while the heart was paced at a rapid rate.

In conclusion, it can be said that in the very simple animal model imitating the acute phase of myocardial ischaemia in man, both re-entry and a focal mechanism localised close to the ischaemic border play a role in the genesis of ventricular arrhythmias. Drugs which further depress the electrical activity of ischaemic cells act against the re-entry mechanism without entirely abolishing it. Further research into the nature of the focal mechanism responsible for the premature impulse which triggers re-entrant arrhythmias may lead to the development of approaches to suppress that component of these arrhythmias.

ACKNOWLEDGEMENT

This study was supported by the Wynand Pon Foundation.

REFERENCES

Adgey, A. A. J. and Webb, S. W. (1979). The treatment of ventricular arrhythmias in acute myocardial infarction. *Br. J. Hosp. Med.*, **1979**, 356-65

Adrian, E. D. (1921). Recovery of excitability. *J. Physiol., Lond.*, **55**, 193-225

Antzelevitch, C., Jalife, J. and Moe, G. K. (1980). Characteristics of reflection as a mechanism of re-entrant arrhythmias and its relation to parasystole. *Circulation*, **61**, 182-91

Baum, R. S., Alvarez, H. and Cobb, L. A. (1974). Survival after resuscitation from out of hospital ventricular fibrillation. *Circulation*, **50**, 1231-5

Capelle, F. J. L. van, Morsink, H., Janse, M. J. and Durrer, D. (1979). Computerised DC epicardial mapping during experimental coronary occlusion. *Proc. I.E.E.E. Conf. Comput. Cardiol.*, 99-102

Cardinal, R., Janse, M. J., Eeden, I. van, Werner, G., Naumann d'Alnoncourt, C. and Durrer, D. (1981). The effects of lidocaine on intracellular and extracellular potentials, activation and ventricular arrhythmias during acute regional ischemia in the intact isolated porcine heart. *Circulation Res.*, **49**, 792-806

Cinca, J., Janse, M. J., Moréna, H., Candell, J., Valle, V. and Durrer, D. (1980). Mechanism and time course of the early electrical changes during acute coronary artery occlusion. An attempt to correlate the early ECG changes in man to the cellular electrophysiology in the pig. *Chest*, 77, 499-505

Cranefield, P. F. (1975). *The Conduction of the Cardiac Impulse: The Slow Response and Cardiac Arrhythmias*, Futura Publishing Co., Mount Kisco, N.Y.

Délèze, J. (1970). The recovery of resting potential and input resistance in sheep heart by knife or laser. *J. Physiol., Lond.*, **208**, 547-62

Downar, E., Janse, M. J. and Durrer, D. (1977). The effect of acute coronary artery occlusion on subepicardial transmembrane potentials in the intact porcine heart. *Circulation*, **56**, 217-24

Gettes, L. S. and Reuter, H. (1974). Slow recovery from inactivation of inward currents in mammalian myocardial fibres. *J. Physiol., Lond.*, **240**, 703-24

Harris, A. S. (1950). Delayed development of ventricular ectopic rhythm following experimental coronary occlusion. *Circulation*, **1**, 1318-28

Hoffman, B. F. (1966). The genesis of cardiac arrhythmias. *Progr. cardiovasc. Dis.*, **8**, 319-29

Jalife, J. and Moe, G. K. (1976). Effect of electrotonic potentials on pacemaker activity of canine Purkinje fibres in relation to parasystole. *Circulation Res.*, **39**, 801-8

Janse, M. J., Cinca, J., Morena, H., Fiolet, J. W. T., Kléber, A. G., de Vries, G. P., Becker, A. E. and Durrer, D. (1979). The 'border zone' in myocardial ischemia. An electrophysiological, metabolic and histochemical correlation in the pig heart. *Circulation Res.*, **44**, 576-88

Janse, M. J., Capelle, F. J. L. van, Morsink, H., Kléber, A. G., Wilms-Schopman, F., Cardinal, R., Naumann d'Alnoncourt, C. and Durrer, D. (1980). Flow of 'injury' current and patterns of excitation during early ventricular arrhythmias in acute regional myocardial ischemia in isolated porcine and canine hearts. *Circulation Res.*, **47**, 151-65

Katzung, B. G., Hondegham, L. M. and Grant, A. O. (1975). Cardiac ventricular automaticity induced by current of injury. *Pflügers Arch. ges. Physiol.*, **360**, 193-7

Kléber, A. G., Janse, M. J., Capelle, F. J. L. van and Durrer, D. (1978). Mechanisms and time course of S-T and T-Q segment changes during acute regional myocardial ischemia in the pig heart determined by intracellular and extracellular recordings. *Circulation Res.*, **42**, 603-13

Lazzara, R., El-Sherif, N. and Scherlag, B. J. (1975). Disorders of cellular electrophysiology produced by ischemia of the canine His bundle. *Circulation Res.*, **36**, 444-53

Lazzara, R., El-Sherif, N., Hope, R. R. and Scherlag, B. J. (1978). Ventricular arrhythmias and electrophysiological consequences of myocardial ischemia and infarction. *Circulation Res.*, **42**, 740-49

Lie, K. I., Wellens, H. J. J., Capelle, F. J. L. van and Durrer, D. (1974). Lidocaine in the prevention of primary ventricular fibrillation. *New Engl. J. Med.*, **291**, 1324-6

McCallister, L. P., Trapudki, S. and Neely, J. R. (1979). Morphometric observations on the effects of ischemia in the isolated perfused rat heart. *J. molec. cell. Cardiol.*, **11**, 619-30

Moe, G. K. (1962). On the multiple wavelet hypothesis of atrial fibrillation. *Archs int. Pharmacodyn. Thér.*, **140**, 740-9

Oosterom, A. van, Boer, R. W. de and Dam, R. Th. van (1979). Intramural resistivity of cardiac tissue. *Med. Biol. Engl.*, **17**, 337-43

Pantridge, J. F., Webb, S. W. and Adgey, A. A. J. (1981). Arrhythmias in the first hours of acute myocardial infarction. *Progr. cardiovasc. Dis.*, **23**, 265-77

Scherlag, B. J., Helfant, R. H., Haft, J. T. and Damato, A. N. (1970). Electrophysiology underlying ventricular arrhythmias due to coronary ligation. *Am. J. Physiol.*, **219**, 1665-72

Scherlag, B. J., El-Sherif, N., Hope, R. R. and Lazzara, R. (1974). Characterisation and localisation of ventricular arrhythmias resulting from myocardial ischemia and infarction. *Circulation Res.*, **35**, 372-83

Schütz, E. (1936). Elecktrophysiologie des Herzens bei einphäsischer Ableitung. *Ergebn. Physiol.*, **38**, 493-620

Stephenson, S. E., Ide, R. K., Parcish, T. F., Bauer, F. M., Johnson, I. T., Kochtizky, M., Anderson, J. S., Hibbitt, L. L., McCarty, J. E., Young, E. R., Wilson, J. R., Meiers, N. H., Neador, C. K., Ball, O. T. and McNeely, A. R. (1960). Ventricular fibrillation during and after coronary artery occlusion. Incidence and protection afforded by various drugs. *Am. J. Cardiol.*, **5**, 77-87

Tennant, R. and Wiggers, C. J. (1935). The effect of coronary occlusion on myocardial contraction. *Am. J. Physiol.*, **112**, 351-61

Wit, A. L., Cranefield, P. F. and Hoffman, B. F. (1972). Slow conduction and reentry in the ventricular conducting system. II. Single and sustained circus movement in networks of canine and bovine Purkinje fibres. *Circulation Res.*, **30**, 11-22

Wojtczak, J. (1979). Contractures and increase in internal longitudinal resistance of cow ventricular muscle induced by hypoxia. *Circulation Res.*, **44**, 88-95

5

Stress-strain-related Depolarisation in the Myocardium and Arrhythmogenesis in Early Ischaemia

Max J. Lab

5.1 INTRODUCTION

There is no entirely satisfactory explanation for the premature excitation that initiates ventricular fibrillation in the very early stages of myocardial ischaemia. The electrophysiological disturbances which accompany the ischaemia, such as differential changes in conduction velocity, re-entry and enhanced automaticity, have been invoked as causing ventricular fibrillation (chapters 3 and 4 in this book). However, correlation does not imply causality. There are severe mechanical disturbances during regional ischaemia and extrasystoles can accompany physical stresses and strains in the normal myocardium. A critical consideration of mechanical causes for extrasystoles during ischaemia is therefore appropriate. This chapter briefly discusses the mechanical generation of threshold excitations and considers the possibility that mechanical changes may induce ectopic impulses in early ischaemia.

5.2 MECHANICALLY INDUCED DEPOLARISATION IN THE NORMAL MYOCARDIUM

Several studies show that three types of mechanical intervention can produce depolarisation in myocardium.

Sustained passive stretch

Although Ling and Gerard in 1949 first successfully used micropipettes for recording intracellular potentials and found no changes in resting membrane potential when they stretched isolated skeletal muscle, Ishiko (1956, 1958) produced small but clear depolarisations with this manoeuvre. Further, Bülbring *et al.* (1956) stretched calcium-deficient skeletal muscle and caused spontaneous activity. In heart muscle mechanically induced changes are more easily demonstrated. Stretch of several isolated preparations of cardiac muscle produce depolarisation, steeper diastolic depolarisation associated with spontaneous activity, and/or threshold depolarisation (Dudel and Trautwein, 1954; Penefsky and Hoffman, 1963; Deck, 1964; Kaufmann and Theophile, 1967; Lab, 1974). Figure 5.1 shows examples of sus-

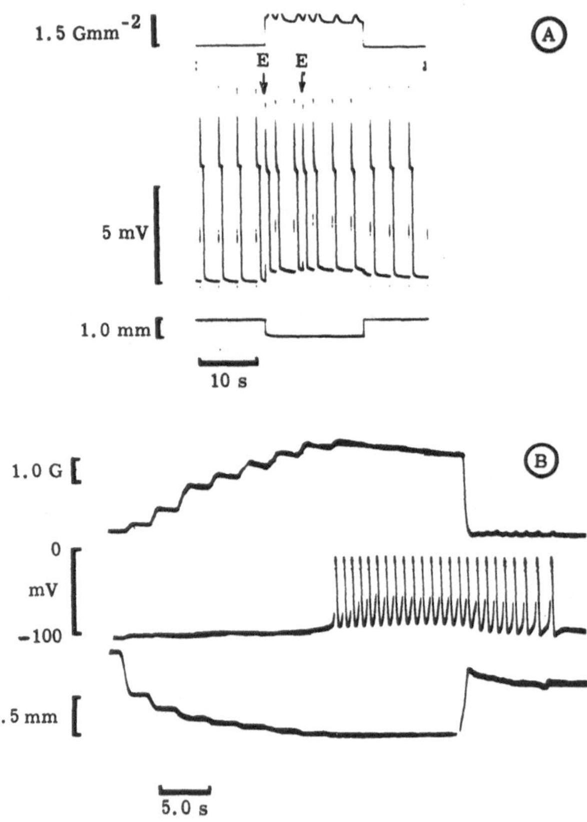

Figure 5.1 Effects of sustained stretch on action potentials from isolated ventricular myocardium. Traces from above down: tension (increase is upward deflection), action potential and length (increase is downward deflection). A, Records from unstretched frog ventricular strip which is regularly stimulated. A stretch causes depolarisation which is accompanied by an extrasystole (E). The sustained increase in length produces a sustained depolarisation and commensurate reduction in spike height. Action potentials recorded via insulation gap technique. (From Lab (1974).) B, Preparation of quiescent cat papillary muscle. Stepwise increases in length produce a small but perceptible depolarisation in the resting membrane potential until pronounced diastolic depolarisations develop to produce spontaneous activity. Action potentials recorded with micro-electrodes. (After Kaufmann and Theophile (1967).)

tained stretch producing depolarisation in ventricular muscle which can then cause threshold excitation. Increases in muscle length of intact ventricles have also produced analogous depolarisations (Lab, 1969, 1978a,b; Boland and Troquet, 1980), sometimes associated with extrasystoles (Lab, 1969, 1978a,b; Covell *et al.*, 1981).

Rapid transient stretch

Rapid transient stretch of frog ventricular strips after the repolarisation phase can induce transient depolarisations associated with extrasystoles (Lab, 1974). These have also been seen in the intact frog ventricle following sudden increases in ventricular volume (Lab, 1978a). Figure 5.2A shows a depolarisation with stretch, which produces an extrasystole when the stretch is delayed beyond the mechanical refractory period. Kluge and Vincenci (1971) have mechanically provoked extrasystoles in Langendorff-perfused rabbit hearts and have also shown refractory periods to mechanical interventions, as did a previous study by Brooks *et al.* (1964). The extrasystoles never produced fibrillation but could do so easily in the presence of acetylstrophanthidin, which also reduced the 'mechanical' refrac-

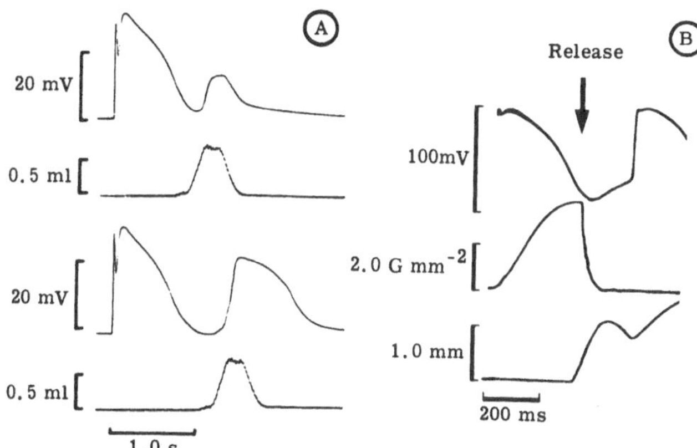

Figure 5.2 Threshold depolarisations produced by different, rapid, mechanical manoeuvres in two preparations of ventricular myocardium. A, An isolated intact frog ventricle is rapidly and transiently injected (stretched) near the end of the repolarisation phase of the action potential (the top trace in each panel). In the upper panel the intraventricular injection, given just before repolarisation is complete, produces a discrete depolarising potential. An injection after completion of repolarisation (lower panel) produces a depolarisation associated with threshold excitation. Action potentials recorded with suction electrodes. (After Lab (1978a).) B, Records, from isolated cat papillary muscle. The muscle begins its contraction isometrically, that is, develops force (middle trace) with no length change (lowest trace). Near the end of the repolarisation phase of the action potential (top trace) the muscle is 'released' and allowed to shorten. This manoeuvre causes the membrane to depolarise to reach threshold for a propagated action potential. Action potentials recorded with micro-electrodes. (After Kaufmann *et al.* (1971).)

tory period. In patients, mechanical perturbations, such as a blow to the chest (Hurst and Logue, 1966), and cardiac catheterisation can also induce threshold depolarisations. Moreover Zoll *et al.* (1976) were able systematically and mechanically to stimulate the heart externally and non-invasively with a 'mechanical thumper'. This device has been used in patients with cardiac arrest.

Mechanical changes during the action potential

In contrast to the foregoing, stretch during the action potential has no effect on the membrane potential of cat papillary muscle. However, the opposite mechanical perturbation, a sudden shortening or 'release' of isometrically contracting muscle at the equivalent time, does produce a depolarising potential. If the release is near the end of the repolarising phase of the action potential, this change in potential resembles a discrete transient depolarisation or early after-depolarisation (Cranefield, 1977). Figure 5.2B is an example of such a transient depolarisation which was accompanied by a propagated extrasystole. In Kluge and Vincenci's study the electrical impulse followed the mechanical impulse by about 40 ms, a latency which they were unable to explain. A release-induced depolarisation is just discernible within 5-10 ms and reaches threshold within 40 ms (Kaufmann *et al.*, 1970, 1971). The latency measurements would be in keeping with the possibility that the myocardium was being released following the compression of the heart with the 'thump'. However, one cannot exclude the mechano-electric link being via the stretch described in the two preceding subsections.

5.3 MECHANICALLY INDUCED DEPOLARISATION IN ISCHAEMIC MUSCLE

The factors predisposing to extrasystoles in ischaemia are thought to be related to altered membrane characteristics which are directly due to the consequences of the reduced blood flow (Hauswirth and Singh, 1978; Cranefield and Wit, 1979; Hoffmann and Rosen, 1981). However, premature excitations may be observed purely with sudden changes in the mechanical conditions of contraction of heart muscle. Tennant and Wiggers (1935) were the first to describe inhomogenous wall motion with coronary occlusion. In this situation ischaemic ventricular muscle is stretched during systole and shortens (that is, is released) during diastole. There are thus analogous mechanical situations to those described in section 5.2, for example the stretch or late release of an isometrically contracting papillary muscle. If this is the case then the mechanical changes which affect still viable muscle during ischaemia would cause depolarisations. Janse *et al.* (1980) have already suggested a role for diastolic depolarisation of viable myocardium, rather than re-entry in ischaemic muscle, in generating the first ectopic beat during early ischaemia. The questions are whether conditions predisposing to the 'contraction-excitation feedback' pertain in ischaemic myocardium and whether this feedback is a hitherto unsuspected cause of early ectopic beats in myocardial ischaemia. Figure 5.3 shows

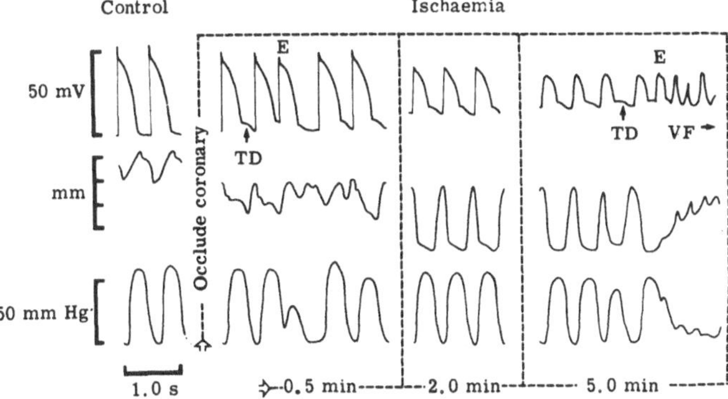

Figure 5.3 Effect of ischaemia on action potential (upper trace), ventricular segment motion (middle trace) and intraventricular pressure (lower trace). In the control panel segment shortening (upward movement of trace) occurs during the action potential, that is, mainly during systole; the configuration of the control action potential was stable over several minutes. After coronary occlusion the shortening occurs predominantly when repolarisation is over (that is, during diastole) and a transient depolarisation (TD) appears, which sometimes seems to reach threshold for an extrasystole (E). The transient depolarisation of the ectopic action potential is not pronounced but the length changes are also small. Continued ischaemia progressively reduces the action potential amplitude and duration while the segment shows holosystolic bulging. The final panel demonstrates an extrasystole precipitating ventricular fibrillation (VF). See text for further discussion. Monophasic action potentials and segment length records as in Lab and Woollard (1978).

monophasic action potentials and epicardial segment motion before and soon after occlusion of a small coronary artery. After occlusion the area becomes dyskinetic and demonstrates paradoxical wall motion; it lengthens during ventricular contraction and actually shortens when the ventricle relaxes. These movements are associated with a transient depolarisation which can reach the threshold for a new propagated action potential. If ventricular fibrillation does not ensue, the multiple extrasystoles disappear within an hour of the onset of ischaemia. It is of interest in this respect that Pirzada *et al.* (1976) showed that ventricular ischaemia produced systolic stretching of the affected segments which reached a maximum after 15 min, remained high during the first hour and thereafter declined towards normal. The time course of these compliancy changes roughly parallels the frequency distribution of ectopic beats. The complex inhomogenous intramural stresses and strains hinder definition of the relationship between mechanical changes and depolarisation in the intact beating ventricle *in situ*. Further, the re-entry mechanism could explain the depolarisation as being the result of electrotonic spread of a delayed action potential in an adjacent area of the heat; the retardation a consequence of the conduction defect because of the ischaemia. In fact, similar transient depolarisations to those reported here have been observed using micro-electrodes, and re-entry mechanisms were invoked to explain these (Czarnecka *et al.*, 1973;

Downar *et al.*, 1977). The nature of suction electrode recording from a large number of cells increases the difficulty in interpretation. One could strengthen the credibility of a stress–strain cause of arrhythmia by demonstrating mechanically induced transient depolarisations and accompanying premature beats in intact hearts while minimising the possibility of re-entry circuits due to ischaemia. In fact this demonstration should be a prerequisite of 'contraction–excitation feedback' as a mechanism causing extrasystoles during ischaemia. The specific requirement still would be 'abnormal' segment motion associated with extrasystoles. This situation appears during ventricular outflow constriction in the frog ventricle (Lab, 1978a) and analogous experiments in the intact dog produce comparable findings. Figure 5.4 (Covell *et al.*, 1981) demonstrates that pulmonary artery occlusion

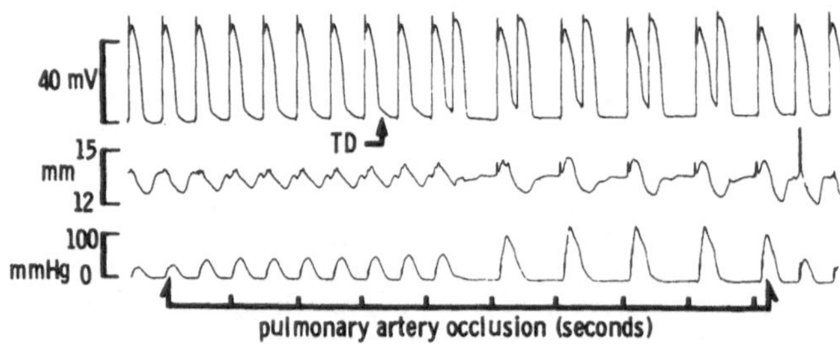

Figure 5.4 Changes in monophasic action potential (top trace), segment length (middle trace) and right intraventricular pressure (bottom trace) during pulmonary artery occlusion. Occlusion increased ventricular pressure and induced coupled extrasystoles. See text for further discussion. TD = transient depolarisation. (After Covell *et al.* (1981).)

increases right ventricular pressure, disturbs segment motion and produces afterdepolarisations (transient depolarisations) on the action potential. The depolarisations progressively increase in size during the occlusion and are associated with right ventricular extrasystoles, which in this case are coupled. The extrasystoles occur too suddenly to be explained by external reflexes or by imbalances in oxygen supply and demand. The results not only support the findings in the ischaemic ventricle but also largely confirm some of the micro-electrode studies in isolated perfused preparations described in section 5.2, indicating that changes in myocardial mechanics may be accompanied by transient depolarisations which can reach threshold.

5.4 MECHANISMS

Proposals for the molecular mechanisms for mechanically induced potentials have been presented (Kaufmann *et al.*, 1971; Lab, 1978a) and discussed in a recent review (Lab, 1982). It is of interest to see how these mechanisms relate to the changes found in ischaemia and to other hypotheses explaining early ectopics.

First, passive mechanical alterations could distort the internal and external membranes and produce permeability changes so that, for example, the membrane potential would move closer to the relevant equilibrium potentials. A non-specific increase in permeability could depolarise the membrane despite the probability that the final potential reached would be more negative than zero (Takeuchi and Takeuchi, 1960). This increase in permeability could augment the ischaemically induced potassium leak. The changes in tension could also distort intracardiac spaces. Changes in potassium movement or accumulation could follow rapidly (Kline and Morad, 1976) and thus influence potassium conductance to alter membrane repolarisation (Weidman, 1956). However, these hypotheses do not easily explain some of the experimental observations described in section 5.2. For example, a release can induce a transient depolarisation but a stretch at the equivalent time does not produce the expected and opposite change in potential (a repolarisation). Another possibility relates to intracellular calcium. Mechanically induced changes in intracellular calcium (Allen and Kurihara, 1981) show analogous alterations to the mechanically induced changes in action potential, and figure 5.5

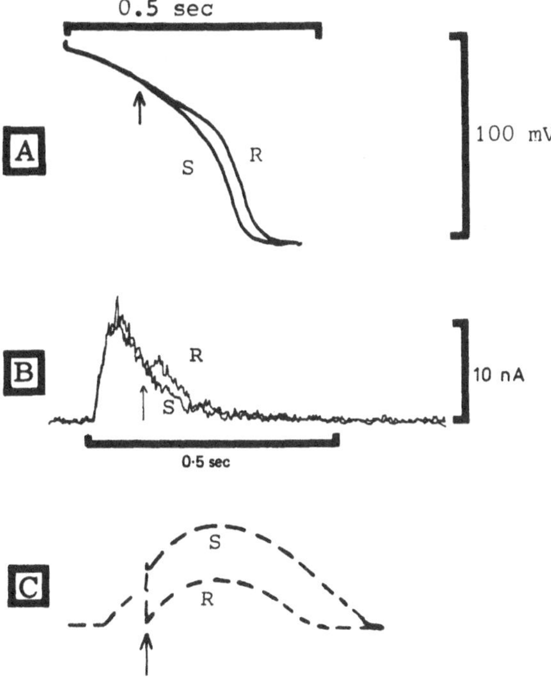

Figure 5.5 Analogous effects on action potential (A) and free sarcoplasmic calcium (B) of mechanical perturbations diagrammatically presented in C as dashed lines. Both records were from cat papillary muscle, but were obtained in different laboratories. Sarcoplasmic calcium, $[Ca^{2+}]_s$, is indicated by the light output (in nanoamperes) of intracellularly injected aequorin. A stretch (S) halfway up developed tension affects neither the action potential nor $[Ca^{2+}]_s$. However, a release (R) at the equivalent time delays the repolarisation and also the fall in $[Ca^{2+}]_s$. (Panel B is after Allen *et al.* (1981).)

demonstrates this similarity. These calcium variations have been invoked to explain the mechanically induced changes in potential (Lab, 1982). Further, lowered pH can increase sarcoplasmic Ca^{2+} in cat papillary muscle (Allen *et al.*, 1981) and this is expected in ischaemia. Myoplasmic calcium can affect outward currents (Isenberg, 1975; Bassingthwaighte *et al.*, 1976), the electromechanical gradient for the inward calcium current (Reuter, 1979) and an electrogenic Na/Ca exchange (Mullins, 1979). The transient depolarisation observed with strophanthidin (Kass *et al.*, 1978) and low potassium (Eisner and Lederer, 1979) may also have similar common explanations.

It appears that during the critical first hour or so of ischaemia there are coincident wall motion disturbances, after-potentials and changes in cyclic AMP (chapter 11) as well as in intracellular Ca^{2+}. It is tempting to speculate that all these findings are causally related to the extrasystoles observed in this period. Pollack (1977) has suggested that stretch accelerates diastolic depolarisation via a cyclic AMP-mediated mechanism, and there are interactions between Ca^{2+} and cyclic AMP pertinent to transmembrane ionic currents and to contraction (Harary *et al.*, 1976; Schneider and Sperelakis, 1975; Reuter and Scholz, 1977; Tsien, 1977; Chapman, 1979; Katz, 1979). Notwithstanding which mechanism is responsible, stress–strain-related ectopics via some sort of contraction excitation feedback may occur regularly in very early myocardial ischaemia. This is a subject that needs further investigation as a triggering cause of the premature beat that, in the appropriate ionic, metabolic and electrophysiological milieu, precedes potentially lethal arrhythmias.

REFERENCES

Allen, D. G. and Kurihara, A. (1981). Length changes during contraction affect the intracellular Ca^{2+} of heart muscle. *J. Physiol., Lond.*, **310**, 75-6P

Allen, D. G., Kurihara, A. and Orchard, C. H. (1981). The effects of reducing extracellular carbon dioxide concentration on intracellular calcium transients in mammalian cardiac muscle. *J. Physiol., Lond.*, **317**, 52P

Bassingthwaighte, J. B., Fry, C. H. and McGuigan, J. A. S. (1976). Relationship between internal calcium and outward current in mammalian ventricular muscle; a mechanism for the control of the action potential duration. *J. Physiol., Lond.*, **262**, 15-37

Boland, J. and Troquet, J. (1980). Intracellular action potential changes induced in both ventricles of the rat by an acute right ventricular pressure overload. *Cardiovasc. Res.*, **14**, 735-40

Brooks, C. McC., Gilbert, J. L. and Suckling, E. E. (1964). Excitable cycle of the heart as determined by mechanical stimuli. *Proc. Soc. exp. Biol. Med.*, **117**, 634

Bülbring, E., Holman, M. and Lüllman, H. (1956). Effects of calcium deficiency on striated muscle of the frog. *J. Physiol., Lond.*, **133**, 101-17

Chapman, R. A. (1979). Excitation-contraction coupling in cardiac muscle. *Progr. Biophys. molec. Biol.*, **35**, 1-52

Covell, J. W., Lab, M. J. and Pavalec, R. (1981). Mechanical induction of paired action potentials in intact heart in situ. *J. Physiol., Lond.*, **320**, 34P

Cranefield, P. F. (1977). Action potentials, afterpotentials and arrhythmias. *Circulation Res.*, **41**, 415-23

Cranefield, P. F. and Wit, A. L. (1979). Cardiac arrhythmias. *A. Rev. Physiol.*, **41**, 459-72

Czarnecka, M., Lewartowski, B. and Prokopczuk, A. (1973). Intracellular recording from the *in situ* working dog heart in physiological conditions and during acute ischaemia and fibrillation. *Acta physiol. pol.*, **24**, 331-7

Deck, K. A. (1964). Anderungen des Rühepotentials und der Kabeleigenschaflen von Purkinje-Fäden bei der dehnung. *Pflügers Arch. ges. Physiol.*, **280**, 131-40

Downar, E., Janse, M. J. and Durrer, D. (1977). The effect of acute coronary artery occlusion on the subepicardial transmembrane potentials in the intact porcine heart. *Circulation*, **56**, 217-24

Dudel, J. and Trautwein, W. (1954). Das Aktionspotential und Mechanogram des Herzmuskels unter dem Einflus der dehnung. *Cardiologie*, **25**, 344-62

Eisner, D. A. and Lederer, W. J. (1979). Inotropic and arrhythmogenic effects of potassium-depleted solutions on mammalian cardiac muscle. *J. Physiol., Lond.*, **294**, 255-77

Harary, I., Renaud, J., Sato, E. and Wallace, G. A. (1976). Calcium ions regulate cyclic AMP and beating in cultured heart cells. *Nature, Lond.*, **261**, 60-1

Hauswirth, O. and Singh, B. H. (1978). Ionic mechanisms in heart muscle in relation to the genesis and pharmacological control of cardiac arrhythmias. *Pharmac. Rev.*, **30**, 5-63

Hoffman, B. F., Cranefield, P. F., Lepeschkin, E., Surawicz, B. and Herrlich, H. C. (1959). Comparison of cardiac monophasic action potentials recorded by intracellular and suction electrodes. *Am. J. Physiol.*, **196**, 1297-301

Hoffman, B. F. and Rosen, M. R. (1981). Cellular mechanisms for cardiac arrhythmias. *Circulation Res.*, **49**, 1-15

Hurst, J. W. and Logue, R. B. (1966). *The Heart, Arteries and Veins*, McGraw-Hill, New York

Isenberg, G. (1975). Is potassium conductance of cardiac Purkinje fibres controlled by Ca^{2+}? *Nature, Lond.*, **253**, 273-4

Ishiko, N. (1956). The effect of stretch on electrical properties of striated muscle of the frog. *J. Physiol., Lond.*, **133**, 101-17

Ishiko, N. (1958). Changes in resting and potentials of striated muscle fibres by stretch. *Kumanato med. J.*, **11**, 18-31

Janse, M. J., van Capelle, F. J. L., Morsink, H., Kleber, A. G., Wilms-Schopman, F. W., Cardinal, R., D'Alnoncourt, C. N. and Durrer, D. (1980). Flow of 'injury' current and patterns of excitation during early ventricular arrhythmias in acute regional myocardial ischaemia in isolated porcine and canine hearts. Evidence for two different arrhythmogenic mechanisms. *Circulation Res.*, **47**, 151-65

Kass, R. S., Lederer, W. J., Tsien, R. W. and Weingart, R. (1978). Role of ionic basis of transient inward current induced by strophanthidin in cardiac Purkinje fibres. *J. Physiol., Lond.*, **281**, 209-26

Katz, A. M. (1979). Role of the contractile proteins and sarcoplasmic reticulum in the response of the heart to catecholamines: an historical review. *Adv. cyclic Nucleotide Res.*, **11**, 303-43

Kaufmann, R. and Theophile, U. (1967). Automatie fordernde Dehnungseffects am Purkinje Faden, Pappilarmuskeln und vorhoftrabekeln von Rhesusaffen. *Pflügers Arch. ges. Physiol.*, **291**, 174-89

Kaufmann, R., Hennekes, R. and Lab, M. J. (1970). The latency period of feedback interaction between mechanical and electrical events in mammalian cardiac muscle. *Pflügers Arch. ges. Physiol.*, **319**, 10

Kaufmann, R., Lab, M. J., Hennekes, R. and Krause, H. (1971). Feedback interaction of mechanical and electrical events in the isolated ventricular myocardium (cat papillary muscle). *Pflügers Arch. ges. Physiol.*, **332**, 96-116

Kline, R. and Morad, M. (1976). Potassium efflux and accumulation in heart muscle. *Biophys. J.*, **16**, 367-72

Kluge, W. F. and Vincenci, F. F. (1971). Mechanically-induced arrhythmias in digitalised hearts. *J. Electrocardiol.*, **4**, 11-18

Lab, M. J. (1969). The effect on the left ventricular action potential of clamping the aorta. *J. Physiol., Lond.*, **202**, 73-4P

Lab, M. J. (1974). Mechano-electric interactions in cardiac muscle. PhD thesis, University of London

Lab, M. J. (1978a). Mechanically dependent changes in action potentials recorded from the intact frog ventricle. *Circulation Res.*, **42**, 519-28

Lab, M. J. (1978b). Depolarization produced by mechanical changes in normal and abnormal myocardium. *J. Physiol., Lond.*, **284**, 143-4P

Lab, M. J. (1982). Contraction-excitation feedback in myocardium: physiological basis and clinical relevance. *Circulation Res.*, **50**, 757-66

Lab, M. J. and Woollard, K. V. (1978). Monophasic action potential, electrocardiograms and mechanical performance in normal and ischaemic epicardial segments of the pig ventricle *in situ*. *Cardiovasc. Res.*, **42**, 519-28

Ling, G. and Gerard, R. W. (1949). The influence of stretch on the membrane potential of the striated muscle fibre. *J. cell. comp. Physiol.*, **34**, 397-405

Mullins, J. J. (1979). The generation of electric currents in cardiac fibres by Na/Ca exchange. *Am. J. Physiol.*, **263**, C103-10

Penefsky, Z. J. and Hoffman, B. F. (1963). Effects of stretch on mechanical and electrical properties of cardiac muscle. *Am. J. Physiol.*, **204**, 433-8

Pirzada, F. A., Ekong, E. A., Vokonas, P. S., Anstein, C. A. and Hood, W. B. (1976). Experimental infarction. XIII. Sequential changes in left ventricular pressure-length relationships in the acute phase. *Circulation*, **53**, 970-5

Pollack, G. H. (1977). Cardiac pacemaking: an obligatory role of catecholamines. *Science, N.Y.*, **196**, 731-8

Reuter, H. (1979). Properties of two inward membrane currents in the heart. *A. Rev. Physiol.*, **41**, 413-24

Reuter, H. and Scholz, H. (1977). The regulation of the calcium conductance of cardiac muscle by adrenaline. *J. Physiol., Lond.*, **264**, 49–62

Schneider, J. A. and Sperelakis, N. (1975). Slow Ca^{2+} and Na^{+} responses induced by isoproterenol and methylxanthines in isolated perfused guinea-pig hearts exposed to elevated K^{+}. *J. molec. cell. Cardiol.*, 7, 249-73

Takeuchi, A. and Takeuchi, V. (1960). On the permeability of the end plate membrane during the action of transmitter. *J. Physiol., Lond.*, **154**, 52-7

Tennant, R. and Wiggers, D. J. (1935). The effect of coronary occlusion on myocardial contraction. *Am. J. Physiol.*, **112**, 351–61

Tsien, R. W. (1977). Cyclic AMP and contractive activity in the heart. *Adv. cyclic Nucleotide Res.*, **8**, 363-420

Weidmann, S. (1956). Shortening of the cardiac action potential due to a brief injection of KCl following the onset of contractility. *J. Physiol., Lond.*, **132**, 157–63

Zoll, P. M., Belgard, A. H., Weintraum, J. J. and Frank, H. A. (1976). External mechanical cardiac stimulation. *New Engl. J. Med.*, **294**, 1274-5

6

Early Arrhythmias and Primary Ventricular Fibrillation after Acute Myocardial Ischaemia in Relation to Pre-existing Coronary Collaterals

W. Meesmann

6.1 INTRODUCTION

For more than 10 years our group has been performing acute experimental coronary occlusions in dogs to study the pathophysiological and therapeutic problems of myocardial ischaemia. These experiments have clearly shown that primary ventricular fibrillation (VF) after acute ligation of a main coronary artery depends not only on the potential size of the ischaemic area and such factors as general experimental conditions, operating technique, narcosis, site of ligation and whether the artery is abruptly or slowly occluded, but especially on the presence of functionally effective pre-existing coronary collaterals (Meesmann *et al.*, 1970).

It is surprising, therefore, that hitherto most authors have not taken collaterals into account in the discussion of their results from acute experimental coronary occlusion. This explains why in the literature the rate of mortality within 1 h after acute occlusion of a main coronary artery of the untreated dog varies between 0 and 100 per cent (Meesmann *et al.*, 1970). One of the reasons why so little attention has been paid to pre-existing coronary collaterals is that, in the case of survival following coronary occlusion, extensive necrosis occurs in the ischaemic area; in addition, the collateral flow directly measured as retrograde coronary flow is very low (Gregg and Fisher, 1963). It should be mentioned in passing that the dog, in contrast to man, has a left coronary preponderance, the region supplied by the circumflex branch of the left coronary artery (LCFX) usually being considerably larger than that supplied by the left anterior descending branch (LAD).

Pre-existing collaterals are coronary connections with arterial or arteriolar characteristics and in dogs are mainly situated in the subepicardial area (Schaper, 1979). They are normally between 40 and 100 μm in diameter, and, more rarely, up to 200 μm in diameter. In dogs the number of these collaterals, and hence their functional importance, varies greatly. On the other hand, pig hearts usually have fewer collaterals or hardly any at all (Schaper, 1979). However, since cardiovascular function is less stable in untrained pigs (Schaper, 1979; Schaper *et al.*, 1971), dogs are still most widely used in studies for examining the consequences of acute coronary artery occlusion.

6.2 METHODS OF DETERMINING CORONARY COLLATERAL FLOW

As yet there is no generally agreed simple and reliable method for determining the extent of functionally effective pre-existing collaterals. The methods that have been used include those described below.

Retrograde coronary flow

For about 50 years retrograde flow (that is, a backflow from an occluded major coronary artery) has been taken as a measure of collateral flow (Anrep and Haüsler, 1928; Mautz and Gregg, 1937; Gregg *et al.*, 1939; Eckstein, 1954; Kattus and Gregg, 1959; Gregg and Fisher, 1963; Herzberg *et al.*, 1966; Elliot *et al.*, 1971; Pasyk *et al.*, 1971). For a long time it was assumed that retrograde flow overestimates true collateral flow by up to 20 per cent. It was thought that the resistance to the collateral flow in the myocardium was considerably higher than that to the free retrograde coronary outflow against air (Kattus and Gregg, 1959; Gregg and Fisher, 1963). More recent experiments have shown, however, that by measuring retrograde coronary flow true collateral flow is not overestimated but underestimated (Schulz *et al.*, 1973).

Retrograde coronary pressure

Retrograde coronary pressure is mainly determined by perfusion pressure, the rate of flow and vascular resistance in the individual coronary artery. However, it is also strongly dependent on extravascular support, especially as ventricular pressure might be passively transmitted to the vascular system. As myocardial capillary blood flow takes place mainly during diastole, only diastolic retrograde coronary pressure is evaluated. Following Schaper (1979) it is therefore logical to relate this coronary pressure to the corresponding diastolic pressure in the aorta near the coronary ostium. This quotient is then termed relative *retrograde coronary pressure.* It should only be used as a functional index for collateral flow when the peripheral coronary blood flow is fairly constant (Schaper, 1979).

This method, and also that described in the preceding subsection, are quantitatively less accurate than their precise data would suggest and are limited in their practical applications. If used in connection with single or multiple acute coronary occlusions (for example, for obtaining temporary coronary flow zero with a pneumatic occlusive cuff or for ^{86}Rb or ^{133}Xe clearance) the effect is functionally the same as using repeated and short two-phase ligations after Harris (1950). The mortality rate following such repeated and acute coronary occlusions is considerably reduced, and usually no VF occurs (see, for example, Pasyk *et al.*, 1971).

Selective regional radio-clearance methods

These methods, which usually depend on the myocardial clearance of either ^{133}Xe or ^{86}Rb require a gamma-ray camera, involve special operative techniques and must be preceded by a coronary occlusion of short duration for intra-coronary application of the isotope if the collateral flow into the total occluded vascular area is to be evaluated.

Radioactive tracer microsphere techniques

This technique is expensive, specialised and requires considerable experience if precise, reproducible collateral flow data are to be obtained. The errors and problems inherent in this technique have been discussed recently by Patterson and Kirk (1980). Even if these errors are avoided, exact collateral flow values obtained in several myocardial samples (epicardium and endocardium) do not really provide precise information about *total* collateral function.

Anatomical methods

Using post-mortem methods (see, for example, Menick *et al.*, 1971) an anatomic anastomotic index can be deduced and the extent of functionally effective collateral flow estimated. These are relatively rough indices which can, however, be applied for answering appropriate questions of limited scope (see, for example, Garza *et al.*, 1974).

Selective retrograde coronary angiography with simultaneous measurement of back pressure

Over the years we have gained much empirical experience using this technique and have related this index of the coronary collateral circulation to survival rates after acute coronary artery ligation. The method is as follows.

After death the hearts are carefully removed and stored under moist conditions in a closed receptacle. Twenty-four hours after removal, cannulae are placed in the three main coronary arteries and the coronary vascular system is perfused with physiological sodium chloride solution under low pressure. The composition of the contrast medium used is as follows: 20 g Unibaryt C (Röhm-Pharma, Darmstadt,

West Germany), 50 ml physiological sodium chloride solution and 3 ml of 12 per cent sterile gelatin. It is essential that the contrast medium (Unibaryt C micro-opaque particles of barium sulphate of approximately 10 μm in diameter) contains gum arabic because only in this form does it *not* pass through the capillaries. The contrast medium is heated to 35-38 °C, sedimentation being prevented by a magnetic stirrer, and is injected over a period of 10 min via an intermediate Windkessel at a constant filling pressure of 120 mmHg. The three main coronary arteries are filled one after the other in a set order while the heart is at room temperature.

At the constant filling pressure the gum arabic causes the barium sulphate to agglomerate quickly, occluding the small vessels as well as the collaterals. This contrast medium penetrates into the arterioles (approximately 20 μm) but does not reach the capillaries. Histologically, all the arterioles are filled.

With this procedure the time available for the retrograde filling of the vascular system of the acutely ligated coronary artery is limited and as a result the extent of filling depends on the number and diameter of the pre-existing collaterals. As orthograde filling proceeds, the back pressures (that is, the retrograde filling pressures developed in the main neighbouring coronary arteries) are continuously measured. The height and steepness of the retrograde pressure developed and the degree of filling determined by X-ray analysis are the established coronary function criteria. After each coronary artery is filled with the contrast medium, X-ray photographs are taken under identical conditions to evaluate the retrograde filling of the non-orthogradely filled coronary vessel areas. These are then finally compared with the complete orthograde filling of all three main coronary arteries.

The following are the evaluation criteria of post-mortem retrograde coronary angiography (Meesman *et al.*, 1970):

State 0	No retrograde contrast whatsoever
State I	Spots or small strips of contrast medium in the main coronary arteries
State II	Fragmentary filling of the main and/or secondary coronary arteries; slight contrast
State III	Continuous filling of the main coronary arteries, with partial filling of large and small secondary arteries; only slight contrast
State IV	Continuous filling of the main coronary arteries with large and small arteries, but only weak filling of the vessels (recognisable by the smaller width and density of the filling contrast)
State V	Complete retrograde filling of the entire arterial system as with orthograde filling

Good correlation of the coronary angiograms with the retrograde pressure curve is a prerequisite for correct evaluation. Correction is necessary in some cases, for example, where there are only some larger collateral vessels with a slow retrograde pressure rise but collateral states for V. *In vivo* measurements in a main ramus of the left coronary artery at normal arterial pressure show that dogs with the most pronounced pre-existing collaterals achieve a systolic back pressure of up to 25 mmHg.

The survival rate after acute high LCFX occlusion almost exactly corresponds to collateral states IV and V; primary VF is rarely seen with this degree of collateral function. In the following discussion dogs with pre-existing, functionally effective collaterals are simply termed dogs with collaterals. In contrast, dogs with collateral states 0-III are termed dogs without collaterals; primary VF is the invariable consequence of high LCFX occlusion in these dogs. In our most recent experiments, determining collateral blood flow in the area of infarction using radioactive tracer microspheres, we found a critical blood flow of about 10 ml per 100 g, corresponding to the border between states III and IV.

Figure 6.1 shows two examples of dogs with collateral states I and IV. The pictures show the good correlation between the empirical evaluation by post-

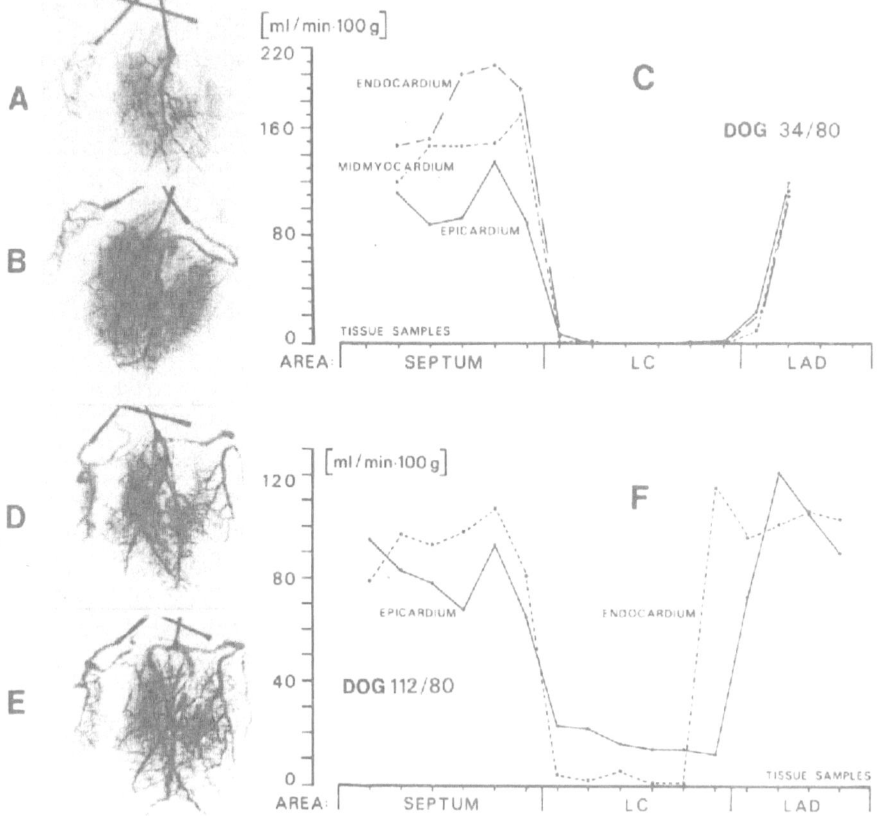

Figure 6.1 Examples of post-mortem selective coronary angiography related to change in blood flow following occlusion of the circumflex branch (LC) of the left coronary artery in dogs with few pre-existing collaterals (state I, above) and with good collateral development (stage IV, below). Blood flows were measured (C and F) with radioactive microspheres given 30 min after occlusion and were performed in collaboration with S. von Krosigk and M. Neumann. In A and D after orthograde injection into the right coronary artery and LAD with nearly complete filling of the circumflex branch; in B and E there is complete orthograde filling of all three main coronary arteries. For full explanation see text.

mortem selective coronary angiography and the results of myocardial collateral blood flow measurements using tracer microspheres.

6.3 SURVIVAL RATE DURING MYOCARDIAL ISCHAEMIA IN RELATION TO PRE-EXISTING CORONARY COLLATERALS

Table 6.1 shows our earlier results, obtained from a total of 62 dogs, of the incidence of VF during the first hour after acute coronary occlusion as related to the function of pre-existing coronary collaterals. All experiments were performed

Table 6.1 Incidence of ventricular fibrillation after acute coronary occlusion; dependence on coronary collaterals (from Meesmann *et al.*, 1970)

	Total	Ventricular fibrillation	
	n	*n*	Per cent
LAD artery			
With collaterals	7	0	0
Without collaterals	9	5	55.6
LFCX artery			
With collaterals	27	1	3.7
Without collaterals	19	19	100

$P < 0.001$.

under morphine-chloralose-urethane narcosis (Meesmann *et al.*, 1970). The data shows that without exception VF after acute LCFX ligation only occurs in dogs without collaterals. These results clearly reveal the most suitable conditions for experiments on dogs to determine the effects of preventive drugs on primary VF in the early arrhythmic phase following coronary occlusion, that is, acute high ligation of the LCFX in dogs *without* effective pre-existing collaterals. On the other hand, the incidence and distribution with time of ventricular premature beats (VPBs) can be best investigated in animals in which the LAD is ligated since here the percentage of surviving animals is greater, even in the absence of collaterals.

6.4 INCIDENCE AND DISTRIBUTION OF EARLY ARRHYTHMIAS IN RELATION TO PRE-EXISTING CORONARY COLLATERALS

In a series of experiments performed by us in 1976 (Komhard *et al.*, 1978; Meesmann *et al.*, 1978b,c) involving various conditions of anaesthesia, it was revealed that following acute coronary occlusion there is a bimodal distribution of arrhythmias in the early phase. This had previously been considered a uniform phase. This was first reported, as far as we know, by Haase and Schiller in 1969; prior to our experiments in 1976 their results had been virtually ignored in the international literature.

Figure 6.2 (top) shows our results after acute LAD occlusion in 65 dogs using three different anaesthetics. Two phases in which VPBs and VF more frequently

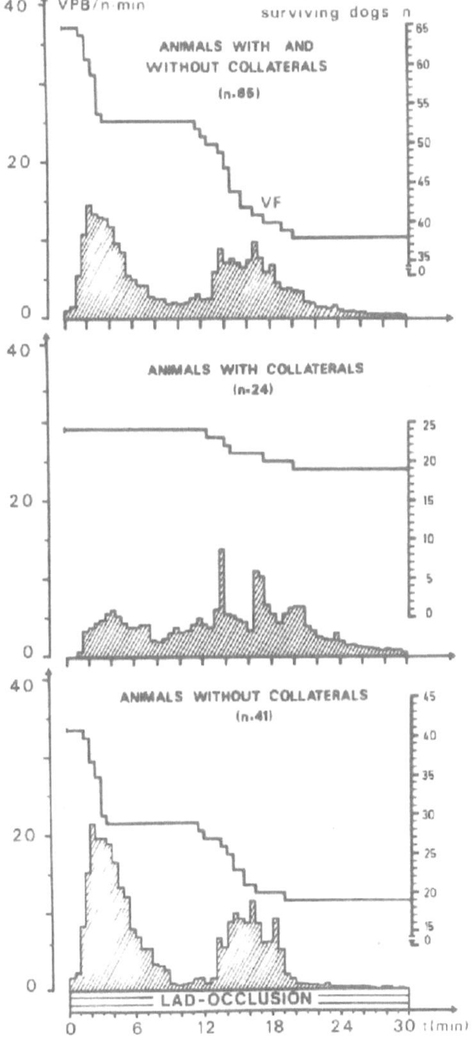

Figure 6.2 The incidence of ventricular premature beats (VPB) and of VF during the first 30 min of acute ligation of the left anterior descending coronary artery (LAD) in a group of 65 mongrel dogs (above). When these animals are subdivided into those with, and those without, pre-existing coronary collaterals a marked difference is observed with regard to the incidence of VF and the distribution of VPBs. A clear differentiation into two distinct groups of VPBs (phases 1a and 1b) is especially seen in those dogs without pre-existing collaterals.

occur can be clearly differentiated. In both the first (1a) and second (1b) phases an unequivocal coincidence in time of peak ventricular ectopic activity (VPBs) and VF is obtained.

The distribution of VPBs in phases 1a and 1b in all animals is shown in table 6.2; 13 animals had no VPBs at all, 16 only in phase 1a, 11 only in phase 1b, and 25 in phases 1a and 1b. Figure 6.3 shows three typical examples of the incidence and distribution of VPBs obtained from three individual dogs.

Table 6.2 Distribution of the VPBs in phases 1a and 1b

	1a + 1b	Only 1a	Only 1b	No VPB	Total
All animals	25	16	11	13	65
Survivors	13	4	8	13	38

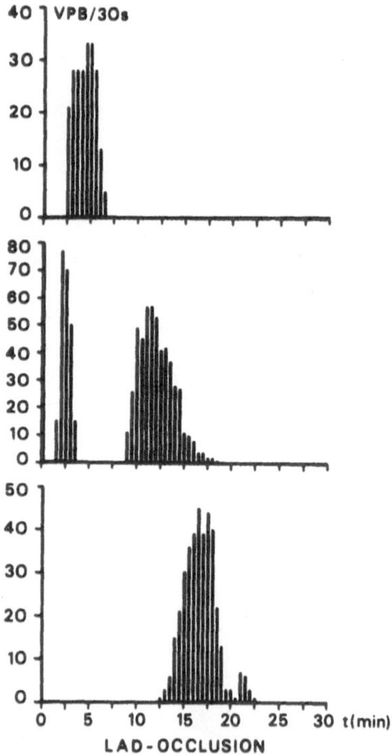

Figure 6.3 The distribution of VPBs in three individual dogs following acute occlusion of the LAD. From the top: showing phase 1a arrhythmias only; showing phase 1a and 1b arrhythmias; showing phase 1b arrhythmias only.

The presence of these two sub-phases becomes even more clearly recognisable when the animals are divided into groups with and without collaterals (figure 6.2). In these animals without coronary collaterals a clearly recognisable peak of the incidence of VPBs and VF is reached between the second and sixth minutes.

Thereafter, VPBs are strongly reduced until phase 1b develops from the 12th minute onwards. Peak ectopic activity is not so pronounced during this phase but it continues for a longer time. In comparison, this distinction between phases 1a and 1b is less marked in animals with functional collaterals. Only five such animals had VF and this occurred only in phase 1b. Table 6.3 shows the precise distribution

Table 6.3 Incidence of ventricular fibrillation after acute LAD occlusion in phases 1a and 1b; dependence on coronary collaterals

VF	Without collaterals	With collaterals	
Phase 1a	12	0	$P < 0.01$ (Phase 1a vs 1b)
Phase 1b	10	5	
No VF	19	19	
Total	41	24	

and incidence of VF following LAD occlusion in phases 1a and 1b as a function of coronary collaterals. Only animals without collaterals died of VF in phase 1a.

Generally animals without collaterals have more VPBs than those with collaterals. Table 6.4 illustrates this difference, which occurs mainly in phase 1a. The median time for the occurrence of VPBs in those animals without collaterals occurs earlier. It is remarkable that after acute coronary occlusion in the dog this early arrhythmic phase almost always stops abruptly after exactly 30 min.

After the completion of these experiments our results were confirmed by Kaplinsky and Dreifus (Kaplinsky *et al.*, 1979) in the United States. From their data the median values of the two phases of VPBs correspond exactly to our own results.

Also noteworthy is the different transition from ventricular ectopic activity to VF in the two phases. This is illustrated in figure 6.4, which shows two typical electrocardiographs after LAD ligation. In the upper example single and multiple

Table 6.4 Mean number of VPBs per 30 s period; *n* and median value

	Phase 1a		Phase 1b	
	Mean number of VPBs per 30 s period, *n*	Median value (min)	Mean number of VPBs per 30 s period, *n*	Median value (min)
Animals with collaterals (n = 24)	3.3 ± 0.7*	5.5 ± 0.3	4.0 ± 0.9	17.6 ± 0.3
Animals without collaterals (n = 41)	11.5 ± 1.8*	4.1 ± 0.1	4.0 ± 0.9	16.4 ± 0.3

*Significant difference, $P < 0.01$.

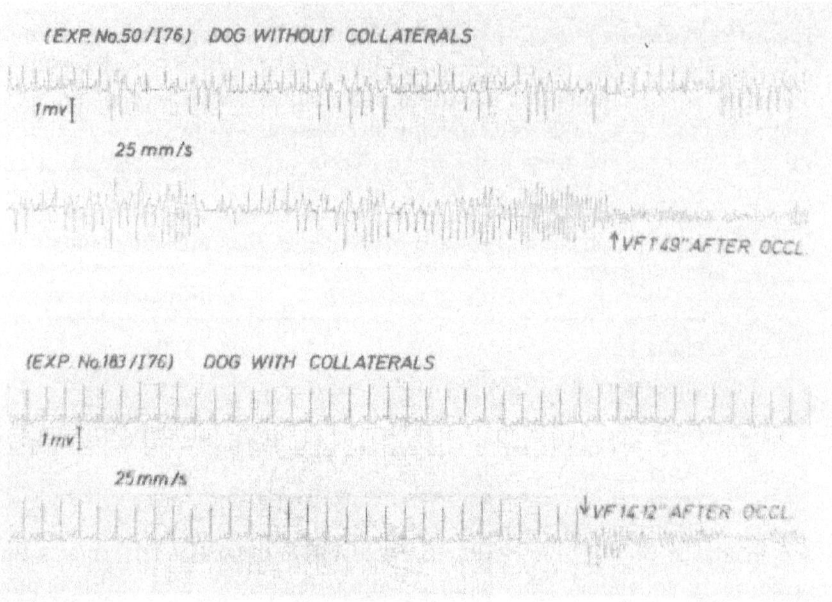

Figure 6.4 The occurrence of VF in (above) a dog without pre-existing coronary collaterals, when it is preceded by marked ectopic activity and (below) in a dog with good pre-existing collaterals, when VF occurred suddenly without being preceded by 'warning' VPBs. (Reproduced with permission from Meesmann *et al.*, in *The Arterial System* (ed. R. D. Bauer and R. Bussel), pp. 275–84, 1978.)

VPBs and ventricular tachycardia occur. This may suddenly stop or, as here, develop into ventricular flutter and then fibrillation. The situation is different in those animals with collaterals, where usually no phase 1a arrhythmias develop. In the lower part of figure 6.4 a VPB suddenly occurs in phase 1b during normal sinus rhythm. A second VPB then arises in the vulnerable phase of the first; this is followed by ventricular flutter of short duration and the rapid development of VF.

This bimodal vulnerability is even more marked following ligation of the LCFX (see figure 9.1 in chapter 9 of this book). Thus all of 19 animals died of VF within 21 min. The onset and peak activity of phase 1a occurs earlier than following ligation of the LAD and the period of sinus rhythm prior to the onset of phase 1b can be clearly recognised (Komhard *et al.*, 1978; Meesmann *et al.*, 1978b,c). Similar results (illustrated in figure 6.5) are also obtained from conscious dogs (Bucher *et al.*, 1978).

A similar distribution of the early arrhythmias resulting from coronary occlusion has also been described in pigs by Hirche *et al.* (1980) and by Parratt and his colleagues in rats (see chapter 18). It thus follows that there are presumably no major species differences with regard to the incidence and genesis of VF and VPBs following acute myocardial ischaemia.

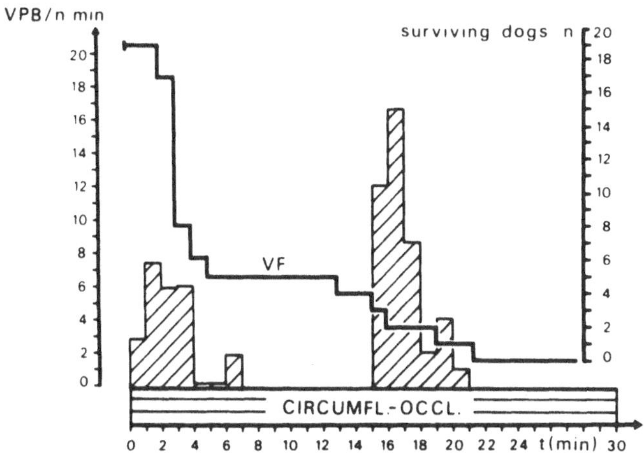

Figure 6.5 The occurrence of ventricular ectopic beats (VPBs) and of ventricular fibrillation following occlusion of the left circumflex coronary artery in dogs without pre-existing coronary collaterals. Compare with the lower part of figure 6.2. (Reproduced with permission from Meesmann *et al.*, in *The Arterial System* (ed. R. D. Bauer and R. Bussel), pp. 275–84, 1978.)

6.5 THE INFLUENCE OF DIFFERENT ANAESTHETICS ON THE DISTRIBUTION OF EARLY ARRHYTHMIAS

The following anaesthetic procedures were used:

(1) Pentobarbitone: 30 mg kg^{-1} i.v. initially and 10 mg kg^{-1} 1 and 2 h later.

(2) Morphine-chloralose-urethane: morphine hydrochloride 3 mg kg^{-1} i.m. premedication and then initially chloralose-urethane 3 ml kg^{-1} administered slowly i.v. (solution containing 20 g chloralose and 250 g urethane in 1000 ml heated up to 50 °C).

(3) Piritramide-nitrous oxide: atropine sulphate 0.5 mg premedication and piritramide (Janssen GmbH, West Germany) 1.25 mg kg^{-1}, then thiopentone (300-500 mg) i.v. followed by inhalation with nitrous oxide and oxygen in the ratio 75 : 25 volume per cent.

Phase 1a arrhythmias are more pronounced in those animals anaesthetised with pentobarbitone. This is especially marked in those animals without collaterals, where the mean number of VPBs per 30 s period in phase 1a under different anaesthetic procedures is significantly different (figure 6.6). In phase 1b the incidence of VPBs per 30 s period under piritramide-nitrous oxide anaesthesia is significantly smaller. The median values in the two phases under the different anaesthetics do not differ significantly. It was not possible to demonstrate with certainty that the three anaesthetic procedures examined exerted a significant influence on the mortality rate following acute coronary occlusion.

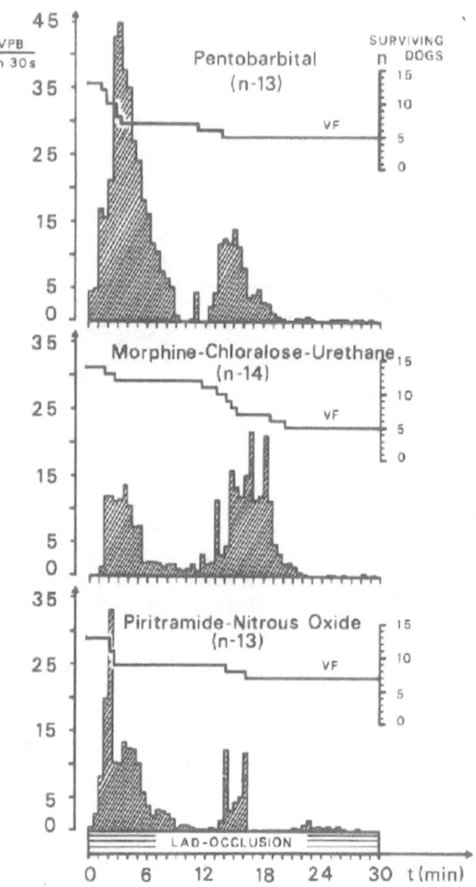

Figure 6.6 The effect of three different premedication and anaesthetic procedures on the incidence of VPBs and of VF in dogs following occlusion of the LAD coronary artery. For details see text.

Thus, compared with the other animals, those anaesthetised with pentobarbitone had a high resting heart rate, attributable to the familiar vagolytic effect of this drug (Nash *et al.*, 1956). In contrast, the possibility cannot be ruled out that vagal stimulation induced by piritramide could have a direct electrophysiologic effect on the slow Ca^{2+} and Na^{+} channels and might reduce the incidence of VPBs in phase 1b through these ionic mechanisms. This effect of anaesthesia on the incidence and distribution of VPBs early in ischaemia, which has also been reported by others (Marshall and Parratt, 1980) could result, in part, from the different haemodynamic effects of anaesthetics and of premedication.

These experiments using different anaesthetics showed a positive correlation between the maximum heart rate during the 30 min ischaemic period (usually reached during the first 10 min) and the number of VPBs per 30 s period in phase

1a (figure 6.7). Similarly, the initiation of VPBs in phase 1a after acute coronary occlusion is also dependent on the initial heart rate ($r = 0.6312; P < 0.01$; figure 6.8).

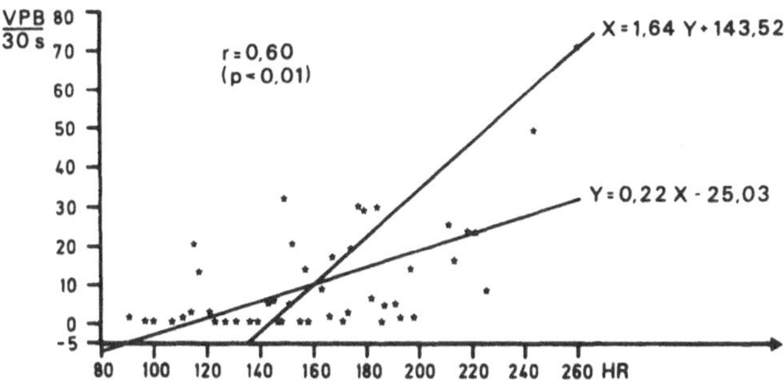

Figure 6.7 The dependence of the frequency of VPBs (phase 1a) following LAD in dogs on resting heart rate.

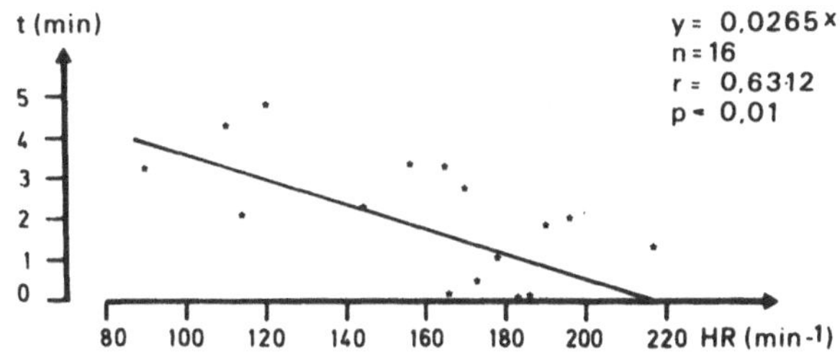

Figure 6.8 Time of onset of early (phase 1a) ventricular arrhythmias following LAD occlusion in relation to the initial heart rate.

6.6 VENTRICULAR FIBRILLATION THRESHOLDS DURING MYOCARDIAL ISCHAEMIA IN RELATION TO PRE-EXISTING COLLATERALS

The electrical ventricular fibrillation threshold (VFT) serves as a good measure of the vulnerability of the myocardium after acute coronary occlusion. It is well known that the VFT decreases following acute coronary occlusion (Wiggers *et al.*, 1940; Shunway *et al.*, 1957; MacLean and Phibbs, 1960; Shinohara, 1968; Han, 1969; Burgess *et al.*, 1971; Axelrod *et al.*, 1973; Schley *et al.*, 1973, 1975; Battle *et al.*, 1974; Verrier *et al.*, 1974; Roland *et al.*, 1975; Meesmann *et al.*, 1976), although the magnitude of this decrease has usually only been determined a few minutes after acute ligation. Consequently, only limited information is available on the time course of changes in VFT which occur following acute coronary occlusion. In determining this time course it should be borne in mind that when coronary occlusion is repeated several times, the extent of the decrease in VFT becomes increasingly less and the duration increasingly shorter. Finally there is no significant decrease in VFT at all (Gülker *et al.*, 1977). In contrast, reperfusion after coronary occlusion leads to an abrupt decrease in VFT within 1 min and this is followed by a rapid increase to control values. This particular time course following reperfusion does not depend upon the number of prior occlusions (Gülker *et al.*, 1977).

Determination of VFT

Since our earlier investigations in 1972-3 (Schley *et al.*, 1973, 1975), we have experimented on a further group of 18 dogs (Meesmann *et al.*, 1976), determining the VFT using stimulus trains of 140 ms duration with square wave pulse currents of 2 ms duration delivered at 3 ms intervals. The impulses were triggered by the R-wave of the electrocardiogram and for each determination of VFT the delay of the stimulus train was reset using an oscilloscope. This ensured that the stimulus train coincided with the vulnerable period of the cardiac cycle and did not extend beyond the end of the T-wave. Stimuli were applied to basic heart beats only. The stimulus intensity was increased in steps of 1 mA, VFT being that stimulus intensity just sufficient to elicit VF. The stimulating electrodes, made of silver chloride plates (diameter 7 mm), were sutured directly on to the epicardium of the right and left ventricles. They were about 30 mm apart and approximately 10 mm outside the area of expected ischaemia. A few seconds after VF, defibrillation was induced by a DC countershock via pericardially attached plate electrodes (diameter 30 mm). Exponentially increasing capacitor steps up to 6.4 W were used. In this way VFT data were easily reproducible every 2 min, differing only by up to ± 2 mA from the mean value.

At first VFT was determined several times prior to acute coronary ligation. Following acute ligation VFT was measured every 2 min and up to 18-20 min. The number of measurements obtained for the various time intervals differ from each other because spontaneous arrhythmias or VF at times made the determination of VFT impossible.

The time course of the VFT during the first hour after acute occlusion of the LAD

This is shown in figure 6.9 (left). A marked difference exists between the time course of VFT after acute coronary occlusion in dogs with and without collaterals. In phase 1a the VFT values temporarily fall from 17 to 5 mA ($P < 0.001$) in dogs without collaterals after acute LAD occlusion and in those with collaterals only from 18 to 13.5 mA ($P < 0.02$). The VFT values of both groups measured between the second and the 10th minutes of LAD occlusion differ significantly. It should be noted that VFT values do not fall again during phase 1b.

Figure 6.10 shows the time course of VFT during protracted LAD occlusion in a dog without collaterals. The VFT changes only a little and for a short time in the phase of critical flow reduction during protracted, finally complete, coronary occlusion. Only sporadic VPBs occur; often no arrhythmias occur at all (Gülker *et al.*, 1975; Krämer and Meesmann, 1978). A comparison of protracted LAD

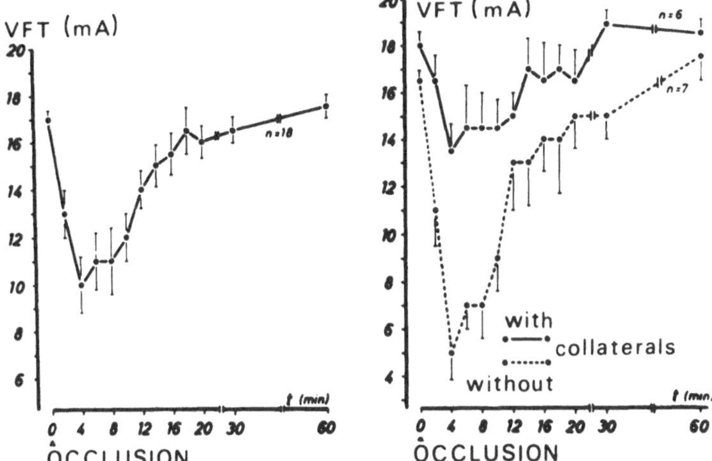

Figure 6.9 Changes in the ventricular fibrillation threshold (VFT) with time following LAD coronary artery occlusion for 30 min in a mixed group of mongrel dogs (left) and in dogs subdivided into those with and those without pre-existing coronary collaterals (right). A decrease in VFT is especially pronounced in those dogs without collaterals and this corresponds (figure 6.2) to the higher incidence in this group of VF. (Reproduced with permission from Meesmann *et al.*, *Cardiovasc. Res.*, **10**, 466–73, 1976.)

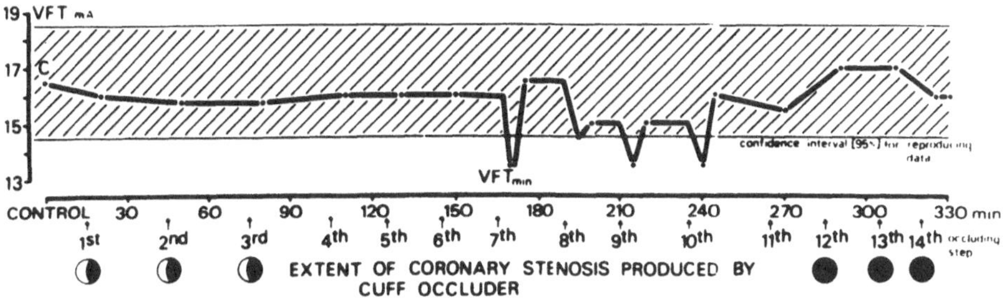

Figure 6.10 The time course of changes in VFT in an individual dog during slow coronary artery occlusion (illustrated schematically below). The shaded area represents the range of reproducibility of control VFT values (pre-occlusion).

occlusions in animals with and without collaterals shows that there is no difference between the time course of VFT. Under such experimental conditions, therefore, the coronary collaterals are of no importance.

6.7 FOCAL BLOCK AND OXYGEN CONSUMPTION DURING MYOCARDIAL ISCHAEMIA IN RELATION TO PRE-EXISTING COLLATERALS

Further experiments were performed in order to determine the occurrence of focal block (FB) in epicardial electrograms following acute occlusion of the distal branches of the LAD. Before VPBs occur the ventricular activation time is significantly prolonged in the epicardial electrograms. If the QRS complex widens over 50 ms a monophasic deformation of QRS termed focal block (FB) occurs. The evaluation of six epicardial electrograms out of the centre of the ischaemic area demonstrates that the FBs are more reliable than is ST elevation as prognostic parameters for ventricular vulnerability. The results of these experiments show that during phase 1a FBs occur significantly earlier, and in more leads of the epicardial ECG, in dogs without collaterals than in those with collaterals. This coincides with the different decreases in VFT as a function of collateral state (Meesmann *et al.*, 1978a; Stephan *et al.*, 1978).

Epicardial electrocardiographic maps were also used to assess the effects of heart rate, myocardial contractility and oxygen consumption on the severity of myocardial ischaemic injury following acute LAD occlusion in dogs and indicate the dependence of the severity of ischaemia on these variables. This dependence is largely influenced by the extent of pre-existing coronary collaterals (Stephan *et al.*, 1975).

6.8 INCIDENCE OF DOGS WITH FUNCTIONALLY EFFECTIVE PRE-EXISTING CORONARY COLLATERALS

Out of a total of 201 dogs, 77 (38.3 per cent) had functionally effective pre-existing coronary collaterals (states IV and V; figure 6.11). However, this ratio was not constant; in 13 individual experimental series the proportion of dogs with collaterals ranged between 16.7 and 60 per cent (Schulz *et al.*, 1972). This remarkable fact further explains the very different mortality rates after acute coronary occlusion reported in the literature.

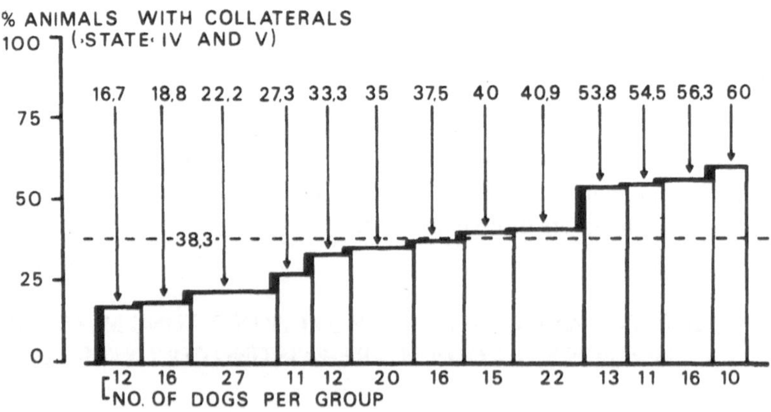

Figure 6.11 Frequency of effective pre-existing coronary collaterals in 13 separate groups of mongrel dogs (see text). (Reproduced with permission from Schulz *et al.*, *Med. Welt*, 23, 1375–6, 1972.)

6.9 CONCLUSIONS

It should be emphasised that effective pre-existing coronary collaterals cannot prevent myocardial infarction following acute coronary artery occlusion. Moreover, the initial morphologic injury patterns remain constant. The experiments outlined above have shown, however, that, with a sufficiently large area of incipient ischaemia, protracted coronary flow reduction up to coronary occlusion and effective pre-existing collaterals both have the same effect; that is, they can prevent a rapid simultaneous development of inhomogeneous electrical instability, which seems to be one of the most important factors triggering early arrhythmias and primary ventricular fibrillation after acute myocardial ischaemia.

On the basis of the experiments reported and other experimental results we are quite certain that the genesis of these two sub-phases is different. This is explained in detail in chapter 9.

We conclude that it is of great importance that all experimental preventive measures (for example, with drugs) taken against the early arrhythmias occurring during myocardial ischaemia have to take into account events occurring, not only during the initial 5-10 min period, but indeed throughout the entire 30 min post-occlusion period. Finally, account must also be taken of the presence of functionally effective pre-existing coronary collaterals.

REFERENCES

Anrep, G. V. and Häusler, H. (1928). The coronary circulation. 1. The effect of changes of the blood pressure and of the output of the heart. *J. Physiol., Lond.*, **65**, 357-73

Axelrod, P. J., Verrier, R. L. and Lown, B. (1973). Extreme vulnerability to ventricular fibrillation with acute coronary occlusion exposed by frequent R/T pulsing. *Am. J. Cardiol.*, **31**, 117

Battle, W. E., Naimi, S., Avital, S., Brilla, A. H., Banas, J. S., Bete, J. M. and Levine, H. J. (1974). Distinctive time course of ventricular vulnerability to fibrillation during and after release of coronary ligation. *Am. J. Cardiol.*, **34**, 42-7

Bucher, P., Dallmer, H., Derks, M. and Meesmann, W. (1978). Prophylaxis of ventricular fibrillation following acute coronary occlusion by chronic oral application of the beta-adrenoceptor blocking agent atenolol in conscious dogs. *Pflügers Arch. ges. Physiol.*, **377**, Suppl. R2

Burgess, M. J., Abildskov, J. A., Millar, M., Geddes, J. S. and Green, L. S. (1971). Time course of vulnerability to fibrillation after experimental coronary occlusion. *Am. J. Cardiol.*, 27, 617-21

Eckstein, R. W. (1954). Coronary interarterial anastomoses in young pigs and mongrel dogs. *Circulation Res.*, 2, 460-5

Eckstein, R. W. (1957). Effects of exercise and coronary artery narrowing in coronary collateral circulation. *Circulation Res.*, **5**, 230-5

Elliot, E. C., Bloor, C. M., Jones, E. L., Mitchell, W. J. and Gregg, D. E. (1971). Effect of controlled coronary occlusion on the collateral circulation in conscious dogs. *Am. J. Physiol.*, **220**, 857-62

Garza, B. A., White, F. C., Bloor, L. M. and Wall, R. E. (1974). Effect of coronary collateral development on ventricular fibrillation threshold. *Basic Res. Cardiol.*, **69**, 371-8

Gregg, D. E. and Fisher, L. E. (1963). Blood supply of the heart. In *Handbook of Physiology*, Sec. 2, Vol. 11, American Physiology Society, Washington, D.C., pp. 1517-84

Gregg, D. E., Thornton, J. J. and Mautz, F. R. (1939). The magnitude, adequacy and source of the collateral blood flow and pressure in chronically occluded coronary arteries. *Am. J. Physiol.*, **127**, 161-75

Gülker, H., Krämer, B., Stephan, K. and Meesmann, W. (1975). Differing effects of acute and protracted coronary occlusion on the time course of the ventricular fibrillation threshold (VFT) of the heart. *Pflügers Arch. ges. Physiol.*, **359**, Suppl. R17

Gülker, H., Krämer, B., Stephan, K. and Meesmann, W. (1977). Changes in ventricular fibrillation threshold during repeated short-term coronary occlusion and release. *Basic Res. Cardiol.*, **72**, 547-62

Haase, M. and Schiller, U. (1969). Zur zeitlichen Parallelität zwischen der Aktivität ectopischer Schrittmacher und dem Eintritt von Kammerflimmern nach Ligatur eines Hauptkoronarastes beim Hund. *Acta biol. med. germ.*, **23**, 413-22

Han, J. (1969). Ventricular vulnerability during acute coronary occlusion. *Am. J. Cardiol.*, **24**, 857-64

Harris, A. S. (1950). Delayed development of ventricular ectopic rhythms following experimental coronary occlusion. *Circulation*, **1**, 1318-28

Herzberg, R. M., Rubio, R. and Berne, R. M. (1966). Coronary occlusion and embolisation. Effects on blood flow in adjacent arteries. *Am. J. Physiol.*, **210**, 169-75

Hirche, Hj., Franz, Ch., Bös, L., Bissig, R., Lang, R. and Schramm, M. (1980). Myocardial extracellular K^+ - and H^+ - increase and noradrenaline release as possible cause of early arrhythmias following acute coronary artery occlusion in pigs. *J. molec. cell. Cardiol.*, **12**, 579-93

Kaplinsky, E., Ogawa, S., Balke, C. W. and Dreifus, L. S. (1979). Two periods of early ventricular arrhythmia in the canine acute myocardial infarction model. *Circulation*, **60**, 397-403

Kattus, A. A. and Gregg, D. E. (1959). Some determinants of coronary collateral blood flow in open chest dog. *Circulation Res.*, **7**, 628-42

Komhard, W., Rehwald, U., Meesmann, W., Stephan, K. and Abendroth, R.-R. (1978). Bimodale Häufigkeitsverteilung der Arrhythmien (VES) und des Klammerflimmerns (KF) in der ersten Arrhythmiephase nach akutem experimentellen Koronarverschluß und ihre Charakteristika. *Z. Kardiol.*, **67**, 220

Krämer, B. and Meesmann, W. (1978). Akuter und protrahierter Koronarverschluß. *Z. allg. Med.*, **54**, 9-14

MacLean, L. D. and Phibbs, C. M. (1960). Relative effect of chronic ischaemia and a myocardial revascularization procedure on the ventricular fibrillation threshold. *Circulation Res.*, **8**, 473-8

Marshall, R. J. and Parratt, J. R. (1980). The early consequences of myocardial ischaemia and their modification. *J. Physiol., Paris*, **76**, 699-715

Mautz, F. R. and Gregg, D. E. (1937). The dynamics of collateral circulation following chronic occlusion of coronary arteries. *Proc. Soc. exp. Biol. Med.*, **36**, 797-801

Meesmann, W., Schulz, F. W., Schley, G. and Adolphsen, P. (1970). Uberlebensquote nach akutem experimentellen Koronarverschluß in Abhängigkeit von Spontankollateralen des Herzens. *Z. ges. exp. Med.*, **153**, 246-64

Meesmann, W., Gülker, H., Krämer, B. and Stephan, K. (1976). Time course of changes in ventricular fibrillation threshold in myocardial infarction. Characteristics of acute and slow occlusion with respect to the collateral vessels of the heart. *Cardiovasc. Res.*, **10**, 466-73

Meesman, W., Gülker, H., Stephan, K., Krämer, B., Komhard, W., Rehwald, U. and Menken, U. (1978a). Arrhythmias, vulnerability and focal blocks in relation to coronary collateral vessels. In *Coronary Heart Diseases: 3rd International Symposium Frankfurt* (ed. M. Kaltenbach, P. Lichtlen, R. Balcon and W.-D. Bussmann), G. Thieme Verlag, Stuttgart, pp. 56-61

Meesmann, W., Stephan, K., Abendroth, R.-R., Menken, U. and Wiegand, V. (1978b). Arrhythmien, insbesondere Kammerflimmern, nach akutem experimentellen Koronarverschluß und Beta-Rezeptoren-Blockern. In *Beta-Blockade 1977, Internationales Symposium* (ed. W. Maurer, A. Schömig, R. Dietz and P. R. Lichtlen), G. Thieme Verlag, Stuttgart, pp. 333-6

Meesmann, W., Wiegand, V., Menken, U., Komhard, W. and Rehwald, U. (1978c). Early mortality due to ventricular fibrillation and the vulnerability of the heart following acute experimental coronary occlusion: possible mechanisms and pharmacological prophylaxis. In *The Arterial System* (ed. R. D. Bauer and R. Bussel), Springer Verlag, Berlin and Heidelberg, pp. 275-84

Menick, F. J., White, F. C. and Bloor, C. M. (1971). Coronary collateral circulation: determination of an anatomical index of functional collateral flow capacity. *Am. Heart J.*, **82**, 503-10

Nash, C. B., Davis, F. and Woodbury, R. A. (1956). Cardiovascular effects of anaesthetic doses of pentobarbital sodium. *Am. J. Physiol.*, **185**, 107-12

Pasyk, S., Bloor, C. M. and Gregg, D. E. (1971). Systemic and coronary effects of coronary artery occlusion in the unanaesthetised dog. *Am. J. Physiol*, **220**, 646-54

Patterson, R. E. and Kirk, E. S. (1980). Apparent improvement in canine collateral myocardial blood flow during vasodilatation depends on criteria used to identify ischemic myocardium. *Circulation Res.*, **47**, 108-16

Roland, J. M., Dashkoff, N., Varghese, P. J. and Pitt, B. (1975). Time course of ventricular fibrillation threshold in infarcted and non-infarcted myocardium after acute coronary ligation. *Fedn Proc. Fedn Am. Socs exp. Biol.*, **34**, 390

Schaper, W. (1979). Collaterals in chronic coronary occlusion. In *Pathophysiology of Myocardial Perfusion* (ed W. Schaper), Elsevier/North Holland, Amsterdam, pp. 415-70

Schaper, W., Flaming, W., Snoeckx, L. and Jagenau, H. (1971). Der Einfluss des körperlichen Trainings auf den Killateralkreislauf des Herzens. *Verh. ges. Kreislforsch.*, **37**, 112-21

Schley, G., Meesmann, W., Mescher, H., Wilde, A. and Wild, U. (1975). Der Einfluss von Spontankollateralen auf die Flimmerschwelle des Herzens nach akutem Koronarverschluss. *Z. Kardiol.*, **64**, 202-11

Schley, G., Meesmann, W., Wilde, A. and Wild, U. (1973). Die Beeinflussung der Flimmerschwelle des Herzens durch Practolol vor und nach akutem experimentellen Koronarverschluss. *Verh. dtsch. Ges. inn. Med.*, **79**, 983-6

Schulz, F. W., Meesmann, W. and Schley, G. (1972). Der Einfluss von Spontankollateralen auf akute experimentelle Myokardinfarkte. *Med. Welt*, **23**, 1375-6

Schulz, F. W., Raff, W. K., Meyer, U. and Lochner, W. (1973). Messung der Kollateraldurchblutung am Hundeherzen mit Hilfe der selektiven Embolisierung eines Koronargefässes. *Pflügers Arch. ges. Physiol.*, **342**, 243-56

Shinohara, Y. (1968). Ventricular fibrillation threshold in experimental coronary occlusion: comparative studies on the effect of GIK-solution and some new antiarrhythmic agents. *Jap. Circulation J.*, **32**, 1269-81

Shunway, N. E., Johnson, J. A. and Stish, R. I. (1957). The study of ventricular fibrillation by threshold determinations. *J. thorac. Surg.*, **34**, 643-53

Stephan, K., Meesmann, W. and Sadony, V. (1975). Oxygen demand and collateral vessels of the heart. *Cardiovasc. Res.*, **9**, 640-8

Stephan, K., Meesmann, W., Menken, U., Rehwald, U. and Komhard, W. (1978). Fokale Blockierung im experimentellen EKG - Vorstufe ventrikulärer Arrhythmien (VES) beim akuten experimentellen Myokardinfarkt. *Z. Kardiol.*, **67**, 221

Verrier, R., Corbalan, R. and Lown, B. (1974). Analysis of vulnerability changes during acute coronary occlusion and release. *Am. J. Cardiol.*, **33**, 174

Wiggers, C. J., Wegria, R. and Pinera, B. (1940). The effects of myocardial ischemia on the fibrillation threshold - the mechanism of spontaneous ventricular fibrillation following coronary occlusion. *Am. J. Physiol.*, **131**, 309-16

7

Early Arrhythmias, Myocardial Extracellular Potassium and pH

Hj. Hirche, R. Friedrich, U. Kebbel, F. McDonald and V. Zylka

7.1 INTRODUCTION

It is well known that following acute coronary artery occlusion ventricular arrhythmias occur in distinct phases (Harris, 1950; Haase and Schiller, 1969; Gettes, 1974; Gülker *et al.*, 1977; Meesmann *et al.*, 1978; Hirche *et al.*, 1980). A first, early phase starts 3-5 min after the onset of occlusion and lasts about 5-10 min. In our studies following occlusion of the distal half of the left anterior descending coronary artery (LAD) in the pig, more than 50 per cent of the animals develop ventricular fibrillation (VF) during this first early phase (phase 1a). This phase 1a is followed by an interval without arrhythmias beginning about 8-10 min after the onset of occlusion and lasting for 4-10 min; 15-20 min after the onset of ischaemia the second early phase of arrhythmias (phase 1b) begins, lasting up to 15 min. About one-third of the animals develop VF during this phase (Hirche *et al.*, 1980). This means that only 15-20 per cent of the control animals survive the 1a and 1b phases (Hirche *et al.*, 1980, 1981c; Zylka *et al.*, 1981). After this second, early phase of arrhythmias an intermediate phase of 4-8 h ensues during which arrhythmias seldom occur; 5-8 h after the onset of infarction a late phase of arrhythmias begins. This lasts 2-4 days with a maximal ectopic activity occurring at about 10-20 h after the onset of ischaemia (Harris, 1950). The reason for this sequence of post-ischaemia ventricular arrhythmias is not yet completely understood.

Among the many factors which have been proposed as causes of early post-ischaemic arrhythmias (phases 1a and 1b) two are of special importance. These are the release of K^+ from the ischaemic cells (Harris *et al.*, 1958; Benzing *et al.*, 1972; Gettes, 1974; Hirche *et al.*, 1976; Bös *et al.*, 1978; Franz *et al.*, 1978; Hill *et al.*, 1978; Meesmann *et al.*, 1978; Wiegand *et al.*, 1979; Hill and Gettes, 1980; Gettes and Hill, 1981; Hirche *et al.*, 1981a) and the myocardial release of noradrenaline from nerve fibres (Gettes, 1974; Franz *et al.*, 1978; Meesmann *et al.*, 1978; Lang *et al.*, 1979; Opie *et al.*, 1979; Wiegand *et al.*, 1979; Hirche *et al.*, 1980, 1981a; Zylka *et al.*, 1981, and reviewed in chapters 8, 9 and 10 of this book). Until recently, the amount of K^+ released from the ischaemic myocardium could only be estimated by measuring coronary arteriovenous K^+ differences (Cherbakoff *et al.*, 1957; Cherry and Myers, 1970; Thomas *et al.*, 1970; Ettinger *et al.*, 1973; Marshall and Parratt, 1975). Since in pigs the major part of the K^+ which is released from the ischaemic myocardial cells accumulates in the interstitial space and is not washed out (as a consequence of the very low collateral flow; Howe *et al.*, 1968), coronary arteriovenous K^+ differences cannot represent the amount of K^+ lost from the intracellular compartment. However, during the last few years it has been shown that the extracellular K^+ ($[K^+]_e$) in the interstitial space of the myocardium can be measured with sufficient accuracy by application of the new technique of ion measurement with ion-selective electrodes (Benzing *et al.*, 1972; Hirche *et al.*, 1976, 1979, 1980, 1981a,b; Bös *et al.*, 1978; Franz *et al.*, 1978; Hill *et al.*, 1978; Hill and Gettes, 1980; Gettes and Hill, 1981). We have previously used this technique to look at K^+ uptake during reperfusion following open-heart surgery performed under cardioplegia and also in skeletal muscle during long-lasting ischaemia. Apart from $[K^+]_e$, the increase of H^+ activity ($[H^+]_e$) in the ischaemic myocardium due to lactic acid (Braasch *et al.*, 1968) and local p_{CO_2} (Case *et al.*, 1979), accumulation has also been measured with different types of ion-selective electrode (Benzing *et al.*, 1972; Hirche *et al.*, 1976, 1979, 1980, 1981b; Cobbe and Poole-Wilson, 1980).

It is the aim of this chapter to review our recent results concerning the release of K^+ from hypoxic myocardial cells and the consequent increase in K^+ activity in the interstitial space as measured with ion-selective electrodes. Ion shifts may correlate with the occurrence of ventricular ectopic beats and VF following acute coronary occlusion. Pigs were chosen as experimental animals because their ventricular arterial pattern resembles that of humans (Fedor *et al.*, 1978) and because there is less individual variation in coronary anatomy in pigs than in dogs (Howe *et al.*, 1968). Furthermore, in the pig heart occlusion of the left anterior descending coronary artery (LAD) causes a transmural infarction whilst in the dog a more subendocardial infarction results (Holland and Brooks, 1975); this may be more difficult to assess using epicardial electrodes.

7.2 CHANGES IN EXTRACELLULAR K^+ AND H^+ FOLLOWING ACUTE CORONARY ARTERY OCCLUSION IN YOUNG DOMESTIC PIGS

Details of the methods employed have been described recently (Hirche *et al.*, 1981c). Following anaesthesia (ketamine and pentobarbitone followed by droperidol and fentanyl) and artificial ventilation, median sternotomy was performed and the heart suspended in a pericardial cradle. Coronary artery occlusion was performed by means of a ligature in the middle portion of the LAD. At the end of the experiments a gross estimate of the extent of the ischaemic region was obtained by separation from the normal perfused myocardium after post-mortem injection of fluorescein.

The type of K^+-selective surface electrodes which were used in these experiments have been described elsewhere (Hirche *et al.*, 1981c). They were calibrated *in vitro* immediately before and after each experiment. The drift of the electrodes was about 0.4 mV h^{-1} and it was assumed to be linear during the experiment. K^+ concentrations were also determined in arterial and coronary venous blood samples. Under control conditions no coronary arteriovenous K^+ differences were observed; this K^+ value was therefore taken as the initial $[K^+]_e$ value of the myocardium (Downey and Kirk, 1968).

The values (36 pigs) for the increase of $[K^+]_e$, measured in the centre of the ischaemic area following acute occlusion of the distal half of the LAD, are given in figure 7.1 and table 7.1. Fifteen seconds after the onset of coronary artery occlusion $[K^+]_e$ started to increase from a control value of 3.9 ± 0.6 mmol l^{-1}. The rate of $[K^+]_e$ increase was maximal after 2 min of ischaemia, reaching a value

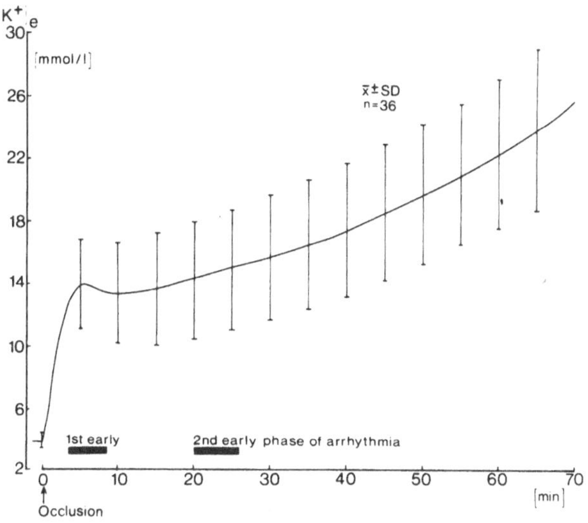

Figure 7.1 Mean values (± S.D.) of the increase of extracellular K^+ concentration ($[K^+]_e$) in the centre of the ischaemic pig myocardium.

of 3.2 mmol l^{-1} min^{-1}. After 3.5 ± 1 min $[K^+]_e$ had increased to 12.9 ± 2.9 mmol l^{-1} and the first early arrhythmic phase (phase 1a) began. Nineteen animals (55 per cent) developed VF during this phase. In the 17 surviving pigs $[K^+]_e$ further increased, reaching 14 ± 2.3 mmol l^{-1} after 5 min. Thereafter, $[K^+]_e$ slightly decreased and after 8.5 min of ischaemia normal sinus rhythm was again observed at a $[K^+]_e$ of 13.5 ± 3.1 mmol l^{-1}. During the following 10-12 min $[K^+]_e$ again increased slowly. After 20 ± 5 min (at a $[K^+]_e$ of 14.3 ± 3.6 mmol l^{-1}) the second early phase (phase 1b) of ventricular arrhythmias began, during which 12 pigs (33 per cent) developed VF. In five animals (14 per cent) which survived, phase 1b ended 26 ± 11 min after the onset of occlusion at a $[K^+]_e$ of 15.2 ± 3.8 mmol l^{-1}.

With regard to the time course of the rate of $[K^+]_e$ increase, three distinct

Table 7.1 Mean value (± S.D.) of the time course of post-ischaemia ventricular arrhythmias and ventricular fibrillation (VF) and corresponding increases of extracellular K^+ concentrations ($[K^+]_e$), extracellular H^+ activity ($[H^+]_e$) and the K^+ equilibrium potential (E_{K^+}) calculated from changes of $[K^+]_e$ and $[K^+]_i$

	Time (min) following acute coronary artery occlusion	$[K^+]_e$ (mmol l^{-1})	$[H^+]_e$ (nmol l^{-1})	E_{K^+} (mV)
Control value (n = 36)	0	3.9 ± 0.3	40 ± 11	−94
Onset of phase 1a	3.5 ± 1	12.9 ± 2.9	175 ± 110	−62
VF in phase 1a (n = 19)	4.5 ± 1	13.8 ± 2.8	250 ± 150	−58.6
End of phase 1a	8.5 ± 4	13.5 ± 3.1	420 ± 240	−59.7
Onset of phase 1b	20.0 ± 5	14.3 ± 3.6	1000 ± 250	−54.6
VF in phase 1b (n = 12)	25.0 ± 10	15.1 ± 3.6	1260 ± 360	−54.5
End of phase 1b (n = 5)	26.0 ± 11	15.2 ± 3.8	1320 ± 410	−54.4
Survivors	40	17.4 ± 4.3	2030 ± 360	−50.7

phases could be distinguished: (1) a phase of rapid $[K^+]_e$ increase which ended after 6 min of ischaemia; (2) a phase during which $[K^+]_e$ decreased slightly (this phase lasted for about 2 min); (3) a phase of further slow $[K^+]_e$ increase.

In contrast to the changing rate of $[K^+]_e$ increase with time, extracellular H^+ activity ($[H^+]_e$) increased at a nearly constant rate (50-60 nmol l^{-1} min^{-1}) during the first 60 min of ischaemia (figure 7.2 and 7.1). Thereafter the rate of $[H^+]_e$ increase became slower; 70 min after the onset of occlusion $[H^+]_e$ had increased

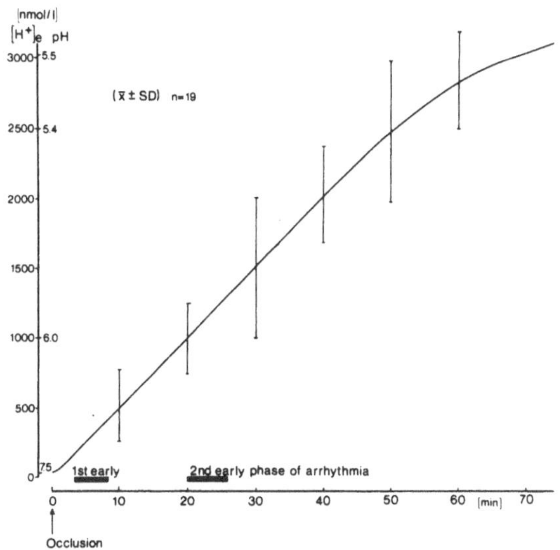

Figure 7.2 Mean values (± S.D.) of the increase of extracellular H^+ activity ($[H^+]_e$) in the centre of the ischaemic pig myocardium. Values taken from Hirche *et al.* (1980) with permission.

to about 3000 nmol l^{-1} (pH 5.6) in the centre of the infarcted zone (Hirche *et al.*, 1980). Soon after the onset of occlusion the ischaemic zone was clearly apparent as a sharply delineated cyanotic area which showed a characteristic ballooning effect during systole. This is because LAD occlusion in the pig causes a transmural infarction. The muscle mass of the ischaemic myocardium was 15 per cent (range 8-25 per cent) of the weight of both ventricles. Heart rate was 120 ± 20 beats min^{-1} before occlusion and increased by only 4 per cent 2 min after the onset of occlusion. Mean arterial blood pressure decreased by 7 per cent (from 80 ± 20 mmHg). Left ventricular dp/dt declined slightly (11 per cent) from 2150 ± 900 mmHg^{-1} s.

7.3 THE MEASUREMENT OF $[K^+]_e$ WITH ION-SENSITIVE ELECTRODES IN THE PIG AND DOG MYOCARDIA

A methodological problem in measurements with ion-selective electrodes in the ischaemic myocardium is the occurrence of DC potentials caused by the inhomogenous depolarisation of hypoxic myocardial cells. These DC potentials alter the standard potential E_0 of the Nernst equation and, since they are also measured by the ion-selective electrodes, they interfere with the signals caused by $[K^+]_e$ changes. The DC potential changes which were measured between the reference electrode outside the heart and the local reference electrodes on the epicardium reached a mean value of 2.5 mV after 5 min of ischaemia and a maximal value of 6 mV 15 min after the onset of occlusion, declining slowly thereafter. Since each $[K^+]_e$ recording was corrected for changes in the standard potential, the values in figure 7.1 represent true increases in $[K^+]_e$.

Other workers have measured $[K^+]_e$ increases in the ischaemic myocardium of pigs with miniature K^+-selective double-barrel electrodes constructed from PVC tubing and PVC-valinomycin matrix membranes (Hill *et al.*, 1978; Hill and Gettes 1980; Gettes and Hill, 1981). Two to five of these K^+ electrodes were inserted into the mid-myocardium of the left ventricular anterior free wall and 5-6 mm below the epicardial surface. An advantage of this type of electrode is the very small distance between the ion-selective and reference electrodes; interference of DC potentials is thus practically avoided. In these studies the increase in $[K^+]_e$ within the ischaemic myocardium also occurred in three phases; an initial rapid $[K^+]_e$ increase beginning within seconds of onset of ligation and lasting 5-15 min, a plateau phase that lasted approximately 15 min and a final phase of slowly rising $[K^+]_e$. Inhomogeneities in $[K^+]_e$ elevations were found between the centre and lateral margins of the mid-myocardial ischaemic zone, between the subendocardium and the subepicardium in the centre of the ischaemic zone and between closely spaced electrodes located in the mid-myocardial centre of the ischaemic zone. $[K^+]_e$ levels during the plateau phase and the maximal rate of $[K^+]_e$ increase were both somewhat lower than in our study (figure 7.1). Whether these differences are due to different types of K^+-selective electrodes used, to variations in anaesthesia or to other reasons is not known. Possibly the insertion of the PVC mini-electrodes causes some tissue damage and therefore measurements are performed in an artificially enlarged interstitial space, with larger diffusion distances for K^+ (see also discussion in Hirche *et al.*, 1980, and in Gettes and Hill, 1981). Nevertheless, both studies are consistent with respect to the time course and magnitude of $[K^+]_e$ rise in the centre of the ischaemic myocardium.

The observation of considerable inhomogeneities of $[K^+]_e$ increases in different layers of the ischaemic myocardium (Gettes and Hill, 1981) is somewhat in contrast to the finding that occlusion of the LAD in the pig heart results in a transmural infarct. Furthermore, no major transmural potential gradients were observed (Kleber *et al.*, 1978) in the ischaemic zone of isolated pig hearts after LAD occlusion.

$[K^+]_e$ measurements have also been performed in the ischaemic dog myocardium (Benzing *et al.*, 1972; Wiegand *et al.*, 1979; Hirche *et al.*, 1981b). Using a somewhat different type of K^+-selective surface electrode, a rapid increase of extracellular K^+ activity was observed ($[K^+]_e$ increased to 10 mmol l^{-1} within 5 min and to about 11.3 mmol l^{-1} after 10 min of ischaemia; Wiegand *et al.*, 1979). Following the initial 10 min of ischaemia no further increase was found. Using an activity coefficient of 0.746 $[K^+]_e$ values of 13.4 and 15.1 mmol l^{-1}

can be calculated. The time course and the extent of this $[K^+]_e$ increase is consistent with our recent results in dogs during severe ischaemia (Hirche *et al.*, 1981b). The fact that $[K^+]_e$ does not further increase after 10 min (in contrast to the pig) is probably due to the higher collateral flow (Howe *et al.*, 1968; Fedor *et al.*, 1978). Consistent with this explanation is the finding of a release of K^+ into coronary venous blood during LAD occlusion in dogs. This has never been observed in pigs (Hirche *et al.*, 1980).

The reason for the different rates of $[K^+]_e$ increase following coronary artery occlusion (figure 7.1) cannot be completely explained at present. It may be assumed that an energy deficit of the membranal Na^+-K^+ pump, and a change in membrane permeability to K^+ (see Hill and Gettes, 1980) play causal roles in the ischaemia-induced $[K^+]_e$ increase. In contrast to the changes in $[K^+]_e$, extracellular p_{CO_2} (Case *et al.*, 1979) and extracellular H^+ ($[H^+]_e$) (shown in figure 7.2 and table 7.1) exhibit almost linear rises during the first hour of ischaemia. The slight transient decrease of $[K^+]_e$ during phase 2 might be caused by a transient reactivation of the Na^+-K^+ pump induced by myocardial catecholamine release soon after the onset of ischaemia (see, for example, Hirche *et al.*, 1980). The changes in $[K^+]_e$ during the first two phases are rapidly reversed by release of the occlusion (Hirche *et al.*, 1979; Hill and Gettes, 1980) whilst the $[K^+]_e$ increase during the slowly rising phase becomes progressively irreversible with time (Hirche *et al.*, 1979), probably because of irreversible disturbances of the local microcirculation. The slowly rising phase seemingly corresponds to the phase of irreversible cell damage which has been shown to occur after 20 min of severe myocardial ischaemia in pigs (literature in Hill and Gettes, 1980).

7.4 CHANGES IN $[Na^+]_e$ AND IN H^+ FOLLOWING ACUTE CORONARY ARTERY OCCLUSION

Recently we have measured extracellular Na^+ concentrations ($[Na^+]_e$) with ion-selective surface electrodes and also the extracellular osmolality ($[Osm]_e$) of the ischaemic myocardium of the pig heart (Hirche *et al.*, 1981b). $[Na^+]_e$ rose from 140 to 160 mmol l^{-1} within the first 10 min of ischaemia, then decreased continuously to reach 120 mmol l^{-1} at 70 min. $[Osm]_e$ increased from 290 to 430 mosmol kg^{-1} after 40 min of ischaemia. Assuming that no H_2O diffused between non-ischaemic and ischaemic areas, the H_2O shift from ECS to ICS was calculated. This revealed a 35 per cent reduction in ECS and 13 per cent increase in ICS after 40 min of ischaemia. The increase in $[K^+]_e$ in our experiments is therefore mainly due to release of K^+ from ICS and the transient increase in $[Na^+]_e$ to a shrinkage of ECS. Intracellular K^+ and Na^+ concentrations ($[K^+]_i$), $[Na^+]_i$) were calculated from $[K^+]_e$ and $[Na^+]_e$ changes and the H_2O shift. $[K^+]_i$ decreased from 137 to 120 mmol l^{-1} and $[Na^+]_i$ increased from 15 to 33 mmol l^{-1} after 40 min of occlusion. K^+ equilibrium potential decreased from −94 mV at 40 min (see also table 7.1). Na^+ equilibrium potential fell from +60 mV to +38 mV after 40 min of ischaemia.

Consistent with these calculations, Kleber *et al.* (1978) observed a decrease of the transmembrane potential in isolated perfused pig hearts after 2.5 min of LAD occlusion. The resting membrane potential then decreased still further and the upstroke velocity, amplitude and action potential duration diminished. By 7 min resting membrane potential had decreased to −65 mV and cells in the centre of the ischaemic zone had become unresponsive. This magnitude of permanent depolarisation of the cell membrane in the ischaemic myocardium, and the corresponding transformation of the action potential from the fast response to the slow response type, is mainly due to the rapid increase of $[K^+]_e$ (Meesmann *et al.*, 1978; Opie *et al.*, 1979; Wiegand *et al.*, 1979).

At present there is only limited data in the literature on measurements with H^+-selective electrodes in the ischaemic myocardium (for example, Cobbe and Poole-Wilson, 1980; Hirche *et al.*, 1976, 1980), although $[pH]_e$ changes up to 1.2 pH units have been reported in dogs after fibrillation. A fall in $[pH]_e$ was apparent within 5 s of the onset of total ischaemia of the isolated interventricular septum of the rabbit heart. $[pH]_e$ fell continuously during ischaemia, the fall after 60 min being 1.41 units (Cobbe and Poole-Wilson, 1980). In our experiments $[H^+]_e$ increased in the centre of the ischaemic zone of pig hearts with an average rate of change of 50-60 nmol l^{-1} min^{-1} during the first 50-60 min of severe ischaemia, reaching about 3000 nmol l^{-1} (pH 5.52; Hirche *et al.*, 1980). Thereafter, $[H^+]_e$ further increased but at a slower rate. Thus the time course of the increase of $[H^+]_e$ (and also that of p_{CO_2}; Case *et al.*, 1979) of the ischaemic myocardium was quite different from that of the $[K^+]_e$ increase.

In our experiments no correlation could be observed between the increase of $[H^+]_e$ and the onset of ectopic activity or VF. Pig hearts undergo VF at widely varying $[H^+]_e$ values (between 50 and 3000 nmol l^{-1}). Therefore, we conclude that an increase in $[H^+]_e$ does not have a direct influence on the occurrence of post-ischaemic ventricular arrhythmias.

7.5 RELATIONSHIP OF $[K^+]_e$ AND NORADRENALINE RELEASE TO EARLY VENTRICULAR ARRHYTHMIAS

A regular finding in our experiments is that, following myocardial ischaemia, ventricular arrhythmias occur in two distinct phases, separated by an intermediate arrhythmia-free phase. Up to now no convincing explanation has been offered for this observation. Apart from the differing rates of $[K^+]_e$ increase, release of myocardial catecholamines may also be involved in this phenomenon (Gettes, 1974; Franz *et al.*, 1978; Hirche *et al.*, 1980, 1981a; Meesmann *et al.*, 1978; Opie *et al.*, 1979). A release of noradrenaline into the coronary sinus has been observed following LAD occlusion in pigs (Franz *et al.*, 1978; Hirche *et al.*, 1980, 1981a;

Zylka *et al.*, 1981). Since noradrenaline is released into coronary sinus blood after coronary occlusion, whereas coronary sinus K^+ levels were not elevated, one must assume that noradrenaline is released from the normally perfused left ventricle via stimulation of cardiac sympathetic reflex mechanisms (Staszewska-Barczak, 1971).

The following known arrhythmogenic actions of catecholamines are of special importance in connection with early post-ischaemia arrhythmias. Myocardial cells which have become inexcitable due to depolarisation by K^+ can be reactivated by the application of catecholamines (Antoni *et al.*, 1963), whilst stimulation of the cardiac sympathetic nerves decreases the ventricular fibrillation threshold (Gettes, 1974, and reviewed in chapters 8-10). These effects of released catecholamines during ischaemia suggest that the resultant electrical inhomogeneity of the heart is a precondition for the occurrence of arrhythmias due to re-entry mechanisms and abnormal automaticity. These might be caused by a combined effect of $[K^+]_e$ and of myocardial noradrenaline release (Gettes, 1974; Franz *et al.*, 1978; Meesmann *et al.*, 1978; Hirche *et al.*, 1980).

This view has received further support from recent investigations on the mode of antiarrhythmic action of lignocaine and prostacyclin (PGI_2), both of which significantly reduce the incidence of VF following LAD occlusion in the pig heart (Hirche *et al.*, 1981a; Zylka *et al.*, 1981). Following the administration of these substances prior to LAD occlusion, the $[K^+]_e$ increase in the ischaemic myocardium was less than under control conditions, and less noradrenaline was released into the coronary sinus. Fluorescence microscopic investigations of adrenergic nerve fibres within the ischaemic myocardium revealed a considerable reduction in catecholamines 3-4 min after LAD occlusion in control animals. However, in pigs treated with PGI_2 or lignocaine an increase in fluorescence intensity within the ischaemic myocardium was observed.

ACKNOWLEDGEMENT

Supported by Deutsche Forschungsgemeinschaft, SFB 68 A 7.

REFERENCES

Antoni, H., Henkel, K. and Fleckenstein, A. (1963). Die Restitution der automatischen Erregungsbilding in Kalium-gelähmten Schrittmacher-Geweben durch Adrenalin. *Pflügers Arch. ges. Physiol.*, 277, 633-49

Benzing, H., Strohm, M. and Gebert, G. (1972). The effect of local ischaemia on the ionic activity of dog myocardial interstitium. In *Vascular Smooth Muscle* (ed. E. Betz), Springer Verlag, Berlin, pp. 172-4

Bös, L., Franz, Chr. and Hirche, Hj. (1978). Cardiac arrhythmia and increase of local myocardial extracellular K^+ activity in pigs. *J. Physiol., Lond.*, **284**, 88P

Braasch, W., Gudbjarnason, S., Puri, P., Ravens, K. G. and Bing, R. J. (1968). Early changes in energy metabolism in the myocardium following acute coronary artery occlusion in anaesthetized dogs. *Circulation Res.*, **23**, 429-38

Case, R. B., Felix, A. and Castellana, F. S. (1979). Rate of rise of myocardial p_{CO_2} during early myocardial ischaemia in the dog. *Circulation Res.*, **45**, 324-30

Cherbakoff, A., Toyama, S. and Hamilton, W. F. (1957). Relation between coronary sinus plasma potassium and cardiac arrhythmia. *Circulation Res.*, **5**, 517-21

Cherry, G. and Myers, M. B. (1970). The relationship to ventricular fibrillation of early tissue sodium and potassium shifts and coronary vein potassium levels in experimental myocardial infarction. *J. thorac. cardiovasc. Surg.*, **61**, 587-98

Cobbe, S. M. and Poole-Wilson, P. A. (1980). The time of onset and severity of acidosis in myocardial ischaemia. *J. molec. cell. Cardiol.*, **12**, 745-60

Downey, H. F. and Kirk, E. S. (1968). Coronary lymph: specific activities in interstitial fluid during uptake of ^{42}K. *Am. J. Physiol.*, **215**, 1177-82

Ettinger, P. O., Regan, T. J., Oldewurtel, H. A. and Khan, M. I. (1973). Ventricular conduction delay and arrhythmias during regional hyperkalaemia in the dog. *Circulation Res.*, **33**, 521-31

Fedor, J. M., McIntosh, D. M., Rembert, J. C. and Greenfield, J. C. (1978). Coronary and transmural myocardial blood flow response in awake pigs. *Am. J. Physiol.*, **235**, H435-44

Franz, Chr., Lang, R., Bös, L., Schramm, M., Bissig, R. and Hirche, Hj. (1978). The release of K^+ and noradrenaline as cause of arrhythmia and ventricular fibrillation following myocardial ischemia in pigs. *Pflügers Arch. ges. Physiol.*, **377**, Suppl. R3

Gettes, L. S. (1974). Electrophysiologic basis of arrhythmias in acute myocardial ischemia. In *Modern Trends in Cardiology*, Vol. 3 (ed. M. F. Oliver), London, Butterworth, pp. 219-46

Gettes, L. S. and Hill, J. L. (1981). The use of K^+ sensitive electrodes to gain an understanding of myocardial ischemia. In *Progress in Enzyme and Ion-selective Electrodes* (ed. D. W. Lübbers, H. Acker, R. P. Buck, G. Eisenmann, M. Kessler and W. Simon), Springer Verlag, Berlin, pp. 171-8

Gülker, H., Krämer, B., Stephan, K. and Meesmann, W. (1977). Changes in ventricular fibrillation threshold during repeated short-term coronary occlusion and release. *Basic Res. Cardiol.*, **72**, 547-62

Haase, M. and Schiller, U. (1969). Zur zeitlichen Parallelität zwischen der Aktivität ektopischer Schrittmacher und dem Eintritt von Kammerflimmern nach Ligatur eines Hauptkoronarastes beim Hund. *Acta biol. med. germ.*, **23**, 413-22

Harris, A. S. (1950). Delayed development of ventricular ectopic rhythm following experimental coronary occlusion. *Circulation*, **1**, 1318-28

Harris, A. S., Toth, L. A. and Hoey, T. E. (1958). Arrhythmic and antiarrhythmic effects of sodium, potassium and calcium salts and of glucose injected into coronary arteries of infarcted and normal hearts. *Circulation Res.*, **6**, 570-9

Hill, J. L. and Gettes, L. S. (1980). Effect of acute coronary artery occlusion on local myocardial extracellular K^+ activity in swine. *Circulation*, **61**, 768-78

Hill, J. L., Gettes, L. S., Lynch, M. R. and Hebert, N. C. (1978). Flexible valinomycin electrodes for on-line determination of intravascular and myocardial K^+. *Am. J. Physiol.*, **235**, H455-9

Hirche, Hj., Gaehtgens, P., Hagemann, H., Kebbel, U., Kleine, H.-J., Schramm, M. and Schumacher, E. (1976). Untersuchungen über die Acidose im ischämischen Hundemyokard mit H^+-sensitiven Minielektroden. *Verh. dt. Ges. Kreislaufforsch.*, **42**, 311-5

Hirche, Hj., Franz, Chr. and Bös, L. (1979). Ion-selective electrodes in cardiac ischemia. In *Heart and Brain Infarct, II* (ed. K. J. Zülch, W. Kaufmann, K. A. Hossmann and V. Hossman), Springer Verlag, Berlin, pp. 104-11

Hirche, Hj., Franz, Chr., Bös, L., Bissig, R., Lang, R. and Schramm, M. (1980). Myocardial extracellular K^+ and H^+ increase and noradrenaline release as possible cause of early arrhythmias following acute coronary artery occlusion in pigs. *J. molec. cell. Cardiol.*, **12**, 579-93

Hirche, Hj., Addicks, K., Deutsch, H. J., Friedrich, R., Griebenow, R., McDonald, F. M. and Zylka, V. (1981a). The effect of lignocaine on the release of K^+ and of noradrenaline from ischemic pig heart. *Pflügers Arch. ges. Physiol.*, **389**, Suppl. R5

Hirche, Hj., Bissig, R., Friedrich, R., Kebbel, U. and Zylka, V. (1981b). Measurement of myocardial extracellular Na^+, K^+, Ca^{2+}, and H^+ using ion-selective electrodes during ischemia. In *Progress in Enzyme and Ion-selective Electrodes* (ed. D. W. Lübbers, H. Acker, R. P. Buck, G. Eisenmann, M. Kessler and W. Simon), Springer Verlag, Berlin, pp. 164-70

Hirche, Hj., Friedrich, R. and Kebbel, U. (1981c). Potassium loss from ischemic myocardium. In *Experimental Myocardial Ischemia and Infarction* (ed. W. Schaper), Marcel Dekker, New York, in press

Holland, R. P. and Brooks, H. (1975). Precordial and epicardial surface potentials during myocardial ischemia in the pig. A theoretical and experimental analysis of the QT and ST segments. *Circulation Res.*, **37**, 471-9

Howe, B. B., Fehn, P. A. and Pensinger, R. R. (1968). Comparative anatomical studies of the coronary arteries of canine and porcine hearts. *Acta anat., Basel*, **71**, 13-21

Kleber, A. G., Janse, M. J., Capelle, F. J. L. van and Durrer, D. (1978). Mechanism and time course of S-T and T-Q segment changes during acute regional myocardial ischemia in the pig heart determined by extracellular and intracellular recordings. *Circulation Res.*, **42**, 603-13

Lang, R., Franz, C., Hirche, Hj. and Kaufmann, W. (1979). Myokardiales Noradrenalin und prähospitale Infarktletalität. *Verh. dt. Ges. inn. Med.*, **85**, 865-7

Marshall, R. J. and Parratt, J. R. (1975). Antiarrhythmic haemodynamic and metabolic effects of 3α-amino-5α-androstan-2β-ol-17-one hydrochloride in greyhounds following acute coronary artery ligation. *Br. J. Pharmac.*, **55**, 359-68

Meesmann, W., Weigand, V., Menken, U., Komhard, W. and Rehwald, U. (1978). Early mortality due to ventricular fibrillation and the vulnerability of the heart following acute experimental coronary occlusion. Possible mechanism and pharmacological prophylaxis. In *The Arterial System. Dynamics, Control, Theory and Regulation* (ed. R. D. Bauer and R. Busse), Springer Verlag, Berlin, pp. 275-84

Opie, L. H., Nathan, R. and Lübbe, W. F. (1979). Biomedical aspects of arrhythmogenesis and ventricular fibrillation. *Am. J. Cardiol.*, **43**, 131-48

Staszewska-Barczak, J. (1971). The reflex stimulation of catecholamine secretion during the acute stage of myocardial infarction in the dog. *Clin. Sci.*, **41**, 419-39

Thomas, M., Shulman, G. and Opie, L. (1970). Arteriovenous potassium changes and ventricular arrhythmia after coronary artery occlusion. *Cardiovasc. Res.*, **4**, 327-33

Wiegand, V., Güggi, M., Meesmann, W., Kessler, M. and Greitschus, F. (1979) Extracellular potassium activity changes in the canine myocardium after acute coronary occlusion and the influence of β-blockade. *Cardiovasc. Res.*, **13**, 297-302

Zylka, V., Addicks, K., Deutsch, H. J., Friedrich, R., Griebenow, R. and Hirche, Hj. (1981). The antiarrhythmic effect of prostacyclin (PGI_2) in severe myocardial ischemia of pig heart. *Pflügers Arch.*, **389**, Suppl. R1.

8

Myocardial Catecholamine Release in Acute Myocardial Ischaemia; Relationship to Cardiac Arrhythmias

R. A. Riemersma

8.1 INTRODUCTION

More than 50 per cent of all deaths from acute myocardial infarction occur within the first 2 h of the onset of symptoms and often before medical help can be activated (Armstrong *et al.*, 1972). The cause of this sudden death is generally considered to be ventricular fibrillation. There is abundant clinical evidence of enhanced sympathetic nervous activity during myocardial infarction (Gazes *et al.*, 1959; Valori *et al.*, 1967; Jewitt *et al.*, 1969, Siggers *et al.*, 1971; Webb *et al.*, 1972; Videbaek *et al.*, 1972; Ceremuzynski *et al.*, 1974; Mueller and Ayres, 1978). Further, plasma catecholamine levels are raised at the earliest measurements after the onset of symptoms and have been correlated with clinical status (Strange *et al.*, 1974; Nadeau and de Champlain, 1979) and with the occurrence of arrhythmias. In general, high plasma noradrenaline concentrations (mainly derived from sympathetic neurones) are found during acute myocardial infarction whereas raised adrenaline levels, reflexly secreted from the adrenal medulla (Ceremuzynski *et al.*, 1969; Staszewska-Barczak, 1971) occur in patients with shock but who do not develop ventricular fibrillation (Mueller and Ayres, 1978). It is the aim of this chapter to re-examine the effects of experimental acute myocardial ischaemia on myocardial noradrenaline metabolism in relation to the development of early serious ventricular arrhythmias.

8.2 MYOCARDIAL CATECHOLAMINE METABOLISM

It is not the purpose of this article to review comprehensively the normal metabolism of myocardial catecholamines; however, for the sake of clarity a brief summary is given. In mammals the main catecholamine found in the post-ganglionic sympathetic nerve fibres is noradrenaline (NA); only small quantities of adrenaline are normally present. Noradrenaline is stored complexed to ATP in the nerve endings inside electron-dense granules. The density of this noradrenergic innervation varies within the myocardium and more fibres can be traced to the atria and specialised conduction system than to the ventricles. These differences are reflected in local myocardial noradrenaline levels, which are higher in the atria than in the ventricles. The noradrenergic nerve fibres originate from the left and the right stellate ganglia. Precise anatomical and physiological studies show that specific fibres innervate small discrete parts of the myocardium (Randall, 1977). The right ventricle and the right atrium are innervated by fibres originating predominately from the right stellate ganglion, whilst the left ventricular wall is mainly innervated from the left side. The effect of electrical stimulation of the cardiac nerves is usually examined using electrophysiological or haemodynamic end points. However, noradrenaline concentrations in coronary venous effluent do exceed those of arterial blood on nerve stimulation (Yamaguchi *et al.*, 1975; R. A. Riemersma and J. C. Forfar, unpublished) although this has not been confirmed in another study (Levy and Blattberg, 1978). Noradrenaline release is inhibited by a wide range of physiologically occurring compounds, such as acetylcholine, adenosine, ATP, certain prostaglandins and also by drugs stimulating α-adrenoceptors; release may be enhanced by β-adrenoceptor stimulation. These effects are considered to be mediated by presynaptic receptors (recently reviewed in detail by Paton, 1979; Langer, 1980). However, the physiological importance and precise mechanisms of presynaptic control remain to be established. Noradrenaline released at these post-ganglionic sympathetic nerve terminals is removed by three main mechanisms. The first, re-uptake into the nerve terminals (re-uptake 1) is quantitatively the most important and has been extensively examined by Iversen (1977). As much as 80–90 per cent of noradrenaline released during sympathetic nerve stimulation may be removed from the synaptic cleft by this high affinity and saturable enzymatic process, which is linked to Na^+, K^+-ATPase. Noradrenaline is then stored in the synaptic vesicles, from which it can be released later. Secondly, some intraneuronal noradrenaline is inactivated by monoamine oxidase, whilst that taken up by extraneuronal tissue is methylated to normetanephrine by catechol-*O*-methyltransferase. Thirdly, what remains of the released noradrenaline 'overflows' into the venous effluent. The main features of catecholamine metabolism are summarised in figure 8.1.

8.3 ARRHYTHMOGENIC EFFECTS OF CATECHOLAMINES

The arrhythmogenic effects of catecholamines have been demonstrated under a wide variety of conditions such as following systemic administration in animals, especially in the presence of acute myocardial ischaemia (Maling and Moran, 1957;

Harris *et al.*, 1971; Kurien *et al.*, 1971) and of certain anaesthetics. Intramyocardial infusions have the same effect (Podzuweit, chapter 11 of this volume). These arrhythmias are prevented, for example, by the prior administration of β-adrenoceptor blocking drugs (Fitzgerald, this volume, chapter 16). However, in contrast to the overwhelming evidence for the arrhythmogenic effects of exogenous catecholamines, the evidence incriminating local myocardial noradrenaline with arrhythmias during acute myocardial ischaemia is largely indirect. For example, chronic cardiac sympathetic denervation leads to depletion of myocardial noradrenaline stores (Schaal *et al.*, 1969; Ebert *et al.*, 1968) and markedly protects against the development of ventricular fibrillation during early ischaemia. In contrast, acute denervation

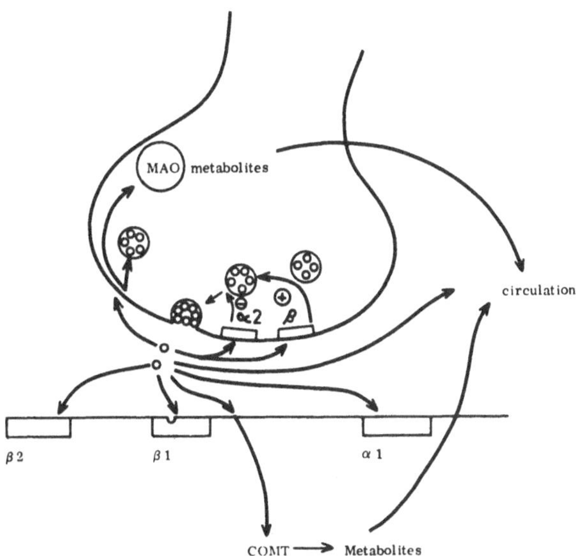

Figure 8.1 Summary of the events at the sympathetic (post-ganglionic) synapse. For details see text. Only catecholamine receptors are indicated.

(which does not deplete myocardial noradrenaline stores) offers no protection (Ebert *et al.*, 1968). Also, left unilateral stellectomy profoundly reduces the incidence of cardiac arrhythmias during myocardial ischaemia (Schwartz *et al.*, 1976), whereas right stellectomy has the opposite effect; stimulation of the stellate ganglion markedly increases the incidence of serious ventricular arrhythmias, whereas cooling has the opposite effect. From the results of these studies it has been suggested that it is the imbalance in sympathetic nervous activity to the myocardium which is the crucial factor; this may have a clinical analogy in the long Q–T syndrome (Schwartz *et al.*, 1975).

8.4 NORADRENALINE RELEASE DURING EARLY MYOCARDIAL ISCHAEMIA

Studies examining the effect of coronary occlusion on catecholamine release have been severely hampered by analytical problems and many methods in use lack both specificity and sensitivity. On the other hand, measurements of tissue levels of noradrenaline have not suffered the same analytical difficulties as those for plasma. The noradrenaline content of the ischaemic myocardium decreases during the first few hours after the onset of ischaemia at a rate of approximately 10 per cent h^{-1} or 0.1 $\mu g\ g^{-1}\ h^{-1}$ (Serrano *et al.*, 1971). Slightly lower rates (3-4 per cent h^{-1}) can be calculated from results given in another study (Mathes and Gudbjarnason, 1971). It is therefore doubtful whether decreased myocardial noradrenaline levels would be demonstrated as early as 30 min after the onset of ischaemia (Didier *et al.*, 1980). After 4 days, myocardial noradrenaline levels become immeasurable in infarcted tissue and remain so thereafter. These findings are consistent with the view that the postganglionic sympathetic nerve terminals are destroyed in the ischaemic myocardium and that this may lead to 'denervation' hypersensitivity (Cha *et al.*, 1970). In the non-infarcted myocardium noradrenaline levels also decrease, although rather more slowly and transiently, reaching a minimum at 12 days; levels are restored to normal at 6 weeks. These studies cannot, of course, provide the answer to the important question under discussion, which is whether enhanced local release of myocardial noradrenaline is the trigger for the early, serious ventricular arrhythmias which are a consequence of acute myocardial ischaemia. Indeed, despite using a radioenzymatic method for the continuous monitoring of noradrenaline in local venous blood draining the ischaemic myocardium, no good evidence has been produced to demonstrate noradrenaline overflow at a time when serious ventricular arrhythmias, such as ventricular tachycardia and fibrillation, occur (see figure 8.2). These findings are similar to those of Marshall and Parratt (1980) and of McGrath *et al.* (1981). They seemingly contradict the earlier observations of Wollenberger's group (Shahab *et al.*, 1972), although a close examination of their data reveals that, in this study using isolated hearts, noradrenaline output from the heart occurred mainly during the reflow (reperfusion) phase and not during occlusion. On the other hand, increased outflow of noradrenaline from the non-ischaemic myocardium has been observed at the time of onset of serious ventricular arrhythmias (10 min after coronary artery ligation) in the pig (Hirche *et al.*, 1980), although it is not clear from this study whether noradrenaline release was related to the development of serious ventricular arrhythmias.

Interpretation of the significance of local venous noradrenaline levels is difficult. Normally, the major fate of released noradrenaline is neuronal re-uptake (Iversen, 1977) and an examination of arteriovenous differences of L-[^{3}H] noradrenaline across the ischaemic and non-ischaemic myocardium shows that acute ischaemia does not inhibit this process (R. A. Riemersma and J. C. Forfar, unpublished observations); it may indeed be accelerated (Preda *et al.*, 1975). In our hands partial (30 per cent) inhibition of neuronal re-uptake using viloxazine did not unmask

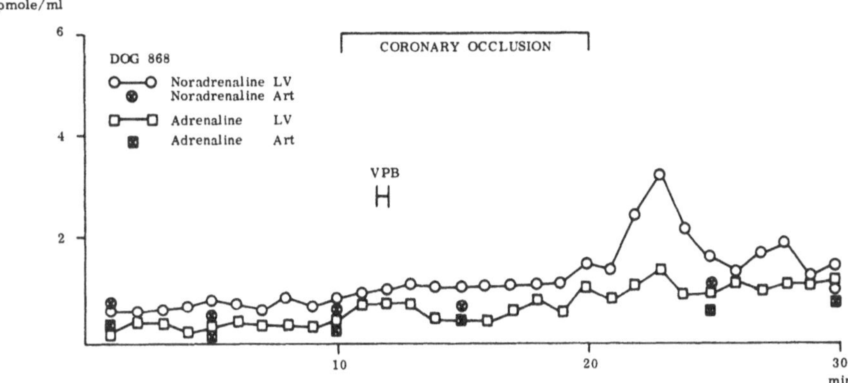

Figure 8.2 An example, in an anaesthetised, open-chest dog, of the effect of acute ligation of the left anterior descending coronary artery on arteriovenous differences of noradrenaline and adrenaline across the ischaemic myocardium. A local venous (LV) catheter was inserted in the vein draining the myocardium supplied by the occluded artery and the continuous withdrawal of venous blood allowed for the analysis of noradrenaline, adrenaline and lactate in blood draining both non-ischaemic (not shown) and ischaemic regions of the left ventricular wall. Despite the occurrence of ventricular premature beats (VPB), no marked overflow of noradrenaline was observed during ischaemia, although there was some evidence of release during the reperfusion phase.

significant noradrenaline overflow into either the ischaemic or non-ischaemic effluent (Riemersma and Forfar, 1981). It would be of interest to repeat such studies with more effective neuronal uptake blocking agents such as desmethylimipramine, although our present view is that it is unlikely that during *early* myocardial ischaemia (when most serious ventricular arrhythmias occur) inhibition of neuronal re-uptake is of much importance. Later (at 60 min of ischaemia) it clearly is important (Schomig *et al.*, 1980).

Thus, most studies have failed to demonstrate a marked overflow of myocardial noradrenaline into the local venous blood draining the ischaemic area at the time of development of serious ventricular arrhythmias. Indeed one study has clearly dissociated local coronary venous noradrenaline or adrenaline levels with the incidence of ventricular fibrillation (see Parratt, 1980). This failure cannot be ascribed to increased inactivation of noradrenaline by deamination and *O*-methylation since identical results have been obtained when the overflow was followed of [^{3}H]noradrenaline plus ^{3}H-labelled metabolites from myocardium prelabelled with [^{3}H]NA (Riemersma and Forfar, 1981; Rochette *et al.*, 1980; Schömig *et al.*, 1980).

This lack of noradrenaline overflow should not be interpreted as indicating that myocardial noradrenaline is not released from the nerve terminals and that it does not stimulate adrenoceptors. Catecholamine-mediated metabolic and electrophysiological effects during acute ischaemia support the view that noradrenaline is indeed released. To date there is no compelling evidence to incriminate enhanced responsiveness at the level of the myocardial adrenoceptor, or of the resultant intracellular consequences.

8.5 MECHANISMS OF NORADRENALINE RELEASE DURING ACUTE ISCHAEMIA

It is widely assumed that myocardial noradrenaline is reflexly released from the efferent sympathetic nerve terminals. Enhanced sympathetic activity has been observed during coronary occlusion in the dog (Malliani *et al.*, 1969; Karlsberg *et al.*, 1979) and in the cat (Brown, 1967; Thoren, 1972). The enhanced contractile and metabolic activity observed in the non-ischaemic myocardium is also reflex in origin (Pashkow *et al.*, 1977). However, no reflex activation of peripheral sympathetic nerves has been demonstrated (Levy and Frankel, 1953; Wegria *et al.*, 1954).

Inhibition of cardiac sympathetic drive after coronary artery ligation has also been observed (Constantin, 1963; Feola *et al.*, 1977). This has been claimed to be the mechanism for the reduced haemodynamic response to stellate ganglion stimulation during myocardial ischaemia (Martins *et al.*, 1980). The afferent limb of this reflex pathway may be vagal afferent fibres (Thoren, 1972).

Whether noradrenaline is directly released from synaptic vesicles by the high extracellular K^+ concentrations found during acute myocardial ischaemia (Hirche *et al.*, 1980) remains to be established but is discussed further in chapter 10. The effects of K^+ on noradrenaline release induced by sympathetic nerve stimulation in other tissues is concentration dependent. At moderately elevated K^+ concentrations (15 mM 1^{-1}) noradrenaline release is inhibited, whilst at high concentrations it is enhanced (Lorenz and Vanhoutte, 1975; Verhaeghe *et al.*, 1977). The effect of noradrenaline on K^+ release is further complicated by the observation that noradrenaline administered in non-pressor doses can *prevent* ischaemia-induced K^+ release (Regan *et al.*, 1970; Hirche *et al.*, 1980). Further work is clearly indicated, particularly on the effect of Ca^{2+} accumulation on noradrenaline release during ischaemia (Flear *et al.*, 1976).

Myocardial acidosis, which develops soon after myocardial ischaemia (Opie *et al.*, 1975; Williamson *et al.*, 1977) may well inhibit noradrenaline release (Puig and Kirpekar, 1971) and neuronal re-uptake (Karpati *et al.*, 1974) and may also interfere with the storage of noradrenaline in the synaptic vesicles (Peach *et al.*, 1970). In the light of these complex interrelationships, the effect of ischaemia on myocardial pH and on noradrenaline release, inactivation and receptor stimulation cannot be easily predicted.

The effect of changes in myocardial metabolism during ischaemia on noradrenaline release also deserves more attention. There is evidence that high concentrations of free fatty acids (in the absence of glucose) may enhance noradrenaline loss during the first 30 min after occlusion, particularly from the ischaemic area (Didier *et al.*, 1980, in a rat isolated heart model). This is presumably due to the Ca^{2+}-ionophoretic property of free fatty acids stimulating noradrenaline release (Stamm and Hulsmann, 1978). This was associated with loss of contractile efficiency, exaggerated enzyme release and a higher incidence of serious ventricular arrhythmias, effects characteristic of adrenoceptor stimulation (Herbacynska-Cedro, 1970; Mjøs, 1973; Waldenstrom *et al.*, 1978). Interestingly, myocardial [^{3}H]noradrenaline was not released following coronary artery ligation in a preparation devoid of arrhythmias (Rochette *et al.*, 1980).

The possible modulation of noradrenaline release by physiologically occurring substances (such as prostaglandins and adenosine) and by drugs has been extensively reviewed (Bevan, 1978; Malik, 1978; Shepherd *et al.*, 1978; Vanhoutte, 1978; Paton, 1979; Langer, 1980) but the physiological importance of these mechanisms has not been established in normal myocardial tissue, let alone during ischaemia. These recent developments will stimulate further research in the field relating adrenergic mechanisms to cardiac arrhythmias. For example, presynaptic control of noradrenaline release has the theoretical advantage over β-blockade in that it does not lead to unopposed α-adrenoceptor stimulation (Sheridan, this volume, chapter 17).

Prostaglandins prevent excessive stimulation of adrenoceptors by noradrenaline mainly by reducing release (Malik, 1978). Indomethacin, which inhibits prostaglandin synthesis, increases myocardial ischaemic injury (Jugdutt *et al.*, 1978) and the incidence of arrhythmias. Aspirin and related drugs have the opposite effect and reduce both myocardial ischaemic injury (Vik-Mo and Mjøs, 1977) and the incidence of serious ventricular arrhythmias (Coker *et al.*, 1981). Whether this difference is due to a more specific effect of thromboxane on ischaemia-induced noradrenaline release remains to be established.

The importance of the interrelationship of vagal activity and sympathetic activity is well recognised and aspects of this in relation to arrhythmias have been discussed (Corr and Gillis, 1978). The importance of this parasympathetic activity depends on the species, anaesthesia and site of coronary artery ligation, as well as on prevailing sympathetic activity. In the cat, which often exhibits enhanced vagal tone after coronary ligation, vagotomy or atropine administration increase the incidence of ventricular fibrillation (Corr and Gillis, 1974) independently of heart rate changes. Unfortunately noradrenaline release was not measured in this study.

Finally, it is possible that metabolites and ions accummulating during ischaemia might modify noradrenaline release. The presynaptic effects of adenosine, K^+ and H^+ (see above) are of particular interest in this respect (see also chapter 10).

8.6 POSSIBLE MECHANISMS THROUGH WHICH NORADRENALINE INDUCES ARRHYTHMIAS

The mechanism of the initiation and exacerbation of early ventricular arrhythmias by *myocardial* noradrenaline is not completely understood. Increased myocardial cyclic AMP (cAMP) levels (rather than enhanced catecholamine β-receptor stimulation) has been proposed as the initiating event leading to arrhythmias (Podzuweit *et al.*, 1976, reviewed in chapter 11). Indeed, increased myocardial cAMP levels have been observed following acute coronary occlusion and *before* the development of ventricular tachycardia and fibrillation (Podzuweit *et al.*, 1978; Corr *et al.*,

1978). This may be due to enhanced adenylate cyclase activation, reduced breakdown by phosphodiesterase, or both. Intramyocardial infusions of noradrenaline are highly arrhythmogenic (chapter 11 of this volume). The question whether cAMP is an independent arrhythmogenic mediator, rather than an accepted second messenger, can only be answered by possible dissociation of β-receptor stimulation from the ischaemia-induced rise in cAMP.

Stimulation of α-adrenoceptors is arrhythmogenic in the cat (Sheridan *et al.*, 1979, and reviewed in chapter 17 of this book), and it has been proposed that the proportional stimulation of α- and β-adrenoceptors is a crucial factor in the genesis of ventricular fibrillation (Lehr *et al.*, 1980).

The detrimental effects of released myocardial noradrenaline could be due to enhanced Ca^{2+} flux, leading to Ca^{2+}-dependent slow potentials, which are important in creating zones with delayed conduction and re-entrant circuits. Although Ca^{2+}-mediated electrophysiological effects are important for the genesis of serious ventricular arrhythmias, an effect on metabolism, for example, on lipolysis and glycogenolysis, cannot be excluded. Although Ca^{2+} loading of mitochondria during ischaemia has been well documented (Kloner *et al.*, 1974), the temporal relationships between Ca^{2+} accumulation, effects on metabolism and ventricular arrhythmias have not been examined.

In experimental studies β-adrenoceptor blockade prevents serious arrhythmias (reviewed by Fitzgerald, in chapter 16), possibly and at least partly by reducing ischaemic injury (Maroko *et al.*, 1971; Serrano *et al.*, 1971; Becker *et al.*, 1975). Noradrenaline release is under presynaptic control and high doses of propranolol and oxprenolol, but not practolol, reduce the amount of noradrenaline released from the well oxygenated dog heart during stellate ganglion stimulation (Nayler and Carson, 1973).

The relevance of these observations for the ischaemic heart remain to be established. They may be of particular importance since both α- and β-adrenoceptor responsiveness alters during acute myocardial ischaemia, at least at postsynaptic level (Moore and Parratt, 1973; Gorman and Sparks, 1980).

β-Adrenoceptor blockade may also modify myocardial ischaemia by effects on metabolism. Thus, myocardial oxygen requirements are higher when plasma free fatty acids, rather than glucose, are utilised as the main substrates and plasma free fatty acid concentrations are certainly lowered after β-blockade. As a result, fatty acid utilisation by the ischaemic heart is diminished (Becker *et al.*, 1975; Riemersma, 1979), with variable effects on glucose utilisation. The reasons for this variability are not known but they may well be related to the residual regional myocardial blood flow, which is known to modify ischaemic myocardial glucose utilisation (Rovetto and Neely, 1977). Oxygen wasting by raised plasma free fatty acid concentrations (by uncoupling ischaemic mitochondrial oxidative phosphorylation) has also been proposed as a mechanism for the induction of arrhythmias (Kurien and Oliver, 1970). This direct effect of raised plasma-free fatty acids on the ischaemic myocardium may be enhanced by catecholamines (Kjekshus *et al.*, 1980). There is also biochemical evidence suggesting enhanced lipolysis of triglycerides in conjunction with energy-requiring resynthesis in the ischaemic heart. Such a cycle would waste the limited ATP resources further (Riemersma, 1979) and could also explain oxygen wastage. The advantage of this hypothesis is that it is not dependent on extrapolation of *in vitro* experiments often performed with high and possibly unphysiological free fatty acid to protein ratios. However, whether altered substrate myocardial metabolism plays an important role in the genesis of serious ventricular arrhythmias still remains to be established (Opie, 1975; Oliver, 1972).

ACKNOWLEDGEMENTS

I am grateful for the support and encouragement of Professor M. F. Oliver and Drs J. C. Forfar and D. C. Russell, and for the secretarial assistance of J. E. Bell.

REFERENCES

Armstrong, A., Duncan, B., Oliver, M. F., Julian, D. G., Donald, K. W., Fulton, M., Lutz, W. and Morrison, S. L. (1972). Natural history of acute coronary heart attacks. A community study. *Br. Heart J.*, **34**, 67-80

Becker, L. C., Ferreira, R. and Thomas, M. (1975). Effect of propranolol and isoprenaline on regional left ventricular blood flow in experimental myocardial ischaemia. *Cardiovasc. Res.*, **9**, 178-86

Bevan, J. A. (1978). Norepinephrine and the presynaptic control of adrenergic transmitter release. *Fedn Proc. Fedn Am. Socs exp. Biol.*, **37**, 187-90

Brown, A. M. (1967). Excitation of afferent cardiac sympathetic nerve fibres during myocardial ischaemia. *J. Physiol., Lond.*, **190**, 35-53

Ceremuzynski, L., Kuch, J., Lawecki, J. and Markiewicz, L. (1974). Adrenergic activity and immunoreactive insulin levels in relation to the clinical course of myocardial infarction. *Cor Vasa*, **16**, 153-61

Ceremuzynski, L., Staszewska-Barczak, J. and Herbaczynska-Cedro, K. (1969). Cardiac rhythm disturbances and the release of catecholamines after acute coronary occlusion in dogs. *Cardiovasc. Res.*, **3**, 190-7

Cha, H. D., Meyers, V. W., Kramar, J. L. and Grinnell, E. H. (1970). Post-infarction myocardial hypersensitivity to naturally occurring humoral agents in dogs. *Am. J. med. Sci.*, **160**, 95-104

Coker, S. J., Ledingham, I. McA., Parratt, J. R. and Zeitlin, I. J. (1981). Aspirin inhibits the early myocardial release of thromboxane B_2 and ventricular ectopic activity following coronary artery occlusion in dogs. *Br. J. Pharmac.*, **72**, 593-5

Constantin, L. (1963). Extracardiac factors contributing to hypotension during coronary occlusion. *Am. J. Cardiol.*, **11**, 205-17

Corr, P. B. and Gillis, R. A. (1974). Role of the vagus nerve in the cardiovascular changes induced by coronary occlusion. *Circulation*, **49**, 86-97

Corr, P. B. and Gillis, R. A. (1978). Autonomic neural influences on the dysrhythmias resulting from myocardial infarction. *Circulation Res.*, **43**, 1-9

Corr, P. B., Witkowski, F. X. and Sobel, B. E. (1978). Mechanisms contributing to malignant dysrhythmias induced by ischemia in the cat. *J. clin. Invest.*, **61**, 109-19

Didier, J. P., Moreau, D. and Opie, L. H. (1980). Effects of glucose and of fatty acids on rhythm, enzyme release and oxygen uptake in isolated perfused working rat heart with coronary artery ligation. *J. molec. cell. Cardiol.*, **12**, 1191-206

Ebert, P. A., Allgood, R. J. and Sabiston, D. C. (1968). The antiarrhythmic effects of cardiac denervation. *Ann. Surg.*, **168**, 728-35

Feola, M., Arbel, E. R. and Glick, G. (1977). Attenuation of cardiac sympathetic drive in experimental myocardial ischemia in dogs. *Am. Heart J.*, **93**, 82-8

Flear, C. T. G., Riemersma, R. A., Nandra, A., Nandra, G. and Talbot, R. (1976). Changes in myocardial water and solutes after ischaemia. *Rec. Adv. Studies cardiovasc. Struct. Metab.*, 7, 297-306

Gazes, P. C., Richardson, J. A. and Woods, E. F. (1959). Plasma catecholamine concentrations in myocardial infarction and angina pectoris. *Circulation*, **19**, 657-61

Gorman, M. W. and Sparks, H. V. (1980). Norepinephrine reduces vascular resistance in ischemic myocardium. *Fedn Proc. Fedn Am. Socs exp. Biol.*, **39**, 531

Harris, A. S., Otero, I. I. and Bocage, A. J. (1971). The induction of arrhythmias by sympathetic activity before and after occlusion of a coronary artery in the canine heart. *J. Electrocardiol.*, **4**, 34-43

Herbaczynska-Cedro, K. (1970). The influence of adrenaline secretion on the enzymes in the heart muscle after acute coronary occlusion in dogs. *Cardiovasc. Res.*, **4**, 168-75

Hirche, Hj., Franz, Chr., Bös, L., Biesig, R., Lang, R. and Schramm, M. (1980). Myocardial extracellular K^+ and H^+ increase and noradrenaline release as possible cause of early arrhythmias following acute coronary artery occlusion in pigs. *J. molec. cell. Cardiol.*, **12**, 579-93

Iversen, L. L. (1977). Uptake processes for biogenic amines. In *Handbook of Psychopharmacology*, Vol. 3 (ed. L. L. Iversen, S. D. Iversen, and S. H. Snyder), Plenum Press, New York, pp. 381-442

Jewitt, D. E., Mercer, C. J., Reid, D., Valori, C., Thomas, M. and Shillingford, J. P. (1969). Free noradrenaline and adrenaline excretion in relation to development of cardiac arrhythmias and heart failure in patients with acute myocardial infarction. *Lancet*, *i*, 635-41

Jugdutt, B. I., Becker, L. C., Bulkley, B. H. and Hutchins, G. M. (1978). Prostaglandin inhibition increases infarct size after coronary artery occlusion in conscious dogs. *Am. J. Cardiol.*, **41**, 359

Karlsberg, R. P., Penkoske, P. A., Cryer, P. E., Corr, P. B. and Roberts, R. (1979). Rapid activation of the sympathetic nervous system following coronary artery occlusion: relationship to infarct size, site and haemodynamic impact. *Cardiovasc. Res.*, **13**, 523-31

Karpati, P., Preda, I. and Endroczi, E. (1974). Effect of acidosis and noradrenaline infusion on ^{14}C-noradrenaline uptake by the rat myocardium. *Acta physiol. hung.*, **45**, 109-14

Kjekshus, J. K., Ellekjaer, R. and Rinde, P. (1980). The effect of free fatty acids on oxygen consumption in man: the free fatty acid hypothesis. *Scand. J. clin. Lab. Invest.*, **40**, 63-70

Kloner, R. A., Ganote, C. E., Whalen, D. A. and Jennings, R. B. (1974). Effect of a transient period of ischemia on myocardial cells. *Am. J. Path.*, **74**, 399-414

Kurien, V. A. and Oliver, M. F. (1970). A metabolic cause for arrhythmias during acute myocardial hypoxia. *Lancet*, *i*, 813-5

Kurien, V. A., Yates, P. A. and Oliver, M. F. (1971). The role of free fatty acids in the production of ventricular arrhythmias after acute coronary artery occlusion. *Eur. J. clin. Invest.*, **1**, 225-41

Langer, S. Z. (1980). Presynaptic receptors and modulation of neurotransmission: pharmacological implications and therapeutic relevance. *Trends Neurosci.*, **3**, 110-2

Lehr, D., Blaiklock, R., Brown, A., Green, M. and Guideri, G. (1980). Alpha-beta adrenergic antagonism in the production of myocardial necrosis and ventricular fibrillation. *Fedn Proc. Fedn Am. Socs exp. Biol.*, **39**, 634

Levy, M. N. and Blattberg, B. (1978). The influence of cocaine and desipramine on the cardiac responses to exogenous and endogenous norepinephrine. *Eur. J. Pharmac.*, **48**, 37-49

Levy, M. N. and Frankel, A. L. (1953). Vasomotor responses to acute coronary occlusion in the dog. *Am. J. Physiol.*, **172**, 427-36

Lorenz, R. R. and Vanhoutte, P. M. (1975). Inhibition of adrenergic neurotransmission in isolated veins of the dog by potassium ions. *J. Physiol., Lond.*, **246**, 479-500

McGrath, B. P., Lim, S. P., Leversha, L. and Shanahan, A. (1981). Myocardial and peripheral catecholamine responses to acute coronary artery constriction before and after propranolol treatment in the anaesthetized dog. *Cardiovasc. Res.*, **15**, 28-34

Malik, K. U. (1978). Prostaglandins-modulation of adrenergic nervous system. *Fedn Proc. Fedn Am. Socs exp. Biol.*, **37**, 204-7

Maling, H. M. and Moran, N. C. (1957). Ventricular arrhythmias induced by sympathomimetic amines in unanaesthetized dogs following coronary artery occlusion. *Circulation Res.*, **5**, 409-13

Malliani, A., Schwartz, P. J. and Zanchetti, A. (1969). A sympathetic reflex elicited by experimental coronary occlusion. *Am. J. Physiol.*, **217**, 703-9

Maroko, P. R., Kjekshus, J. K., Sobel, B. E., Watanabe, T., Covell, J. W., Ross, J. and Braunwald, E. (1971). Factors influencing infarct size following experimental coronary artery occlusions. *Circulation*, **43**, 67-82

Marshall, R. J. and Parratt, J. R. (1980). The early consequences of myocardial ischaemia and their modification. *J. Physiol., Paris*, **76**, 699-715

Martins, J. B., Kerber, R. E., Marcus, M. L., Laughlin, D. L. and Levy, D. M. (1980). Inhibition of adrenergic neurotransmission in ischaemic regions of the canine left ventricle. *Cardiovasc. Res.*, **14**, 116-24

Mathes, P. and Gudbjarnason, S. (1971). Changes in norepinephrine stores in the canine heart following experimental myocardial infarction. *Am. Heart J.*, **81**, 211-9

Moore, G. and Parratt, J. R. (1973). Effect of noradrenaline and isoprenaline on blood flow in the acutely ischaemic myocardium. *Cardiovasc. Res.*, 7, 446-57

Mjøs, O. D. (1973). Mechanical versus metabolic regulation of myocardial oxygen consumption. *Biomedicine*, **18**, 9-12

Mueller, H. S. and Ayres, S. M. (1978). Metabolic responses of the heart in acute myocardial infarction in man. *Am. J. Cardiol.*, **42**, 363-71

Nadeau, R. A. and Champlain, J. de (1979). Plasma catecholamines in acute myocardial infarction. *Am. Heart J.*, **98**, 548-54

Nayler, W. G. and Carson, V. (1973). Effect of stellate ganglion stimulation on myocardial blood flow, oxygen consumption and cardiac efficiency during beta-adrenoceptor blockade. *Cardiovasc. Res.*, 7, 22-9

Oliver, M. F. (1972). Metabolic response during impending myocardial infarction. *Circulation*, **45**, 491-500

Opie, L. H. (1975). Metabolism of free fatty acids, glucose and catecholamines in acute myocardial infarction. *Am. J. Cardiol.*, **36**, 938-53

Opie, L. H., Bruyneel, F. and Owen, P. (1975). Effects of glucose, insulin and potassium infusion on tissue metabolic changes within first hour of myocardial infarction in the baboon. *Circulation*, **52**, 49-57

Paton, D. M. (ed.). (1979). *The Release of Catecholamines from Adrenergic Neurons*, Pergamon, Oxford

Parratt, J. R. (1980). Beta-adrenoceptor blockade and early post-infarction dysrhythmias. In *The Clinical Impact of Beta-adrenoceptor Blockade* (ed. D. M. Burley and G. F. B. Birdwood), Ciba Laboratories, Horsham, Surrey, pp. 29-49

Pashkow, F., Holland, R. and Brooks, H. (1977). Early changes in contractility and coronary blood flow in the normal areas of the ischemic porcine heart. *Am. Heart J.*, **93**, 349-57

Peach, M. J., Ford, G. D., Azzaro, A. J. and Fleming, W. W. (1970). The effects of acidosis on chronotropic responses, norepinephrine storage and release in isolated guinea-pig atria. *J. Pharmac. exp. Ther.*, **172**, 289-96

Podzuweit, T., Lubbe, W. F. and Opie, L. H. (1976). Cyclic adenosine monophosphate, ventricular fibrillation, and antiarrhythmic drugs. *Lancet*, *i*, 341-2

Podzuweit, T., Dalby, A. J., Cherry, G. W. and Opie, L. H. (1978). Cyclic AMP levels in ischaemic and non-ischaemic myocardium following coronary artery ligation: relation to ventricular fibrillation. *J. molec. cell. Cardiol.*, **10**, 81-94

Preda, I., Karpati, P. and Endsoczi, E. (1975). Myocardial noradrenaline uptake after coronary occlusion in the rat. *Acta physiol. hung.*, **46**, 99-106

Puig, M. and Kirpekar, S. M. (1971). Inhibitory effects of low pH on norepinephrine release. *J. Pharmac. exp. Ther.*, **176**, 134-8

Randall, W. C. (1977). Sympathetic control of the heart. In *Neural Regulation of the Heart* (ed. W. C. Randall), Oxford University Press, Oxford, pp. 45-94

Regan, T. J., Markov, A., Oldewurtel, H. A. and Burke, W. M. (1970). Myocardial metabolism and function during ischaemia: response to 1-noradrenaline. *Cardiovasc. Res.*, **4**, 334-42

Riemersma, R. A. (1979). Metabolic aspects of acute myocardial ischaemia. PhD thesis, University of Edinburgh, pp. 452-60

Riemersma, R. A. and Forfar, J. C. (1981). Myocardial norepinephrine release during acute coronary occlusion. *Fedn Proc. Fedn Am. Socs exp. Biol.*, **40**, 646

Rochette, L., Didier, J.-P., Moreau, D. and Bralet, J. (1980). Effect of substrate on release of myocardial norepinephrine and ventricular arrhythmias following reperfusion of the ischaemic isolated worked rat heart. *J. cardiovasc. Pharmac.*, **2**, 267-79

Rovetto, M. J. and Neely, J. R. (1977). Carbohydrate metabolism. In *Pathophysiology and Therapeutics of Myocardial Ischaemia* (ed. A. A. Lefer), Spectrum Publications, London, pp. 169-91

Schaal, S. F., Wallace, A. G. and Sealy, W. C. (1969). Protective influence of cardiac denervation against arrhythmias of myocardial infarction. *Cardiovasc. Res.*, **3**, 241-94

Schömig, A., Dietz, R., Rascher, W., Strasser, R. and Kübler, W. (1980). Noradrenaline release from the ischaemic myocardium. *Circulation*, **62**, Suppl. 3, 669

Schwartz, P. J., Periti, M. and Malliani, A. (1975). The long Q-T syndrome. *Am. Heart J.*, **89**, 378-90

Schwartz, P. F., Stone, H. L. and Brown, A. M. (1976). Effects of unilateral stellate ganglion blockade on the arrhythmias associated with coronary occlusion. *Am. Heart J.*, **92**, 589-99

Serrano, P. A., Chavaz-Lara, B., Bisteni, A. and Sodi-Pallares, D. (1971). Effect of propranolol on catecholamine content of injured cardiac tissue. *J. molec. cell. Cardiol.*, **2**, 91-7

Shahab, L., Wollenberger, A., Krause, E.-G. and Genz, S. (1972). The effect of acute ischaemia on catecholamines and cyclic AMP levels in normal and hypertrophied myocardium. In *Effect of Acute Ischaemia on Myocardial Function* (ed. M. F. Oliver, D. G. Julian, and K. W. Donald), Churchill Livingstone, Edinburgh, pp. 97-108

Shepherd, J. T., Lorenz, R. R., Tyce, G. H. and Vanhoutte, P. M. (1978). Acetylcholine inhibition of transmitter release from adrenergic nerve terminals mediated by muscarinic receptors. *Fedn Proc. Fedn Am. Socs exp. Biol.*, **37**, 191-4

Sheridan, D. J., Penkoske, P. A. and Corr, P. B. (1979). Specific antiarrhythmic effectiveness of α-adrenergic blockade. *Am. J. Cardiol.*, **43**, 372

Siggers, D. C., Salter, C. and Fluck, D. C. (1971). Serial plasma adrenaline and noradrenaline levels in myocardial infarction using a new double isotope technique. *Br. Heart J.*, **33**, 878-83

Stamm, H. and Hülsmann, W. C. (1978). The role of endogenous catecholamines in the depressive effects of free fatty acids on isolated, perfused rat hearts. *Basic Res. Cardiol.*, **73**, 208-19

Staszewska-Barczak, J. (1971). The reflex stimulation of catecholamine secretion during the acute stage of myocardial infarction in the dog. *Clin. Sci.*, **41**, 419-39

Strange, R. C., Vetter, N., Rowe, M. J. and Oliver, M. F. (1974). Plasma cyclic AMP and total catecholamines during acute myocardial infarction in man. *Eur. J. clin. Invest.*, **4**, 115-9

Thoren, P. (1972). Left ventricular receptors activated by severe asphyxia and by coronary artery occlusion. *Acta physiol. scand.*, **85**, 455-63

Valori, C., Thomas, M. and Shillingford, J. P. (1967). Free noradrenaline and adrenaline secretion in relation to clinical syndromes following myocardial infarction. *Am. J. Cardiol.*, **20**, 605-17

Vanhoutte, P. M. (1978). Adrenergic neuroeffector interaction in the blood vessel wall. *Fedn Proc. Fedn Am. Socs exp. Biol.*, **37**, 181-6

Verhaeghe, R. H., Vanhoutte, P. M. and Shepherd, J. T. (1977). Inhibition of sympathetic neurotransmission in canine blood vessels by adenosine and adenine nucleotides. *Circulation Res.*, **40**, 208-15

Videbaek, J., Christensen, N. J. and Sterndorff, B. (1972). Serial determination of plasma catecholamines in myocardial infarction. *Circulation*, **46**, 846-55

Vik-Mo, H. and Mjøs, O. D. (1977). Effects of sodium salicylate and acetylsalicylic acid on epicardial ST-segment elevation during coronary artery occlusion in dogs. *Scand. J. clin. Lab. Invest.*, **37**, 287-94

Waldenstrøm, A. P., Hjalmarson, A. C. and Thornell, L. (1978). A possible role of noradrenaline in the development of myocardial infarction. *Am. Heart J.*, **95**, 43-51

Webb, S. W., Adgey, A. A. J. and Pantridge, J. F. (1972). Autonomic disturbance at onset of acute myocardial infarction. *Br. med. J.*, *ii*, 89-92

Wegria, R., Frank, C. W., Misrahy, G. A., Wang, H.-H., Miller, R. and Case, R. B. (1954). Immediate hemodynamic effects of acute coronary artery occlusion. *Am. J. Physiol.*, **177**, 123-7

Williamson, J. R., Steenbergen, C., Rich, T. and Deleeuw, G. (1977). The nature of ischaemic injury in cardiac tissue. In *Pathophysiology and Therapeutics of Myocardial Ischaemia* (ed. A. M. Lefer), Spectrum Publications, London, pp. 193-225

Yamaguchi, N., Champlain, J. de and Nadeau, R. (1975). Correlation between the response of the heart to sympathetic stimulation and the release of endogenous catecholamine into the coronary sinus of the dog. *Circulation Res.*, **36**, 662-8

9

The Possible Role of the Sympathetic Nervous System in the Genesis of Early Post-ischaemia Arrhythmias

W. Meesmann

9.1 INTRODUCTION

Numerous experimental and clinical findings indicate the decisive importance of the sympathetic nervous system in the early phase of myocardial ischaemia. However, it has not yet been fully established how local activation of the cardiac sympathetic system triggers ventricular arrhythmias and ventricular fibrillation (VF) or which particular phase of early ventricular ectopic activity (that is, phase 1a or phase 1b, chapter 6) is especially initiated by sympathetic activation. This has been investigated in the present experiments in two main ways (1) studies with β-adrenoceptor blocking drugs and (2) experiments with 6-hydroxydopamine to locally deplete myocardial noradrenaline stores.

9.2 STUDIES WITH β-ADRENOCEPTOR BLOCKING AGENTS

Previous investigations

Many investigators have studied the influence of β-adrenoceptor blocking agents on the effects of experimental coronary occlusion (Fearon and Ansten, 1966; Kaumann and Aramendia, 1968; Lown and Ruberman, 1970; Bocage *et al.*, 1971; Lown and Wolf, 1971; Pasyk *et al.*, 1971; Khan *et al.*, 1972; Sehti *et al.*, 1973; Corr and Gillis, 1975; Menken *et al.*, 1979). However, none of these studies have taken into account the presence of pre-existing coronary collaterals; many have involved small numbers of animals and in all of them, including our own previous experiments (Stephan *et al.*, 1972; Stephan and Meesmann, 1974; Abendroth *et al.*, 1977), the β-blocking agents were injected intravenously immediately prior to coronary occlusion. Nevertheless, a marked positive effect on survival by these drugs has been generally revealed (Abendroth *et al.*, 1977; Meesmann *et al.*, 1978a,b, and chapter 16 of this book).

Effects of atenolol

These studies (see also Meesmann *et al.*, 1978a,b; Menken *et al.*, 1979) were particularly concerned with the effects of chronic oral administration of different doses of the β-adrenoceptor blocking agent and with whether this treatment had any influence on the incidence and distribution with time of ventricular premature beats (VPBs) occurring as a result of coronary artery ligation. They were performed in anaesthetised dogs (urethane and chloralose) and also in conscious dogs; only dogs with effective pre-existing collaterals were evaluated (Menken *et al.*, 1979). Our experience from earlier experiments was that steady state conditions, with sufficiently constant atenolol plasma levels, could best be achieved by chronic oral administration for several days before coronary occlusion. Such conditions are also more comparable to the situation of a patient with acute myocardial infarction treated prophylactically with a β-blocking drug. As a measure of the β-blockade existing at the time of coronary occlusion the percentage inhibition of isoprenaline-induced tachycardia was determined and, in addition, plasma atenolol levels at the moment of ligation were measured. There were four separate atenolol-treated groups. Twenty dogs were given a dose of 10 mg kg^{-1} orally for 5 days and, after anaesthesia, the left circumflex coronary artery (LCFX) was ligated either 6 h or 18 h after the last oral dose. Two other groups (16 dogs) received a dose of 2 mg kg^{-1} for 5 days and the LCFX artery was ligated 6 h after the last dose; 10 of these dogs were not subjected to anaesthesia.

The main results are outlined in table 9.1. It can be seen that all 19 animals in the first control (anaesthetised) group died of VF; six of the seven dogs in the control (untreated) conscious group likewise died of VF. Atenolol markedly protected against the development of VF following LCFX occlusion provided the occlusion was performed 6 h after the last oral dose (table 9.1). Although there was no protection 18 h after the last dose, all these animals survived the early post-occlusion period (phase 1a) but died in VF during phase 1b.

The incidence and temporal distribution of VPBs and the mortality from VF of the anaesthetised control group and the atenolol groups (A and B; table 9.1) is shown in figure 9.1. All 19 control animals died of VF and there was the characteristic distribution of VPBs during phases 1a and 1b (chapter 6). In the atenolol-pretreated animals there were clearly fewer VPBs than in the control group during phase 1a. Of these 12 atenolol-treated animals (without collaterals) VPBs occurred in only seven, one of which, together with another without previous VPBs, died of VF at the beginning of phase 1b.

The results of the study in conscious dogs are illustrated in figure 9.2. In contrast to anaesthetised animals (figure 9.1) the incidence of VPBs is higher in phase 1a and phase 1b begins somewhat earlier. Of the 10 conscious dogs pretreated with atenolol, only two died in phase 1a and one died at the beginning of phase 1b. In

Table 9.1 Preventive effects of atenolol and ICI 89406 on primary VF after acute circumflex occlusion

Groups	Atenolol once daily for 5 days, orally (mg kg^{-1})	Interval between last dose and occlusion	*n*	VF	Plasma concentration (μg ml^{-1})	Percentage inhibition of isoprenaline-induced tachycardia, 1 μg kg^{-1} i.v. (%)
Control, anaesthetised		–	19	19	–	–
Control, conscious			7	6		
Atenolol A, anaesthetised	10	18 h	5	5	0.15	42
Atenolol B, anaesthetised	10	6 h	6	1	0.82	77
Atenolol C, anaesthetised	2	6 h	6	1	0.34	59
Atenolol, conscious	2	6 h	10	3	0.34	59
ICI 89406, i.v.	0.3 or 0.5	30 min	8	8	0.03	40

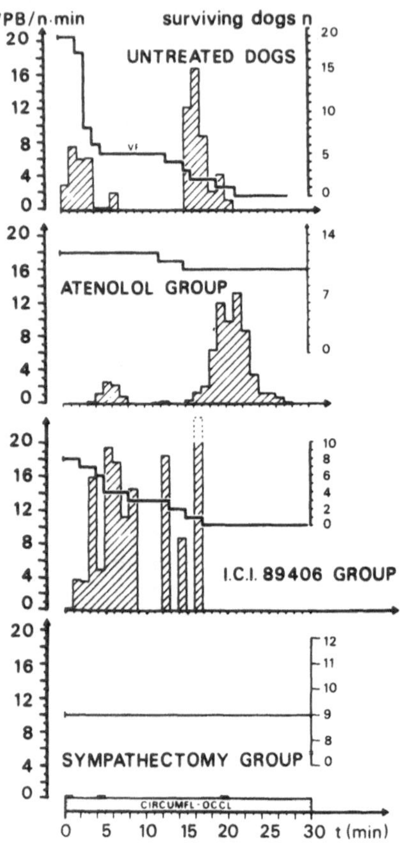

Figure 9.1 The number of ventricular premature beats per minute (shaded columns) and the number of dogs surviving acute coronary artery ligation (circumflex branch) in dogs, without pre-existing coronary collaterals, treated with saline (controls, above), atenolol, the β-blocker ICI 89406 and with 6-hydroxydopamine (pharmacological sympathectomy group). Notice the reduced incidence of VF in the atenolol group and its abolition in the sympathectomised dogs. For details, see text.

comparison with the control group of conscious dogs, this improved survival rate of the atenolol-treated dogs is highly significant. As in earlier investigations of Pasyk *et al.* (1971) and Theroux *et al.* (1976), there was no painful reaction in these conscious dogs as a result of acute coronary occlusion. Thus, there were no limb movements, no salivation, vomiting, whining or respiration disturbances through the entire occlusion period, including the severe arrhythmic phases.

Clearly, a critical degree of β-blockade, reflected by the plasma concentration of the drug and the inhibition of isoprenaline-induced tachycardia, is necessary for the prevention of VF. The lower degree of β-adrenoceptor blockade in group A (table 9.1) is insufficient to protect these animals from VF. However, VF occurs later than in anaesthetised control group dogs (that is, in phase 1b). The higher degree of β-adrenoceptor block in groups B and C, and also in the conscious dogs,

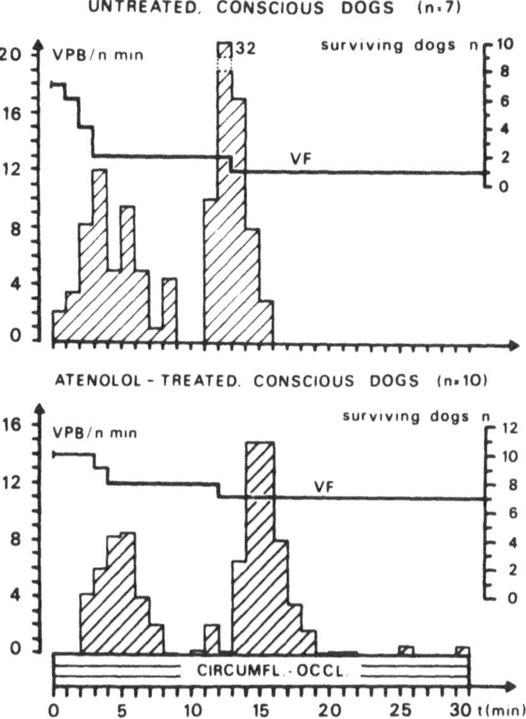

Figure 9.2 Acute circumflex coronary artery occlusion in conscious dogs treated either with saline (above) or atenolol (below); the number of ventricular ectopic beats and the mortality. Notice the reduced incidence of VF in the atenolol group. For details see text.

almost totally protects these animals from VF. Only one animal out of six in group B and in group C, and three out of 10 of the conscious atenolol-treated dogs died of VF, mainly in phase 1b. These results are highly significant, as is the finding that only seven of the 12 dogs in groups B and C had VPBs.

The ventricular fibrillation threshold (VFT) serves as a good measure of the vulnerability of the myocardium after acute coronary occlusion (see chapter 6). The results of studies to examine the effect of chronic oral atenolol on the time course of VFT following LAD occlusion are outlined in figure 9.3. At any given time VFT in the atenolol-pretreated group was significantly higher than in the control group and again a significant decrease in VFT was only found during phase 1a. As in the earlier experiments with untreated animals, VFT had already reached pre-occlusion values, for the treated and the untreated animals, by 12 min (the time phase 1b arrhythmias normally occur).

These results thus clearly demonstrate that, under strict experimental conditions in both anaesthetised and conscious dogs, atenolol markedly reduces primary VF following acute coronary occlusion. These results also show that to be certain of obtaining this protective effect a dosage scheme must be applied that guarantees

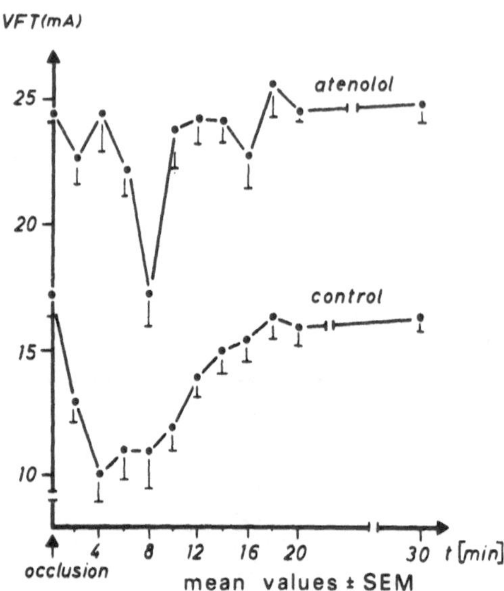

Figure 9.3 Alterations in the ventricular fibrillation threshold (VFT) following acute LAD occlusion (at time 0) in dogs pretreated with saline (control) and atenolol. Notice (1) the recovery of VFT despite the continuing presence of ischaemia and (2) the marked increase in VFT induced by atenolol both before and during the occlusion.

a sufficient degree of β-adrenoceptor blockade all through the day. This may explain the lack of efficacy of some β-blocking drugs in clinical trials. On the other hand, these experimental results are in excellent agreement with the recent clinical study with timolol demonstrating a significant reduction in mortality rate, especially sudden cardiac death, during administration of a sufficiently high daily dosage of this β-blocking agent (Norwegian Multicenter Study Group, 1981).

Effects of ICI 89406

This study was designed to examine whether a β_1-blocking agent with pronounced intrinsic sympathomimetic activity (ISA) was also effective in reducing early post-occlusion arrhythmias. Earlier studies with ICI 89406 revealed that the undesirable negative inotropic effects that result from β-blockade in experimental myocardial infarction may be avoided by a β-blocking drug (like ICI 89406) which has marked ISA.

The experimental conditions were the same as with atenolol but, because of poor absorption by the oral route, the drug was administered intravenously. First, inhibition of isoprenaline-induced tachycardia after various cumulative doses of the compound was examined and on the basis of these results ICI 89406 was administered, in a dosage of 0.3–0.5 mg kg^{-1}, 30 min before acute high ligation of the LCFX. These experiments were performed under morphine–chloralose–urethane narcosis. The main results are illustrated in figure 9.4. Of 11 dogs, only three, which

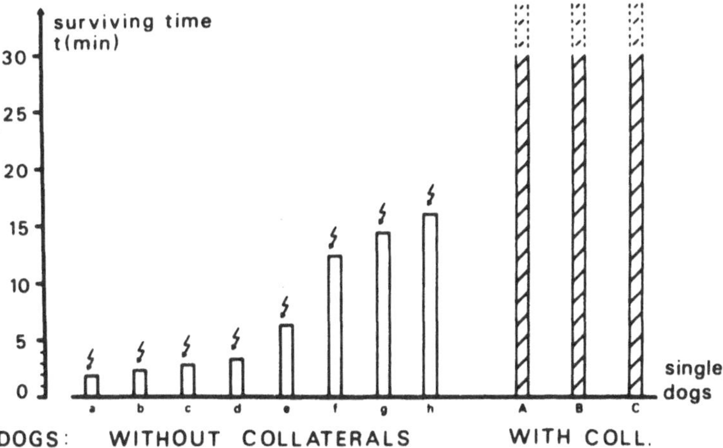

Figure 9.4 The effect of ICI 89406 on survival time in dogs, with and without pre-existing coronary collaterals, following circumflex artery occlusion. Dosage of ICI 89406 was either 0.5 mg kg^{-1} (d, e, g, A, B) or 0.3 mg kg^{-1} (a, b, c, f, C). Crooked arrows indicate onset of VF.

had pre-existing collaterals, survived; the other eight animals without collaterals died of VF, five in phase 1a and three in phase 1b. The differences in the incidence and distribution of the VPBs and in mortality (VF) between the untreated controls, the atenolol group and the ICI 89406 group are clearly evident from figure 9.1. In the dogs pretreated with ICI 89406 the incidence of VPBs in phase 1a was significantly higher than in the controls. This might result from the marked ISA of the compound. This dramatic difference between the two β-blockers is difficult to explain except on the basis of ISA. There were certainly no marked haemodynamic differences between the control group, the atenolol-treated group and the ICI 89406-treated groups, although the heart rate (92 ± 6 beats min^{-1}) was slightly lower in the atenolol-treated group than in the conscious controls (119 ± 9 beats min^{-1}); the heart rate of the ICI 89406-treated group (anaesthetised dogs) was the same as the controls. Also, there was no difference in the degree of β-blockade as indicated from the effects on isoprenaline-induced tachycardia. We can only conclude that ISA in some way contributes to the non-effectiveness of this particular β-blocker.

9.3 STUDIES INVOLVING REGIONAL CHEMICAL MYOCARDIAL SYMPATHECTOMY

It was the purpose of further investigations to differentiate between the diverse components of the sympathetic nervous system with regard to their role in initiating early arrhythmias and/or primary VF during acute myocardial ischaemia.

Our basic hypothesis was as follows:

(1) Only those sympathetic neurones releasing catecholamines locally in the ischaemic myocardium are important in initiating the early VPBs and primary VF following acute coronary occlusion.

(2) Catecholamines (CA) released by the adrenal medulla as a result of a general reflex stimulation of the sympathetic nervous system are of no importance for the initiation of these early arrhythmias because of the low CA uptake from arterial blood within the ischaemic area compared with the high local synaptic concentration of CA released in the ischaemic area.

A differentiation between the effects of catecholamines released locally in the ischaemic myocardium and that of circulating catecholamines is possible by preferentially depleting areas of myocardium subsequently made ischaemic using the technique of regional chemical sympathectomy. This would induce postsynaptic hypersensitivity to circulating catecholamines and also to any noradrenaline released in the adjacent normal myocardium which might diffuse into the ischaemic zone.

Previous investigations

Earlier investigations have involved chronic surgical denervation of the total heart (Ebert *et al.*, 1970; Jones *et al.*, 1978), left stellectomy (Schwartz and Stone, 1980), reserpine pretreatment and cervical vagotomy (Ebert *et al.*, 1970) or chemical sympathectomy of the whole left ventricle (Sehti *et al.*, 1973). Clear results can not be obtained when the occluded coronary artery is the LAD if pre-existing collaterals are not taken into account. This is the case with all of these studies. Furthermore, some of the studies used the gradual production of a thrombus to occlude the coronary artery (Sehti *et al.*, 1973) and, when chemical sympathectomy was used (Sehti *et al.*, 1973), the method of administration was such that detectable amounts of CAs were still present.

In order to examine the influence, on early post-ischaemic arrhythmias, of local catecholamine release in the infarcted area, experiments were performed on 33 dogs under conditions such that only a selected regional area of the left ventricle was chemically sympathectomised. For this, a special form of intracoronary injection of 6-hydroxydopamine (6-OHDA) was used (Trippe *et al.*, 1981). A microcatheter was placed in the LCFX at a previous operation and an inflatable cuff-occluder was implanted proximal to this catheter. Several days after the operation intracoronary injections of 6-OHDA were commenced and, 1 s prior to injection, LCFX flow was interrupted for 40–60 s in order to improve 6-OHDA accumulation in the noradrenergic nerve endings. Of the 22 dogs, seven had collaterals and two were incompletely depleted. All 13 remaining dogs were without collaterals and only these were evaluated.

The noradrenaline content in the LCFX area was 1.5 per cent of normal (mean 0.62 $\mu g\ g^{-1}$ wet weight). Using the glyoxyl acid method (De la Torre and Surgeon, 1976) it was demonstrated that there was no fluorescence of the sympathetic nerve fibres and endings in the area supplied by the LCFX. In the area supplied by the LAD there was only a partial reduction of catecholamine content and there was a normal fluorescent response of the nerve fibres. Table 9.2 shows the time course of the experiments. After the operation for implantation of the catheter, the first and second chemical sympathectomies were performed with an interval of 2-3 days between. Finally, the coronary artery was occluded for 30 min.

Table 9.2 Time course of experiments with acute circumflex occlusion after regional myocardial sympathectomy with 6-OHDA

Sterile operation		1st chemical sympathectomy, circumflex area		2nd chemical sympathectomy, circumflex area		Acute circumflex occlusion (30 min)
	7–14 days		2–3 days		2–3 days	
Piritramide–N_2O anaesthesia + pancuronium				Morphine–chloralose–urethane anaesthesia		
					+ heparin	

6-OHDA: 1.2 mg kg^{-1} dissolved in 1.5 ml saline containing 1.5 mg ascorbic acid. One second prior to injection, circumflex coronary flow was interrupted for 40–60 s to improve 6-OHDA accumulation into adrenergic nerves of this ventricular region.

Results following regional myocardial sympathectomy

Haemodynamic data from the untreated and sympathectomised dogs demonstrated that the reduced contractile state of the LCFX area was compensated by the remaining, partially depleted left ventricle. The haemodynamic effects of LCFX occlusion (increase in heart rate and LVEDP) in these animals was similar to those observed in the controls.

The results obtained from the 13 animals without functionally effective pre-existing collaterals are outlined in figure 9.5. VPBs which occurred only in phase 1a were few in number, and only two dogs died of VF (in phase 1a). The incidence of VPBs was pronounced in four of the 13 dogs which had a wide LCFX area and appeared to be incompletely sympathectomised. If these dogs are disregarded, we are left with a group of nine dogs, completely sympathectomised and without functionally effective pre-existing collaterals. The results are remarkable and show that all of these dogs survived acute LCFX occlusion almost without any arrhythmias. An example of an electrocardiogram from one of these animals is illustrated in figure 9.6. Whilst serious and typical ischaemic changes arise (widening of the QRS complex and ST-segment elevation) there were no ischaemic arrhythmias at all.

Figure 9.1 summarises the results obtained from untreated, atenolol-pretreated and ICI 89406-pretreated, and sympathectomised dogs. There are clearly a number of important differences between these groups.

A number of conclusions can be drawn from these sympathectomy experiments:

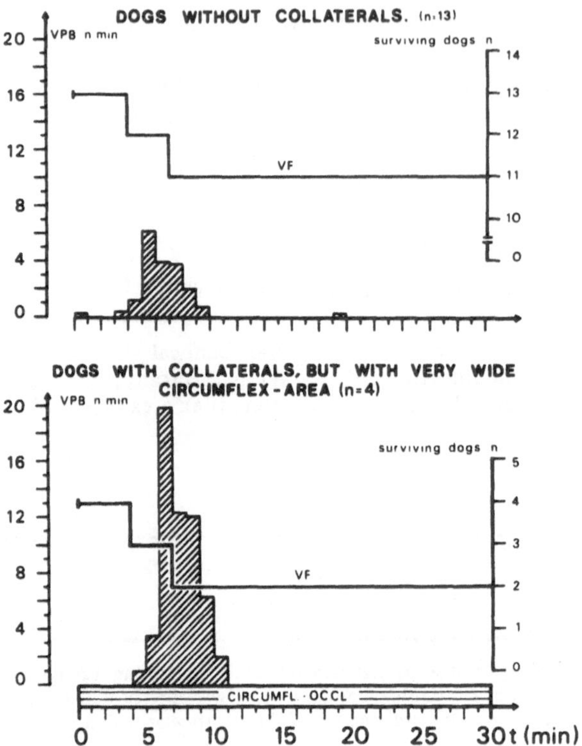

Figure 9.5 The effect of regional chemical sympathectomy (area supplied by left circumflex artery) in the incidence of VF (that is, number of dogs surviving) and on number of ventricular premature beats in dogs without (above) and with (below) pre-existing coronary collaterals.

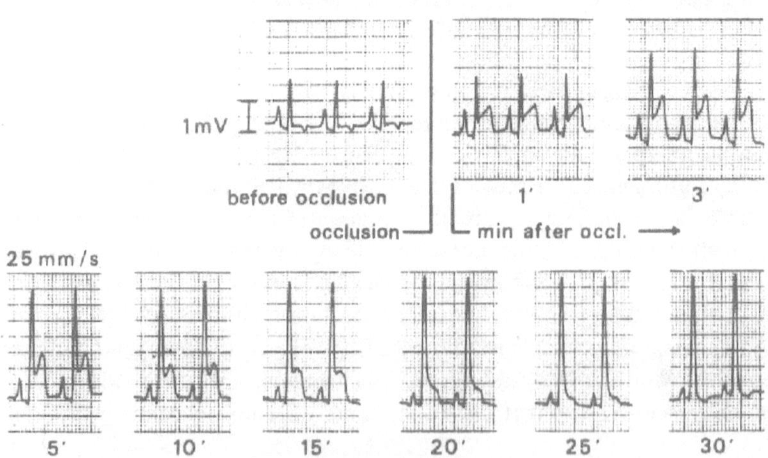

Figure 9.6 Changes in limb lead electrocardiograph (lead II) in a dog, without significant coronary collaterals, subjected to circumflex artery occlusion following regional (chemical) sympathectomy of the area supplied by that vessel. There is typical electrocardiographic evidence of ischaemia (ST-segment elevation, QRS widening) but no arrhythmias resulted.

(1) Following acute, high LCFX ligation, complete regional chemical sympathectomy of the potential infarction area prevents the development of ventricular fibrillation and almost completely prevents the genesis of ventricular arrhythmias.

(2) With incomplete regional sympathectomy VF and VPBs are strongly reduced and develop exclusively in phase 1a.

(3) Only noradrenaline locally released in the ischaemic myocardium causes VPBs and VF in the first (1a and 1b) arrhythmic phases following acute coronary occlusion; a higher noradrenaline concentration appears to be necessary to elicit the phase 1b arrhythmias.

9.4 GENERAL CONCLUSIONS

These summarised results show that chronic oral β-adrenoceptor blockade almost completely prevents VF and VPBs following acute coronary occlusion, even when this is the largest coronary artery (LCFX) and even when the hearts are without functionally effective pre-existing collaterals. It is particularly important, however (table 9.1), that adequate levels of the drug are maintained throughout the entire vulnerable period. It would seem that phase 1a is the most vulnerable early period following coronary artery occlusion, particularly in the conscious dog. This is certainly the period when the incidence of VPBs, and particularly VF, is very high. This is also the only time that a decrease in VFT can be observed. The results of the atenolol study show that, in order to prevent the vulnerable phase 1b arrhythmias, a much higher dose of β-blocking agent is required than for suppression of phase 1a arrhythmias.

The results from the chemically sympathectomised study can be interpreted in the same way. Thus, if a small amount of catecholamines remains in the infarction area, then VPBs and VF occur in phase 1a only (lower part, figure 9.5) and to elicit excitability at this time requires a much higher local concentration of catecholamines. These results clearly demonstrate an important role for locally released noradrenaline in the genesis of early ventricular arrhythmias resulting from acute myocardial ischaemia, especially during phase 1a. These results are much in accord with those described in the following chapter.

REFERENCES

Abendroth, R.-R., Meesmann, W., Stephan, K., Schley, G. and Hübner, H. (1977). Effects of the β-blocking agent atenolol on arrhythmias, especially ventricular fibrillation, and on fibrillation threshold after acute experimental coronary artery occlusion. *Z. Kardiol.*, **66**, 341-50

Bocage, A. J., Otero, H. and Harris, A. S. (1971). Preventive effect of beta adrenergic blockade with practolol on early ventricular arrhythmias after coronary occlusion. *Circulation*, **43/44**, Suppl. 11, 142

Corr, P. B. and Gillis, R. A. (1975). Effect of autonomic neural influence on the cardiovascular changes induced by coronary occlusion. *Am. Heart J.*, **89**, 766-74

De la Torre, F. C. and Surgeon, J. W. (1976). A methodological approach to rapid and sensitive monoamine histofluorescence using a modified glyoxylic acid technique: the SPG method. *Histochemistry*, **49**, 81-93

Ebert, A., Vanderbeek, R. B., Allgood, R. J. and Sabiston, D. C. (1970). Effect of chronic cardiac denervation on arrhythmias after coronary artery ligation. *Cardiovasc. Res.*, **4**, 141-7

Fearon, R. E. and Ansten, W. G. (1966). Beta-adrenergic blockade in experimental myocardial infarction. *Am. Heart. J.*, **72**, 790-6

Jones, C. E., Beck, L. V., DuPont, E. and Barnes, G. E. (1978). Effects of coronary ligation on the chronically sympathectomised dog ventricle. *Am. J. Physiol.*, **235**, H429-34

Kaumann, A. J. and Aramendia, P. (1968). Prevention of ventricular fibrillation induced by coronary ligation. *J. Pharmac. exp. Ther.*, **164**, 326-32

Khan, M. J., Hamilton, J. T. and Manning, G. W. (1972) Early arrhythmias following experimental coronary occlusion in conscious dogs and their modification by β-adrenoceptor blocking drugs. *Am. Heart J.*, **86**, 357-8

Lown, B. and Ruberman, W. (1970). The concept of modern pre-coronary care. *Mod. Concepts cardiovasc. Dis.*, **39**, 97-102

Lown, B. and Wolf, M. (1971). Approaches to sudden death from coronary heart disease. *Circulation*, **44**, 130-43

Meesmann, W., Stephan, K., Abendroth, R.-R., Menken, U. and Wiegand, V. (1978a). Frühe Arrhythmien insbesondere Kammerflimmern, nach akutem experimentellen Koronarverschluß und Beta-Rezeptoren Blocker. In *Beta-Blockade 1977. Internationales Symposium Rottach-Egern* (ed. W. Maürer, A. Schömig, R. Dietz and P. R. Lichtlen), Georg Thieme Verlag, Stuttgart, pp. 244-54

Meesmann, W., Wiegand, V., Menken, U., Komhard, W. and Rehwald, U. (1978b). Early mortality due to ventricular fibrillation, and the vulnerability of the heart following acute coronary occlusion: possible mechanisms and pharmacological prophylaxis. In *The Arterial System. Dynamics, Control Theory and Regulation* (ed. R. D. Bauer and R. Busse), Springer Verlag, Berlin and Heidelberg, pp. 275-84

Menken, U., Wiegand, V., Bucher, P. and Meesmann, W. (1979). Prophylaxis of ventricular fibrillation after acute experimental coronary occlusion by chronic beta-adrenoceptor blockade. *Cardiovasc. Res.*, **13**, 588-94

Norwegian Multicenter Study Group (1981). Timolol-induced reduction in mortality and reinfarction in patients surviving acute myocardial infarction. *New Engl. J. Med.*, **304**, 801-7

Pasyk, S., Bloor, C. M., Khouri, E. M. and Gregg, D. E. (1971). Systemic and coronary effects of coronary artery occlusion in the unanaesthetized dog. *Am. J. Physiol.*, **220**, 646-54

Schwartz, P. J. and Stone, H. L. (1980). Left stellectomy in the prevention of ventricular fibrillation caused by acute myocardial ischaemia in conscious dogs with anterior myocardial infarction. *Circulation*, **62**, 1256-65

Sehti, V., Haider, B., Ahmed, S. S., Oldewurtel, H. A. and Regan, T. J. (1973). Influence of β-blockade and chemical sympathectomy on myocardial function and arrhythmias in acute ischaemia. *Cardiovasc. Res.*, **7**, 740-7

Stephan, K., Meesmann, W. and Tüttemann, J. (1972). Akute Koronarligatur unter β-Rezeptorenblocker mit Practolol. *Pflügers Arch. ges. Physiol.*, **335**, Suppl. R8

Stephan, K. and Meesmann, W. (1974). Beeinflussung der frühen Arrhythmien nach akutem Koronarverschluß durch β-Blockade mit Practolol. *Z. Kardiol.*, **63**, 603-11

Theroux, P., Ross, J., Franklin, D., Kemper, W. S. and Sasayama, S. (1976). Regional myocardial function in conscious dogs during acute coronary occlusion and responses to morphine, propranolol, nitroglycerin and lidocaine. *Circulation*, **53**, 302-14

Trippe, W., Walter, R., Sautter, R., Martin, C., Krosig, K. S. von, Neumann, M. and Meesmann, W. (1981). Einfluß der regionalen myokardialen Sympathektomie auf die ventrikulären Arrhythmien und das Kammerflimmern nach akutem Koronarverschluß. *Z. Kardiol.*, **70**, P141

10

Noradrenaline Release in Acute Myocardial Ischaemia, a Fluorescence-histochemical and Biochemical Study

T. Abrahamsson, S. Holmgren and O. Almgren

10.1 THE EVIDENCE FOR EARLY NORADRENALINE RELEASE IN ACUTE MYOCARDIAL ISCHAEMIA

One of the factors which has been considered as important for the development of serious ventricular arrhythmias in acute myocardial ischaemia is increased regional sympathetic activity in the ischaemic myocardium (Corr and Gillis, 1978; Hjalmarson, 1980). Although early activation of cardiac efferent sympathetic nerves during experimental myocardial ischaemia has been reported by several investigators (Brown and Malliani, 1971; Bosnjak *et al.*, 1979), there are only a few experimental observations which actually demonstrate an increased release of noradrenaline (NA) from the acutely ischaemic myocardium. For example, a sharp increase in coronary venous NA following reperfusion of the ischaemic myocardium was reported by Shahab *et al.* (1969) and a more modest release of NA has been reported following acute coronary artery occlusion (Lammerant *et al.*, 1966; Dutta and Booker, 1970). More recent studies have, however, been unable to demonstrate an early ischaemia-induced release of NA into the coronary venous circulation at the time of pronounced ventricular ectopic activity (Rogg and Bucher, 1979; Marshall and Parratt, 1980; McGrath *et al.*, 1981). Differences in experimental design and coronary artery anatomy may partly explain this apparent discrepancy. In addition, NA released in the ischaemic myocardium may only in part diffuse into venous blood because of neuronal re-uptake, extraneuronal uptake and catabolism. There is certainly strong evidence for a decrease in tissue NA content in the ischaemic myocardium after a period of 0.5-2.5 h in the rat (Gromova, 1977; Abrahamsson *et al.*, 1981, and this chapter) and somewhat later in the dog (Russel *et al.*, 1961; Mathes and Gudbjarnason, 1971).

Most evidence suggesting an early increase in noradrenaline release in the ischaemic myocardium is indirect, for example, the increase in cyclic AMP which occurs in the ischaemic region shortly after coronary artery ligation (reviewed in chapter 11) and the demonstration that chronic sympathectomy depletes myocardial NA storage and also reduces the incidence of early ventricular fibrillation after coronary occlusion (Ebert *et al.*, 1968). Further, chemical sympathectomy by 6-hydroxydopamine reduces the incidence and severity of ventricular arrhythmias following acute coronary artery occlusion (Sethi *et al.*, 1973; Sheridan *et al.*, 1980) and pretreatment with either β-adrenoceptor or α-adrenoceptor blocking drugs (reviewed in chapters 16 and 17) reduces the frequency of ventricular fibrillation in acute experimental myocardial ischaemia.

In myocardial ischaemia there are several possible mechanisms which could result in increased NA release. It may be mediated by increased cardiac efferent nervous activity, either as part of a general reflex sympathetic activation (Staszewska-Barczak, 1971; Karlsberg *et al.*, 1979) or by a local cardiac reflex (Brown and Malliani, 1971; Bosnjak *et al.*, 1979). NA release may also result from direct, local effects on sympathetic neurones by factors such as increased extracellular potassium, acidosis and hypoxia (Shahab and Wollenberger, 1967; Hausler *et al.*, 1968). Energy deficiency within the neurone may also contribute (Wakade and Furchgott, 1968).

The aim of the present study was to clarify the extent of NA release early in myocardial ischaemia and the mechanisms involved in this release. We used acute left coronary artery occlusion in the anaesthetised rat as a model of myocardial ischaemia and studied ischaemia-induced changes in cardiac noradrenergic terminals by means of biochemical and fluorescence-histochemical techniques. In order to identify the importance of efferent sympathetic nerve traffic for the early release of NA in the ischaemic myocardium we also included studies with the ganglion blocking agent chlorisondamine, which would inhibit sympathetic nerve discharge to the heart.

10.2 EXPERIMENTAL PROCEDURES

Male rats (body weight 300-400 g) of the Wistar strain were anaesthetised with pentobarbitone (60 mg kg^{-1} i.p.) and artificially ventilated. Heart rate and arterial blood pressure were continuously recorded and a left thoracotomy performed through the fourth intercostal space. A loose ligature was tied around the left coronary artery and vein a few millimetres distal to the aortic root. After a 10 min period, chlorisondamine (0.1 mg kg^{-1}) or saline was given i.v. and 15 min after drug administration the ligature was tied (occlusion) or pulled a little (sham-operated). For the determination of NA the rats were killed at 0, 0.5 and 2.5 h after occlusion. At the end of the experiments trypan blue (1 ml of a 1 per cent solution) was injected intravenously. If the surface of the left ventricle remained uncoloured in the ligated animals, the occlusion was regarded as complete and the experiment was accepted as valid. The mortality rate of the experimental procedure was less than 10 per cent (control) or 20-30 per cent (after chlorisondamine).

Noradrenaline assay

The heart was rapidly removed and the left (LV) and right (RV) ventricle free walls were separated. The tissues were immediately frozen on dry ice and stored at $-70\,^{\circ}\mathrm{C}$ until analysed. Analysis of NA was performed by reverse phase liquid chromatography and by electrochemical detection (S. Holmgren, T. Abrahamsson and O. Almgren, unpublished; Eriksson and Persson, 1982).

Fluorescence histochemistry

Rats with coronary artery occlusion were killed at various times after ligation and pieces of the intraventricular septum and left (figure 10.1) and right ventricles were

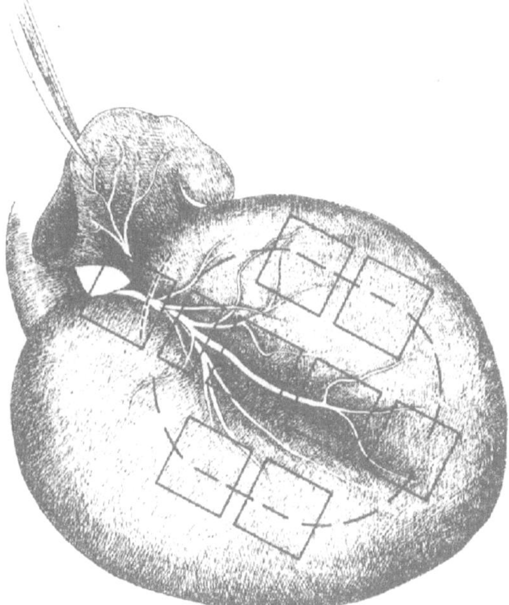

Figure 10.1 Schematic illustration of the rat heart showing the left atrium, left ventricle and the left coronary artery. The site of coronary artery ligation is indicated by the dashed line and the area *not* stained by trypan blue at the end of the experiment ('ischaemic area') is demonstrated by the dashed circle. Tissue pieces for fluorescence histochemistry were dissected out from the left ventricular free wall as shown by the squares.

treated according to the Hillarp-Falck technique for fluorescence histochemistry (Falck and Owman, 1965) to visualise myocardial catecholamines. The freeze-dried pieces of tissue were treated with paraformaldehyde vapour (saturated to 70 per cent) at 80 °C for 1 h and embedded in paraffin wax. Tissue section of 7 μm were mounted in Entellan (Merck) and viewed in a Leitz Ortholux microscope with top light illumination and a barrier filter at 460 nm. Photographs were taken with a Leitz Orthomat automatic camera on Kodak Tri-X film.

10.3 NORMAL ADRENERGIC INNERVATION OF THE RAT VENTRICLES

Large bundles of sympathetic, specifically fluorescent nerve fibres were observed superficially on the ventricles. The ventricular tissue was evenly innervated only by varicose fluorescing fibres running along the muscle fibres (figures 10.2(a), 10.3(a)). An aggregation of fibres occurred especially around smaller arteries (figure 10.4(b)) and arterioles (figure 10.4(a)), while the bigger arteries (figure 10.4(c)) and the veins showed a relatively sparse innervation. Innervation of the smaller arteries and arterioles showed a bipolar distribution around the vessel in cross-section (figure 10.4(a)).

10.4 INNERVATION PATTERN AFTER OCCLUSION OF THE LEFT CORONARY ARTERY

A time-dependent decrease in fluorescence of the noradrenergic terminals was observed in the ischaemic area after ligation of the left coronary artery. Thirty minutes after ligation the terminals of the ischaemic area fluoresced only weakly and appeared to be reduced in number (figure 10.5). However, no area was completely devoid of visible terminals. After 2.5 or 5 h of ischaemia the centre of the occluded area lacked detectable fluorescence for catecholamines (figures 10.2(b), 10.3(b)) and showed only a non-specific yellow fluorescence in scattered small (mast) cells and a weak autofluorescence lining the blood vessels. Often the depletion was restricted to the mid-portion (about 80 per cent) of the thickness of the myocardium with the subepicardium and, less often, the subendocardium still showing innervation by fluorescing terminals.

A thin (100–500 μm wide) 'border zone' occurred between the non-fluorescing centre of the ligated area and the surrounding normally fluorescent areas. This 'border zone' varied in appearance. Most commonly the terminals in this region were fewer than normal but those present showed a normal intensity of fluorescence (figure 10.6(a)). Often the border was very sharp between the area of normal fluorescence and that totally devoid of fluorescing terminals. Occasionally, a normal number of terminals were present in the border zone but they were diffuse and spread out, as if leaking catecholamines (figures 10.6(b), 10.7) The disappearance

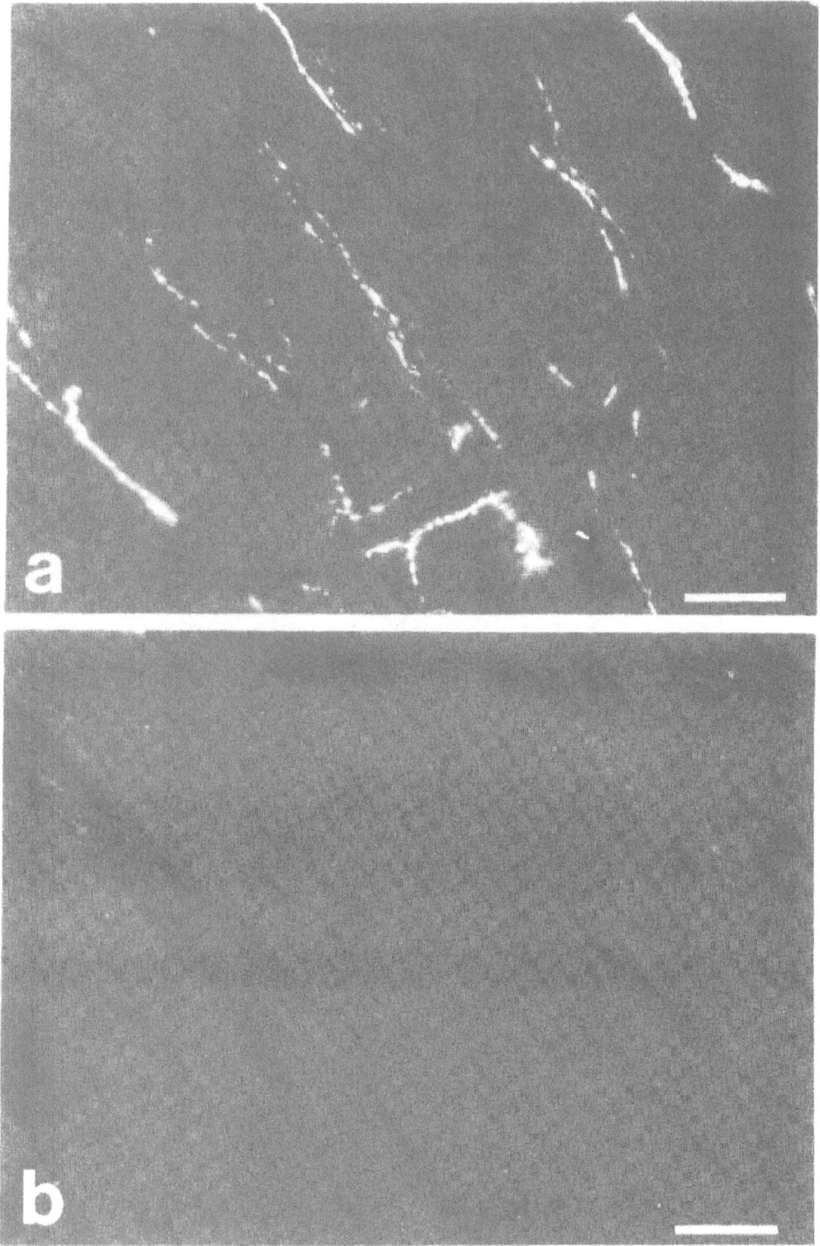

Figure 10.2 Longitudinal section of the myocardium of the rat left ventricle. (a) Normal innervation; strands of varicose fibres showing a fluorescence specific for catecholamines run in the same general direction as the muscle fibres. (b) The appearance of the centre of the ischaemic area 2.5 h after ligation of the left coronary artery. No terminals containing specific fluorescence can be seen. Calibration bars 50 μm.

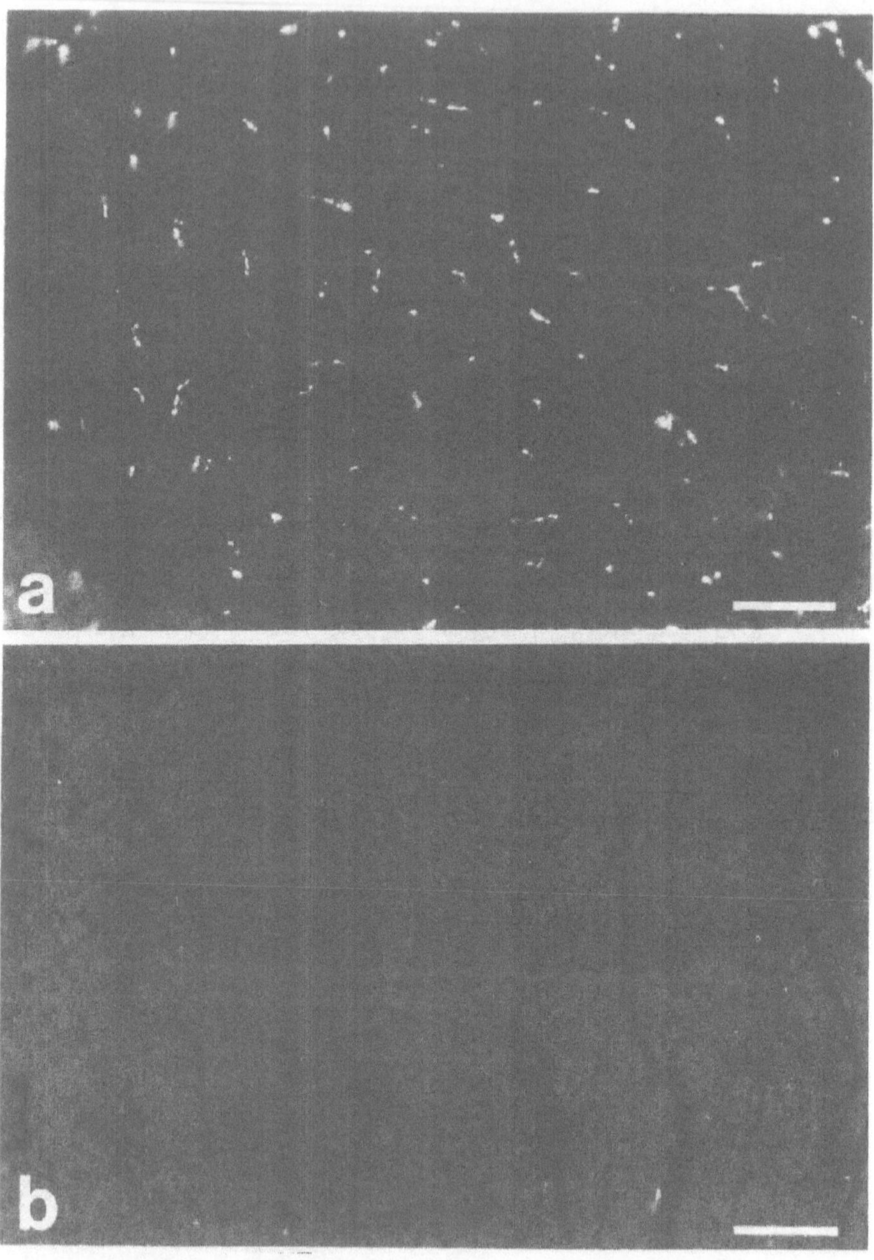

Figure 10.3 Transverse section of the myocardium (myocardial fibres) of the rat left ventricle. (a) Normal innervation. The adrenergic varicose fibres are (like the myocardial fibres) mainly cut in cross-section. Probably only the fibres where the section is going through a varicosity are seen in the picture; a section through the part of the axon between two varicosities probably gives too small an area of fluorescence to be seen. The density of innervation is therefore probably somewhat higher than that appearing in the picture. (b) Cross-section of myocardial fibres in the centre of the ischaemic area 2.5 h after ligation of the left coronary artery. The tissue is completely devoid of specifically fluorescing nerve terminals. Calibration bars 50 μm.

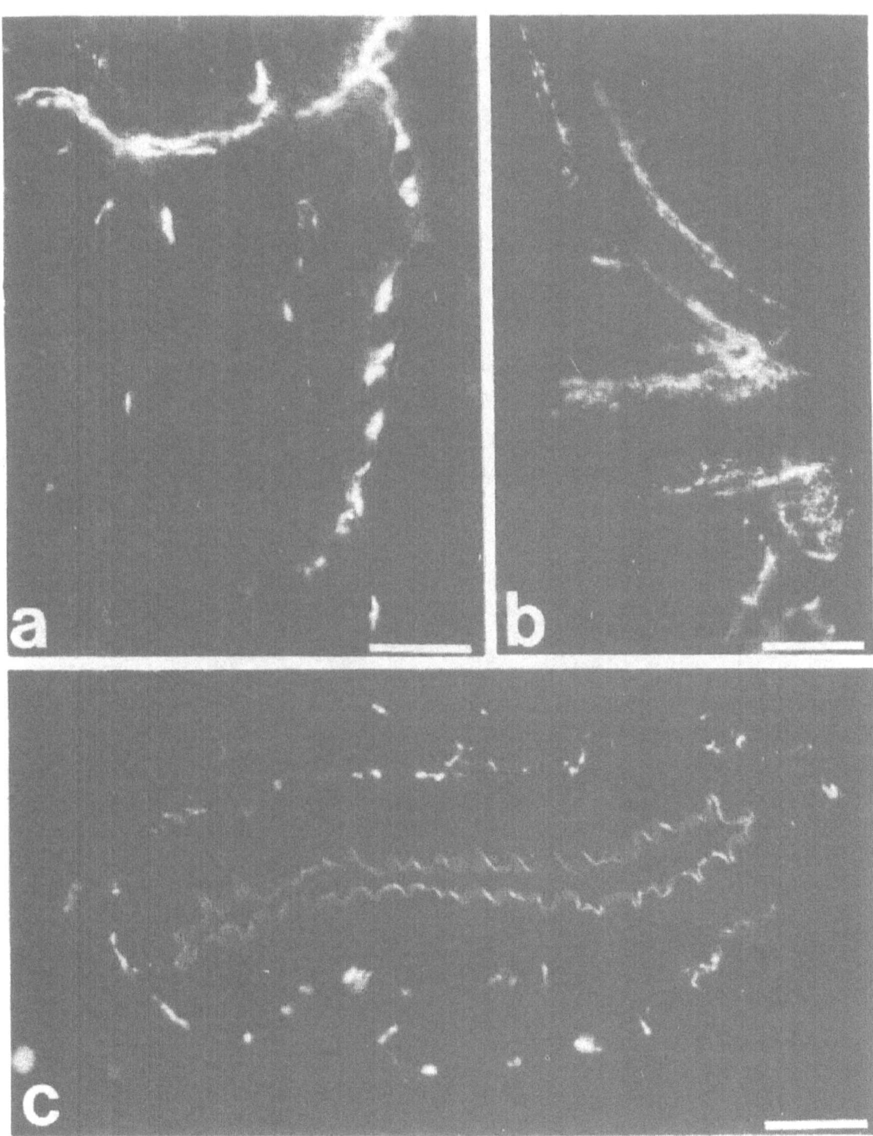

Figure 10.4 The pictures show the density of adrenergic innervation around myocardial vessels of different size. (a) A row of arterioles in cross-section showing the dense innervation around these vessels. Note the bipolar distribution of the nerve net around each vessel. (b) Nerve fibres around a branching small artery. (c) Cross-section of the left coronary artery close to the apex of the ventricle. The innervation of the bigger arteries is relatively sparse compared to that of the smaller arteries and arterioles. No fibres are seen to penetrate the media, while small bundles of fibres run along the vessel and in the adventitia. Calibration bars 50 μm.

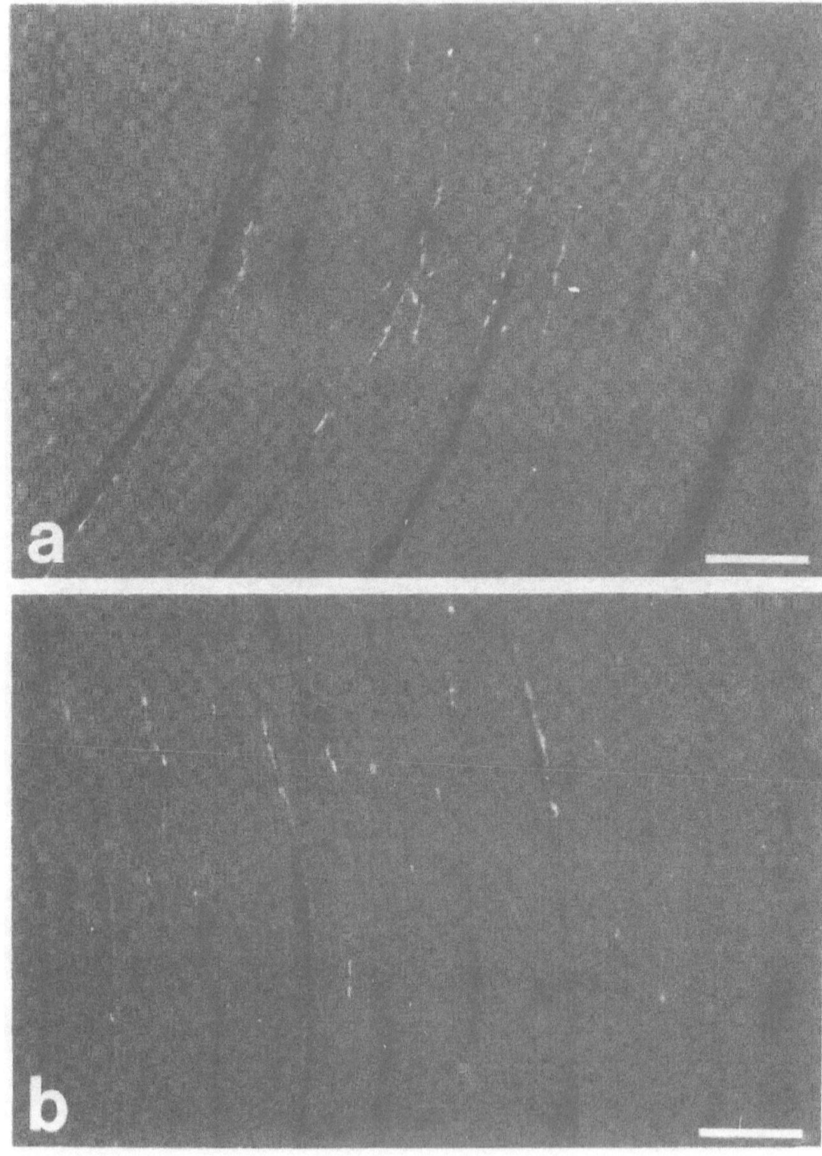

Figure 10.5 Sections of the centre of the ischaemic area of the rat left ventricle 0.5 h after ligation of the left coronary artery. The number of terminals showing specific fluorescence is somewhat reduced and the intensity of fluorescence of those still present is markedly less than that of control tissues. However, no area of the ventricles were found to be *completely* devoid of specifically fluorescent terminals 0.5 h after the ligation. Calibration bars 50 μm.

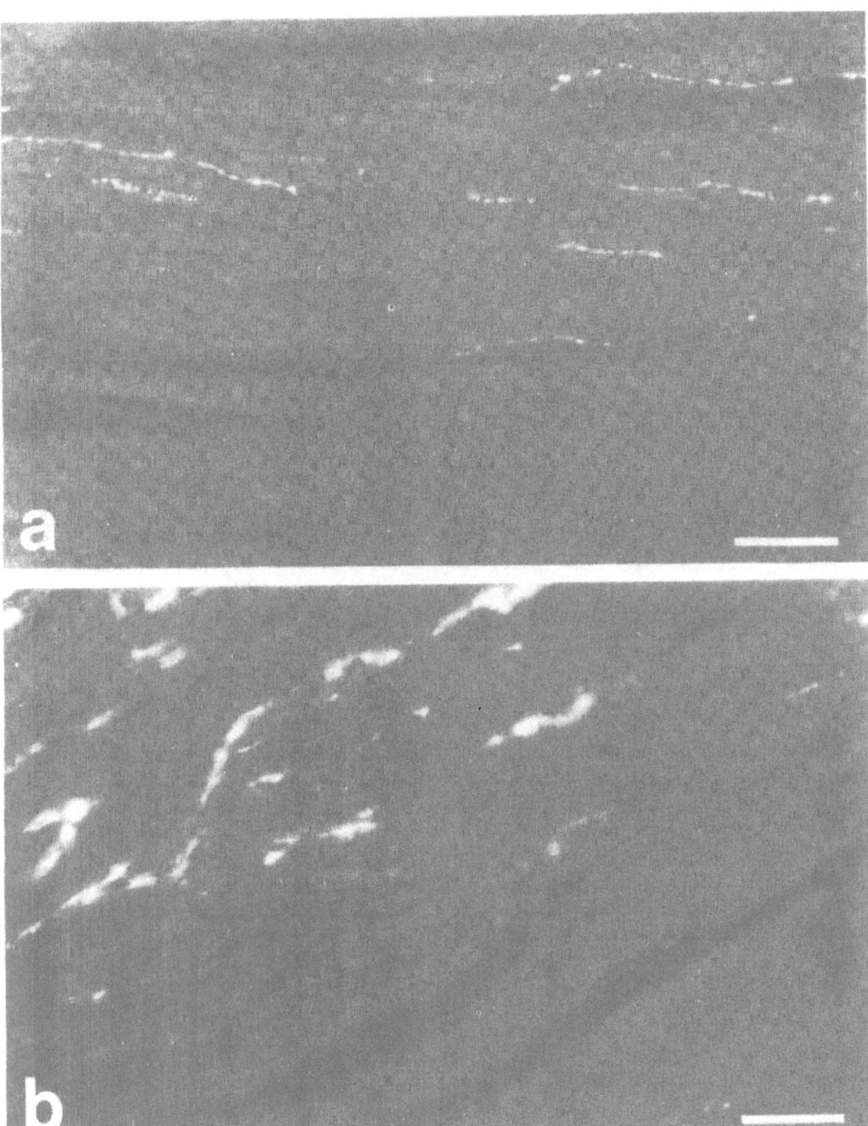

Figure 10.6 The 'border zone', a 100–500 μm wide area between the empty centre of the ischaemic area and the surrounding essentially normal tissues. (a) The most common feature of the border zone is a more or less reduced number of fluorescent terminals which otherwise have a normal appearance. (b) Occasionally parts of the border zone contain terminals with a diffuse 'leaking' appearance. Calibration bars 50 μm.

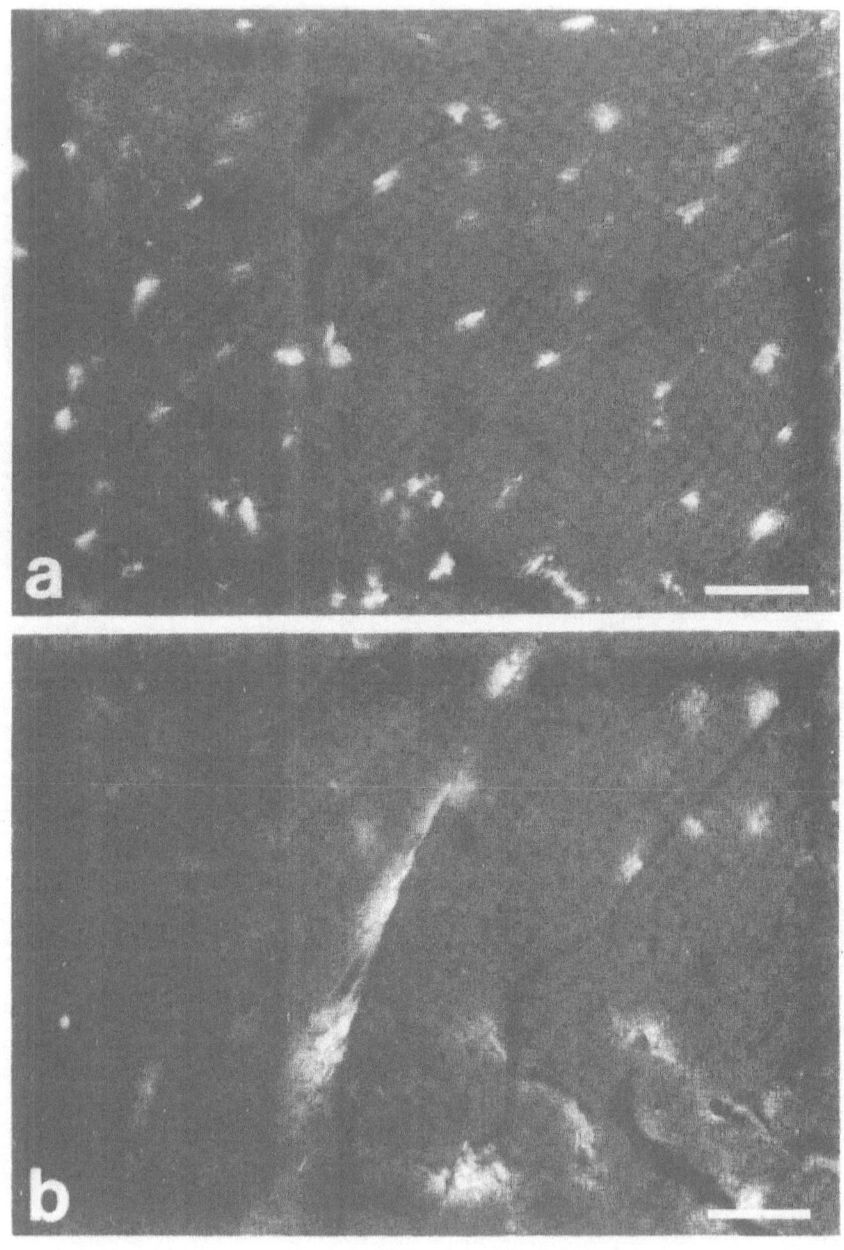

Figure 10.7 Pictures from areas of 'leaking' terminals in the border zone between the totally non-fluorescent ischaemic centre and the surrounding normal tissues. The pictures show two different stages of 'leakage'. In (b) it can also be noted that the specific fluorescence remains longer around the small myocardial vessels than in the myocardial muscle tissue. Calibration bars 50 μm.

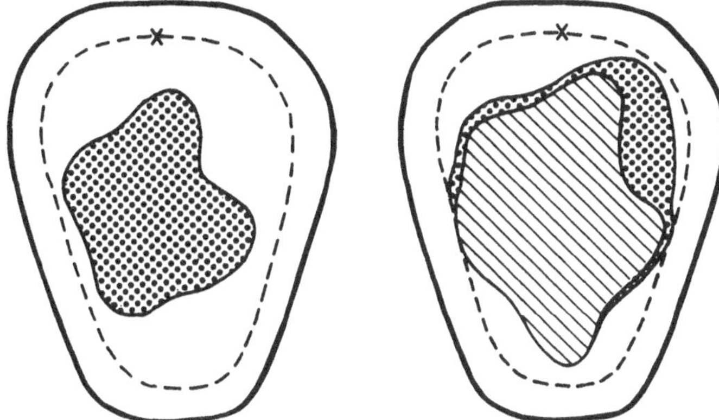

Figure 10.8 Schematic illustration of the rat left ventricular free wall demonstrating the approximate areas with reduced catecholamine fluorescence. The site of coronary artery ligation is indicated by the cross and the area not stained by trypan blue at the end of the experiment (ischaemic area) is demonstrated by the dashed circle. The dotted area represents myocardium with reduced fluorescence intensity and the dashed area shows regions completely devoid of catecholamine fluorescence. The areas represent the maximal distribution observed, which was located in the mid-portion of the thickness of the myocardium. The hearts presented in the figure are typical for saline-treated rats 0.5 h (to the left) and 2.5 h (to the right) after left coronary artery ligation.

of fluorescing terminals seemed to be more rapid in the myocardial tissue than around the blood vessels. The approximate sizes of the non-fluorescent area and the weakly fluorescent area (or border zone) after ligation are shown in figure 10.8.

Pretreatment of the animals with the ganglion blocking agent chlorisondamine did not change the effect of ligation compared to controls in four experiments, while in two experiments the area of decreased fluorescence was considerably less than in the controls.

10.5 VENTRICULAR NORADRENALINE CONTENT

The effect of chlorisondamine treatment and left coronary artery ligation on NA levels in the ventricular myocardium are summarised in figure 10.9. In the saline-treated rats a slight decrease in the LV NA content was observed after 0.5 h. This occurred both in sham-operated and ligated rats and amounted to 11 per cent (n.s.) and 16 per cent ($P < 0.05$) respectively. By increasing the time period of ischaemia to 2.5 h a marked reduction in the NA levels occurred. The NA content of RV was not significantly reduced during the experimental period.

In the chlorisondamine-treated rats, the LV NA content was unchanged 0.5 h after coronary artery ligation. However, an ischaemic period of 2.5 h caused a

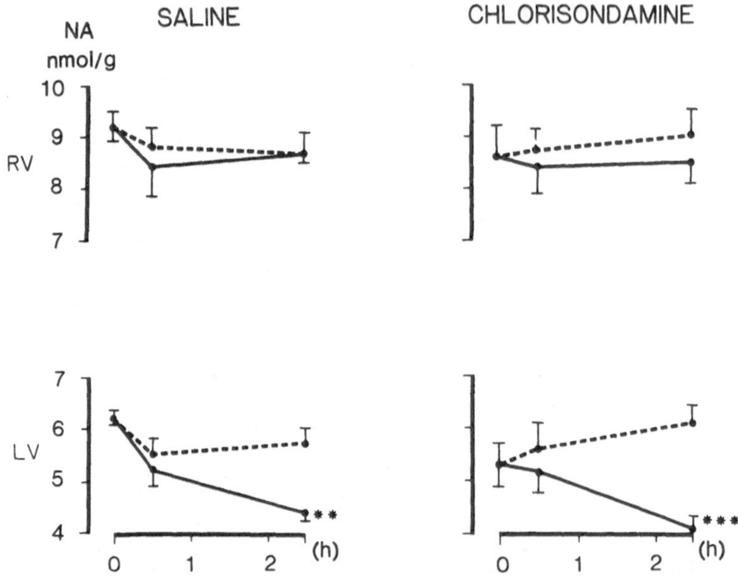

Figure 10.9 Noradrenaline (NA) content of the rat ventricular myocardium following sham operation (dashed line) or left coronary artery ligation (solid line) in saline- and chlorisondamine-treated animals. The myocardial NA content is expressed as nanomoles per gram tissue wet weight (mean ± S.E.), and is plotted against time (h) after sham operation or coronary artery occlusion. Abbreviations and symbols: RV, right ventricular free wall; LV, left ventricular free wall. $^{**}P < 0.02$ and $^{***}P < 0.002$ compared to sham-operated controls (Mann Whitney, two-tailed test).

reduction in LV NA content to the same level as in saline treated animals. In the sham-operated rats there was a tendency towards increased tissue NA content especially in the LV.

10.6 DISCUSSION

The noradrenergic innervation of the normal rat heart has been extensively studied. In general, there is a moderate density of adrenergic fibres, the atria being more densely innervated than the ventricles (Nielsen and Owman, 1968; Winckler, 1969). In a number of species the right ventricle has been reported to have a more dense innervation than the left (Nielsen and Owman, 1968; Angelakos *et al.*, 1969). A typical aggregation of fibres into a rather dense plexus around the arteries has also been described (Dahlström *et al.*, 1965; Nielsen and Owman, 1968; Krokhina, 1969; Winckler, 1969). In agreement with previous observations in the rat

(Winckler, 1969), we found the smaller arteries and arterioles to be heavily innervated, the plexa of these small vessels presenting a characteristic bipolar distribution.

In the rat, occlusion of the left coronary artery, a few millimetres distal to its origin, leads to an infarct involving a large part of the LV (Fishbein *et al.*, 1980; Spadaro *et al.*, 1980). In the isolated perfused rat heart, the acute flow reduction caused by left coronary ligation is most pronounced in the centre of the LV (Kannengiesser *et al.*, 1975). In the present study, ligation of the left coronary artery produced a decrease in the NA content of the ischaemic myocardium. This was demonstrated both by determination of tissue NA content and by the reduction in myocardial catecholamine fluorescence.

In the saline-treated control rats, a reduced catecholamine fluorescence was found in the centre of the LV 30 min after left coronary artery occlusion. After 2.5 and 5 h large areas of the ischaemic myocardium were completely devoid of fluorescent terminals. These findings are in agreement with the reported early disappearance of catecholamine fluorescence from the ischaemic dog myocardium (Vasku *et al.*, 1978). In contrast, previous fluorescence-histochemical studies in ischaemic rat hearts have not found such an early and pronounced decrease in myocardial catecholamine fluorescence (Penttilä *et al.*, 1974; Paessens and Borchard, 1980). These authors demonstrated the presence of small myocardial areas with a slight reduction in fluorescence 2-4 h after coronary artery occlusion. Large areas totally devoid of catecholamine fluorescence were not observed until after 12-24 h. This discrepancy cannot be explained at present, but a sex difference may be involved. In the present study we used male rats, whilst in both the above-cited studies female rats were used. Such a possible sex difference would be interesting in view of marked difference in incidence of myocardial infarction between men and women in the lower age groups (Pisa, 1980) and by the higher severity of arrhythmias following coronary artery occlusion in male rats (A. S. Harris, K. A. Kane and J. R. Parratt, unpublished) compared to female rats.

In the control group, after 30 min of ischaemia, small areas predominantly located in the centre of the LV were found to have a reduced catecholamine (CA) fluorescence. However, since at this time the tissue NA content was also slightly reduced in sham-operated rats, this decrease may reflect enhanced sympathetic nervous activity to the heart caused by the experimental preparation. Coronary artery occlusion for 2.5 h caused a marked reduction in the NA content of the left ventricle at a time when large areas of the ischaemic myocardium completely lacked CA fluorescence.

The degree of reduction in NA tissue content measured in the ischaemic myocardium was perhaps less than would be expected from the histochemical findings. However, neurones in areas lacking CA fluorescence may still contain some 5-10 per cent of the normal NA content. This is undetectable by the histochemical technique used (Sachs and Jonsson, 1973). In addition, the approximate areas with decreased or no fluorescent intensity (figure 10.8) represent the maximal distribution observed, which was located in the mid-region of the ventricular wall. In the outer epicardium and the subendocardium immediately adjacent to the ventricular cavity, normal or only slightly affected fluorescent terminals could be seen. Remaining CA fluorescence was also observed around small arteries and arterioles within the area with otherwise reduced fluorescence. The border between the normally fluorescent myocardial tissue and the areas where this fluorescence disappeared was generally quite sharp. With increased duration of ischaemia this border moves outward from the centre, but retains its sharp appearance. This observation suggests that the disappearance of fluorescence from each individual varicosity under the influence of ischaemia is a rapid process. The fluorescence disappearance after axotomy is also rapid (Malmfors and Sachs, 1965). With the present method we were unable to determine whether or not there was an increased fluorescence in adjacent myocardium; such an increase has been previously described (Paessens and Borchard, 1980) and is perhaps due to uptake into viable myocardium of NA released from 'leaking' nerve terminals in the ischaemic region.

The occasional observation of terminals in the border zone with a more diffuse fluorescence is an interesting finding. A similar appearance of adrenergic terminals may be seen after combined axotomy and the administration of a monoamine oxidase inhibitor (Malmfors, 1965). Thus, the diffuse terminals observed in our study may have been in the process of 'leaking' their monoamines, possibly due to a lack of sufficient energy for intraneuronal amine storage and for the membrane amine pump mechanisms. Monoamine oxidase, the main if not the only intraneuronal monoamine-catabolising enzyme, requires molecular oxygen for its action and its activity may therefore also be reduced in the ischaemic region (Blaschko, 1952). The fact that this picture was only occasionally seen may be due to the short time-span of the process (which would reduce the chances of observing leaking terminals) but another possibility is that the conditions required for such transmitter leakage are only occasionally met. If, for example, monoamine oxidase is fully active at the time when the transmitter-retaining properties of the neurone are lost, most of the transmitter would be inactivated by intraneuronal deamination. This explanation appears unlikely, however, as monoamine oxidase seems to be more sensitive to oxygen lack than the membrane processes of the adrenergic neurones (Malmfors, 1965). Furthermore, it is conceivable that ischaemia may sensitise certain terminals to some kind of fixation artefact. However, if the finding of such 'leaking' terminals is a true phenomenon, it is tempting to speculate that they are related to intense myocardial adrenoceptor activation and perhaps associated with the occurrence of ventricular arrhythmias and infarct development.

In the early stage of myocardial infarction in man, higher centres in the central nervous system are alerted and this may significantly influence autonomic output. Even in the anaesthetised animal basal reflex changes in sympathetic activity will occur (Malliani *et al.*, 1969; Brown and Malliani, 1971; Bosnjak *et al.*, 1979), although these may be blunted by anaesthesia. In the present study a ganglionic blocking agent was used to investigate whether the rapid release of myocardial NA following acute ischaemia can be explained solely by such reflex sympathetic activation or whether a local release from nerve terminals in the ischaemic area contributes. In the chlorisondamine group, the changes observed in CA fluorescence in the acutely ischaemic myocardium were essentially the same as in untreated rats. However, the size of the regions with reduced catecholamine fluorescence and the areas devoid of fluorescing terminals were more variable in the chlorisondamine group, both 0.5 and 2.5 h after coronary artery ligation. This clearly indicates that because a reduction in the CA fluorescence of the ischaemic myocardium was still observed after treatment with chlorisondamine, a locally mediated, nerve impulse-independent release of NA from the ischaemic sympathetic nerve terminals plays an important role. Our tentative conclusion from all these studies is that NA release in the ischaemic region is initially mediated by increased cardiac sympathetic drive and that later NA is also released by local factors such as reduced cellular pH and elevated extracellular K^+.

REFERENCES

Abrahamsson, T., Almgren, O. and Svensson, L. (1981). Local noradrenaline release in acute myocardial ischaemia: influence of catecholamines synthesis inhibition and β-adrenoceptor blockade on ischaemic injury. *J. cardiovasc. Pharmac.*, **3**, 807-17

Angelakos, E. T., King, M. P. and Millard, R. W. (1969). Regional distribution of catecholamines in the hearts of various species. *Ann. N.Y. Acad. Sci.*, **156**, 219-40

Blaschko, H. (1952). Amine oxidase and amine metabolism. *Pharmac. Rev.*, 415-58

Bosnjak, Z. J., Zuperku, E. J., Coon, R. L. and Kampine, J. P. (1979). Acute coronary artery occlusion and cardiac sympathetic afferent nerve activity. *Proc. Soc. exp. Biol. Med.*, **161**, 142-8

Brown, A. M. and Malliani, A. (1971). Spinal sympathetic reflexes initiated by coronary receptors. *J. Physiol., Lond.*, **212**, 685-705

Corr, P. B. and Gillis, R. A. (1978). Autonomic neural influences on the dysrhythmias resulting from myocardial infarction. *Circulation Res.*, **43**, 1-9

Dahlström, A., Fuxe, K., Mya-Tu, M. and Zetterström, B. E. M. (1965). Observations on adrenergic innervation of dog heart. *Am. J. Physiol.*, **209**, 689-92

Dutta, S. N. and Booker, W. M. (1970). Possible myocardial adaption to acute coronary occlusion: relation to catecholamines. *Archs int. Pharmacodyn. Thér.*, **185**, 5-12

Ebert, P. A., Allgood, R. J. and Sabiston, D. C. (1968). The antiarrhythmic effects of cardiac denervation. *Ann. Surg.*, **168**, 728-35

Eriksson, B. M. and Persson, B. A. (1982). Determination of catecholamines in rat heart tissue and plasma samples by liquid chromatography and electrochemical detection. *J. Chromatogr.*, **228**, 143-54

Falck, B. and Owman, C. (1965). A detailed methodological description of the fluorescence method for the cellular demonstration of biogenic monoamines. *Acta Univ. lund*, sect. II, no. 7, 1-32

Fishbein, M. C., Hare, C. A., Gissen, S. A., Spadaro, J., Maclean, D. and Maroko, P. R. (1980). Identification and quantification of histochemical border zones during the evolution of myocardial infarction in the rat. *Cardiovasc. Res.*, **14**, 41-9

Gromova, E. G. (1977). The changes of catecholamine content in the animal organs in experimental myocardial infarction under the influence of malaben. *Bull. eksp. Biol. Med., U.S.S.R.*, 7, 49-51

Hausler, G., Thoenen, H., Haefely, W. and Hurlimann, A. (1968). Electrical events in cardiac adrenergic nerves and noradrenaline release from the heart induced by acetylcholine and KCl. *Naunyn-Schmiedebergs Arch. Pharmak. exp. Path.*, **201**, 389-411

Hjalmarson, A. (1980). Myocardial metabolic changes related to ventricular fibrillation. *Cardiology*, **65**, 226-47

Kannengiesser, G. J., Lubbe, W. F. and Opie, L. H. (1975). Experimental myocardial infarction with left ventricular failure in the isolated perfused rat heart. Effects of isoproterenol and pacing. *J. molec. cell. Cardiol.*, 7, 135-51

Karlsberg, R. D., Penkoske, P. A., Cryer, P. E., Corr, P. B. and Roberts, R. (1979). Rapid activation of the sympathetic nervous system following coronary artery occlusion; relationship to infarct size, site and haemodynamic impact. *Cardiovasc. Res.*, **13**, 523-31

Krokhina, E. M. (1969). The adrenergic component of the effector heart innervation. *Acta anat.*, **74**, 214-27

Lammerant, J., Delterdt, P. and De Schryver, C. (1966). Direct release of myocardial catecholamines into the left heart chambers; the enhancing effect of acute coronary occlusion. *Arch. int. Pharmacodyn. Thér.*, **163**, 219-26

McGrath, B. P., Lim, S. P., Leversha, L. and Shanahan, A. (1981). Myocardial and peripheral catecholamine responses to acute coronary artery constriction before and after propranolol treatment in the anaesthetised dog. *Cardiovasc. Res.*, **15**, 28-34

Malliani, A., Schwartz, P. J. and Zanchetti, A. (1969). Reflex activity of single preganglionic sympathetic fibres during coronary occlusion. *Experientia*, **25**, 152-3

Malmfors, T. (1965). Studies on adrenergic nerves. The use of rat and mouse iris for direct observations on their physiology and pharmacology at cellular and subcellular levels. *Acta. physiol. scand.*, **64**, Suppl. 248, 1-93

Malmfors, T. and Sachs, C. (1965). Direct studies on the disappearance of the transmitter and changes in the uptake-storage mechanisms of degenerating adrenergic nerves. *Acta. physiol. scand.*, **64**, 211-23

Marshall, R. J. and Parratt, J. R. (1980). The early consequences of myocardial ischaemia and their modification. *J. Physiol., Paris*, **76**, 699-715

Mathes, P. O. and Gudjarnason, S. (1971). Changes in norepinephrine stores in the canine heart following experimental myocardial infarction. *Am. Heart J.*, **81**, 211-9

Nielsen, K. C. and Owman, C. (1968). Differences in cardiac adrenergic innervation between hibernators and non-hibernating mammals. *Acta physiol. scand.*, Suppl. 316, 1-30

Paessens, R. and Borchard, F. (1980). Morphology of cardiac nerves in experimental infarction of rat hearts. *Virchows Arch. A, Path. Anat. Histol.*, **386**, 265-78

Penttilä, A., Kormano, M., Ahonen, A., Juntunen, J. and Harkönen, M. (1974). The effects of left coronary artery ligation on rat heart muscle. Angiographic, morphologic and chemical studies. *Ann. Acad. scient. Fenn. A:V Med.*, **161**, 1-60

Pisa, Z. (1980). Sudden death: a worldwide problem. In *Sudden Death* ed. (H. E. Kulbertus and H. J. J. Wellens), Martinus Nijhoff, The Hague, pp. 3-10

Rogg, H. and Bucher, U. M. (1979). Effects of an isolated myocardial ischaemia in dogs on plasma catecholamines in the systemic and local coronary venous blood. *Naunyn-Schmiedebergs Arch. Pharmac.*, **307**, R42

Russel, R. A., Crafoord, J. and Harris, A. S. (1961). Changes in myocardial composition after coronary artery ligation. *Am. J. Physiol.*, **200**, 995-8

Sachs, C. and Jonsson, G. (1973). Quantitative microfluorimetric and neurochemical studies on degenerating adrenergic nerves. *J. Histochem. Cytochem.*, **21**, 902-11

Sethi, V., Haider, B., Ahmed, S. S., Oldewurtel, H. A. and Regan, T. J. (1973). Influence of beta blockade and chemical sympathectomy on myocardial function and arrhythmias in acute ischaemia. *Cardiovasc. Res.*, 7, 740-7

Shahab, L. and Wollenberger, A. (1967). Freisetzung von Noradrenalin aus dem isolierten durchströmten Herzen bei akuter Anoxie und nach Gabe von Stoffwechselgiften. *Acta biol. med. germ.*, **19**, 939-59

Shahab, L., Wollenberger, A., Hause, M. and Schiller, U. (1969). Noradrenalineabgabe aus dem Hundenherzen nach vorubergehender Okklusion einer Koronararterie. *Acta biol. med. germ.*, **22**, 135-43

Sheridan, D. J., Penkoske, P. A., Sobel, B. E. and Corr, P. B. (1980). Alpha-adrenergic contributions of dysrhythmia during myocardial ischemia and reperfusion in cats. *J. clin. Invest.*, **65**, 161-71

Spadaro, J., Fishbein, M. C., Hare, C., Pfeffer, M. A. and Maroko, P. R. (1980). Characterisation of myocardial infarcts in the rat. *Archs Path. Lab. Med.*, **104**, 179-83

Staszewska-Barczak, J. (1971). The reflex stimulation of catecholamine secretion dring the acute stage of myocardial infarction in the dog. *Clin. Sci.*, **41**, 419-39

Vasku, J., Dolezel, S., Sladek, T., Urbanek, E., Filkuka, J., Krcek, L. and Hartmannova, B. (1978). Monoaminergic metabolic activity in experimentally infarcted myocardium. *J. molec. cell. Cardiol.*, Suppl. 1, 10

Wakade, A. R. and Furchgott, R. F. (1968). Metabolic requirements for the uptake and storage of norepinephrine by the isolated left atrium of the guinea pig. *J. Pharmac. exp. Ther.*, **163**, 123-35

Winckler, J. (1969). Über die adrenergen Herznerven bei Ratte und Meerschweinchen. *Z. Zellforsch. mikrosk. Anat.*, **98**, 106-21

11

Early Arrhythmias Resulting from Acute Myocardial Ischaemia; Possible Role of Cyclic AMP

T. Podzuweit

11.1 INTRODUCTION

In 1964, Breckenridge showed that global brain ischaemia produced by decapitation caused a rapid increase in cerebral cyclic AMP (cAMP). Later, Wollenberger *et al.* (1969) found that cAMP also increases in the ischaemic heart. We proposed that this increase of myocardial cAMP might be a critical event in the genesis of ventricular arrhythmias and fibrillation (Podzuweit *et al.*, 1976). Prior to this hypothesis several other metabolic causes of arrhythmias had been suggested, such as the liberation of potassium ions from the heart (Harris *et al.*, 1954), the intracellular accumulation of free fatty acids and fatty acyl CoA (Kurien and Oliver, 1970; Liedtke *et al.*, 1978), lactic acidosis (Wissner, 1974), a decrease in glycolytical ATP production and local (Ebert *et al.*, 1970) and systemic (Clark and Cummings, 1956; Maling and Moran, 1957) catecholamine activity. Some of these hypotheses have been described in earlier chapters.

The value of the cAMP hypothesis was confirmed recently by the finding that the catecholamine-cAMP-Ca^{2+} system induces classical ventricular tachycardia in the intact non-ischaemic heart (Podzuweit, 1980; Podzuweit *et al.*, 1980). The factors responsible for cAMP accumulation in the myocardium remain elusive, although increasing emphasis is being placed on the role of adrenergic influences. The aim of the present paper is firstly, to review the evidence that supports the cAMP hypothesis and, secondly, to discuss arrhythmogenic and antiarrhythmic influences, including cholinergic intervention, which may have a bearing on cAMP and arrhythmias.

11.2 METHODS

Animal experiments

Baboons

Eleven Cape Chacma baboons (14-30 kg body weight) of either sex were immobilised by intramuscular injection of 25 mg phencyclidine hydrochloride and anaesthetised with pentobarbitone. Ventilation with room air from a Harvard respirator was controlled according to intermittent measurements of arterial blood gases. Limb lead electrocardiogram (lead II) and aortic blood pressure were recorded continuously. The chest was opened by mid-sternal incision and the heart was suspended in a pericardial cradle. The anterior descending coronary artery was then dissected. During the minute preceding ligation, two to three mini-drill biopsies (see below) were taken from different sites of the left ventricle. This was followed by abrupt ligation of the dissected artery two-thirds from its origin. At intervals throughout the experiments, repetitive biopsies were taken from the ischaemic and non-ischaemic zones of the left ventricle. There was no perforation of the ventricular wall. The ischaemic zone was delineated visually. Myocardial levels of creatine phosphate were used to confirm classification of biopsies as either ischaemic or non-ischaemic. The experiments were terminated shortly after the heart developed spontaneous ventricular fibrillation or 1 h following coronary artery ligation.

Dogs

Thirteen male mongrel dogs (20-30 kg body weight) were premedicated with 45 mg morphine sulphate (subcutaneous injection) and 75 mg promazine hydrochloride by intramuscular injection. Two dogs were studied without premedication. Anaesthesia was induced and maintained by an intravenous infusion of pentobarbitone. In seven dogs the anterior descending coronary artery was ligated two-thirds from its origin. In eight dogs proximal ligation of the anterior descending coronary artery was performed. Other experimental details were the same as for baboons.

Pigs

White Landrace Cross pigs (20-30 kg body weight) of either sex were studied. Anaesthesia was induced by injecting thiopentone sodium (20 mg kg^{-1} body weight) into a dorsal ear vein. Deep anaesthesia was maintained by intermittent infusion of pentobarbitone sodium into the femoral vein. A Manley respirator was used for mechanical respiration. Twenty-three experiments were used for arrhythmia analysis. In 15 additional experiments myocardial biopsies were taken. These biopsies were not taken sequentially, but at the end of an experiment (see Table 11.2). Other experimental detail was the same as for baboons. Myocardial maps of metabolites were obtained using pig hearts quick-frozen *in situ* (see below).

A unifocal subepicardial infusion technique was used for the chemical induction of ventricular arrhythmias in the *in situ* pig heart (figure 11.1). A 26 gauge hypodermic needle attached to Portex PP 25 tubing was inserted 1-5 mm into the left or right ventricular subepicardium. For the respective infusion of arrhythmogenic

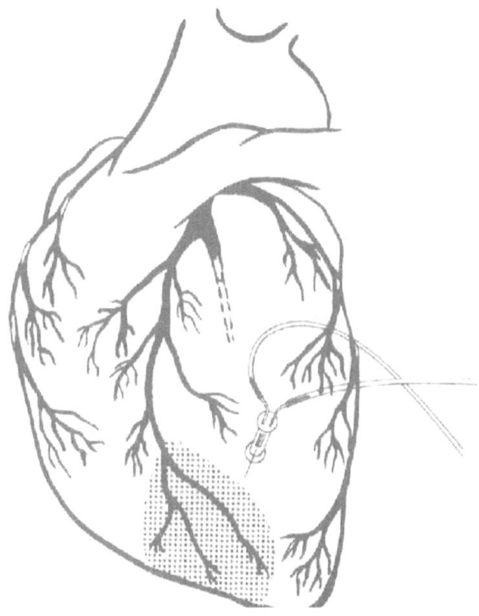

Figure 11.1 Induction of ventricular arrhythmias in the pig, first by abruptly ligating the anterior descending coronary artery two-thirds of the way from its origin and secondly by infusing agents which increase myocardial cAMP subepicardially close to the visible edge of ischaemia (shaded area).

and antiarrhythmic agents a double- or triple-inlet needle was used. Continuous infusion of agents precipitating arrhythmias was started using a Gilson Minipuls 2 peristaltic pump and the infusion rate was 10 μl min^{-1}. The chemicals were dissolved in either 150 mM or 2.5 mM $CaCl_2$-150 mM NaCl prepared from analytical grade salts and freshly distilled water. These solutions were neutralised with sodium hydroxide and the ionic composition was checked with the aid of flame photometry and atomic absorption spectrophotometry. Infusion of agents into the ischaemic heart was begun after the post-ligation arrhythmias had ceased, between 60 and 90 min post-ligation.

Rats

Male Long-Evans rats (200-350 g body weight), fed *ad libitum*, were anaesthetised with ether and given 200 units of heparin intravenously. Hearts were rapidly excised, arrested in ice-cold perfusion buffer and mounted on a Langendorff perfusion apparatus. The perfusion fluid was Krebs-Henseleit bicarbonate buffer ($K^+ = 5.9$ mmol l^{-1}) gassed with 95 per cent O_2 : 5 per cent CO_2 at 37 °C to maintain pH at 7.4. The substrates used were as follows: 11 mM glucose, 5 mM pyruvate, 5 mM acetate, 0.5 mM octanoate, 0.5 mM palmitate–0.1 mM bovine albumin, 0.9 mM palmitate-0.25 mM albumin, 0.9 mM palmitate-0.25 mM albumin plus 11 mM glucose, or 0.9 mM palmitate-0.25 mM albumin plus 22 mM glucose. Conjugation of palmitate to albumin was performed at ambient temperature using a Branson 12 ultrasonic bath. Each litre of conjugate was dialysed three times against 10 times its volume of substrate-free Krebs-Henseleit buffer at 4 °C. The dialysed and filtered conjugate was then split and one part supplemented with either 11 or 22 mM glucose. Perfusion was retrograde from a reservoir of 100 cm H_2O during normal perfusion. Ischaemic perfusion was effected by reducing the perfusion pressure to 20 cm H_2O. In reperfusion experiments the normal 100 cm H_2O perfusion pressure was reinstated after ischaemic 20 cm H_2O pressure perfusion. In all experiments there was a 15 min pre-perfusion period with substrate at 100 cm H_2O. This was followed by either ischaemic or normal perfusion, and reperfusion, with the respective substrates. The ischaemic period lasted either 30 or 45 min. The reperfusion period was 10-30 min. The electrocardiogram was recorded from one electrode on the metal aortic cannula and a wire hooked into the right ventricle. Aortic pressure pulses were recorded using a Statham pressure transducer. Observations of heart rate and coronary flow were made in 5 min intervals throughout the experiments. At the end of experiments hearts were quick-frozen by automatic freeze-clamping (see below).

Biopsy techniques

Drill biopsy

The drill biopsy technique of Pool *et al.* (1968) was modified by attaching a flange to the inside and outside of the hollow cutter to prevent perforation of the ventricular wall (figure 11.2(a)). The cutting tip of the drill was exchangeable to yield 10-50 mg of tissue. The sampling was rapid (less than 1 s elapsed from the time the biopsy tool touched the heart to the start of cooling the biopsy) and only caused superficial bleeding. Liquid nitrogen was used as refrigerant. There was no difference in the biopsy contents of ATP, creatine phosphate, lactate and cAMP when liquid nitrogen was replaced by melting Freon 502.

Core-drilling of frozen hearts

A biopsy technique was developed for hearts quick-frozen *in situ* with the aid of liquid nitrogen. The heart was contained in a plastic cradle made of surgical drapes to separate the freezing heart from the adjacent tissues. After 15 min immersion in liquid nitrogen the frozen heart was removed from the chest and transferred to a liquid nitrogen bath. These hearts were then biopsied while immersed in liquid nitrogen. Six millimetre deep biopsies were retrieved using an automated drill-press and special cutters coated with diamond dust (Gebr. Brasseler, Fabrik für Dental-instrumente Komet, Lemgo, FRG) (figure 11.2(b)). More experimental detail is provided in the captions to the tables and figures.

Automatic freeze-clamping

Isolated perfused rat hearts were quick-frozen using an automatic freeze-clamping device (Podzuweit *et al.*, 1978a). The clamp was triggered by a push-button-operated solenoid valve. Opposed pneumatic pistons fitted with aluminium caps previously cooled in liquid nitrogen (figure 11.2(c)) were used to compress the rat myocardium to a 2 mm thick wafer. The freezing time for such wafers was calculated to be 0.9 s.

Biochemical analysis

Myocardial biopsies were analysed for ATP, creatine phosphate, lactate, cAMP and cyclic GMP (cGMP). The frozen biopsies were weighed and extracted into 0.5 ml ice-cold 5 per cent (w/w) perchloric acid using an Ultra-Turrax blender. The extracts were centrifuged for 2 min in an Eppendorf model 5412 centrifuge at 8000*g*. The supernatants were neutralised with 5 N KOH and the $KClO_4$ precipitates removed by centrifugation to yield clear extracts. The metabolites were measured from these extracts without further purification. cAMP and cGMP were measured by protein binding and radioimmunoassay, respectively. Lactate was measured fluorometrically by a modification of the method of Hohorst *et al.* (1959). ATP and creatine phosphate were assayed either by the firefly bioluminiscence method of Stanley and Williams (1969) or fluorometrically by means of the hexokinase/glucose-6-phosphate dehydrogenase reaction. Metabolite levels of dog, pig and baboon myocardium were expressed as moles per gram wet weight. Rat heart metabolite levels were expressed in terms of fresh weight (= dry weight × 5) to correct for oedema formation. The appropriate correction factor was obtained by drying a known weight of rat myocardium at 90 °C.

Statistical analysis

Results were expressed as mean values ± S.E.M. or S.D. for the number of observations. *P* values were calculated by comparing means according to the method of Scheffe (1959), following single classification analysis of variance or using Student's *t* test for unpaired observations.

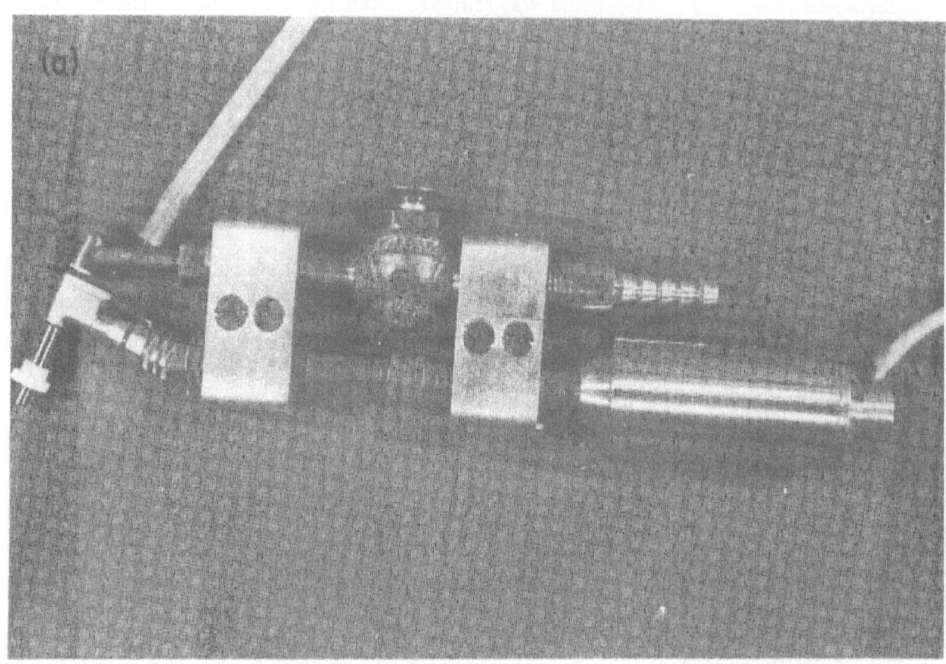
(a)

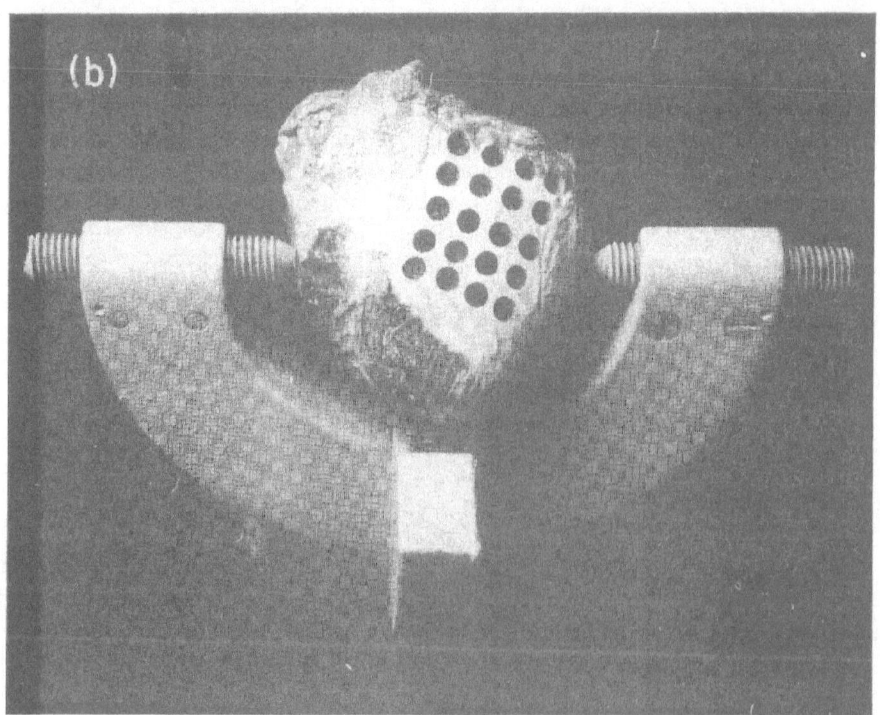
(b)

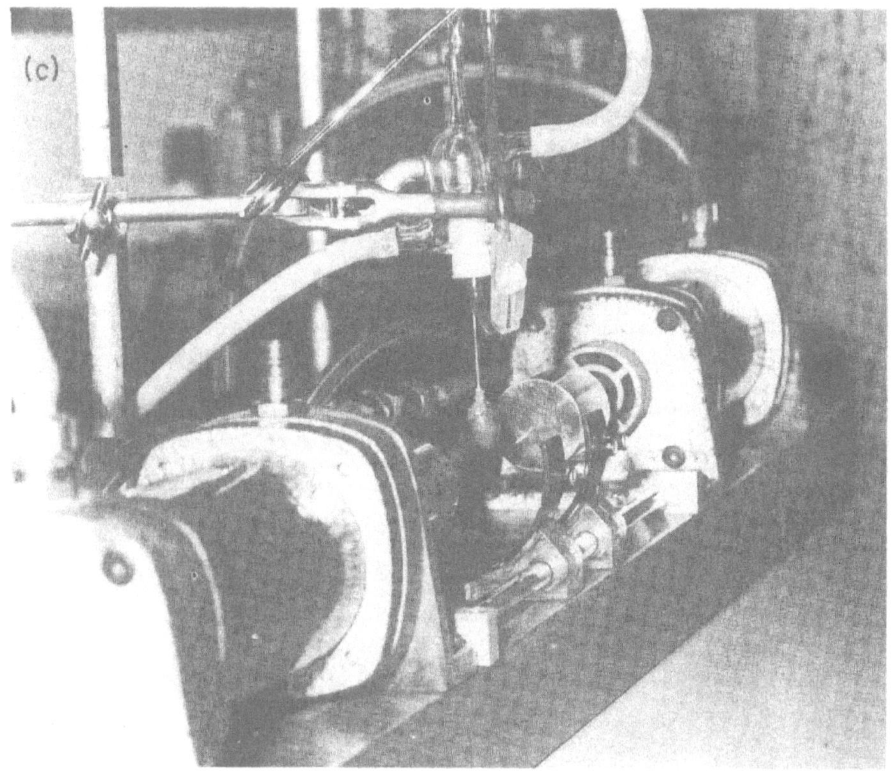

Figure 11.2 Myocardial biopsy techniques.

(a) Drill biopsy device according to Pool *et al.* (1968) assembled from the following parts: Minitech dental engine, type 'regulable' TR 650, including disposable motor TR 610 (Dentimex, Zeist, Netherlands), contra-angle shank 195 (Kaltenbach & Voigt, Biberach, FRG), standard air cut-off valve (local supplier). The device is shown with the vacuum line but the pressure line has been dismantled. The device can be operated with a foot control switch.

(b) Pig heart with ligation of the anterior descending coronary artery two-thirds of the way from its origin, quick-frozen with the aid of liquid refrigerant and biopsied while immersed in liquid nitrogen. The heart is presented within a spherical aluminium clamp. The dark area represents infarcting myocardium.

(c) Pneumatic quick-freeze clamping device mounted on a cast-iron base. An isolated perfused rat heart is situated between the aluminium clamps, previously cooled in liquid nitrogen. On opening a solenoid valve compressed air causes the pistons to collide. Frozen rat heart wafers of 2 mm thickness are obtained. The calculated freezing time was 0.95 s (Podzuweit *et al.*, 1978a).

11.3 RESULTS

Myocardial ischaemia and ventricular fibrillation in the baboon

Ligation of the anterior descending coronary artery two-thirds of the way from its origin precipitated ventricular fibrillation within 35-55 min in eight out of 11 baboons. A single experiment is shown in figure 11.3. After a period of steady

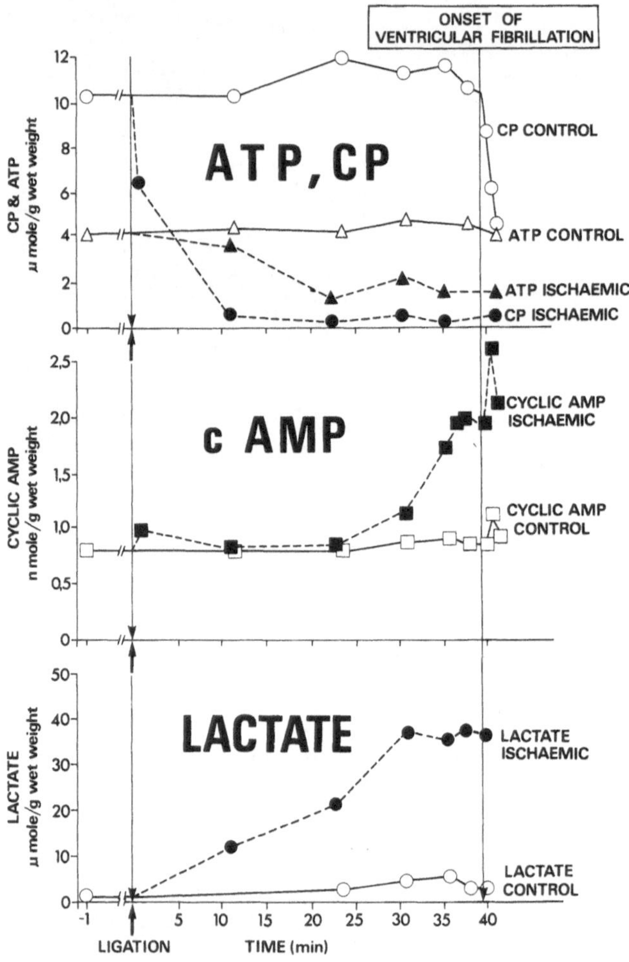

Figure 11.3 Levels of ATP, creatine phosphate, cAMP and lactate in the non-ischaemic (open symbols) and ischaemic (closed symbols) myocardium following abrupt ligation of the anterior descending coronary artery (two-thirds of the way from its origin) in an 18 kg male baboon. Note the late increase of cAMP in the ischaemic myocardium starting about 10 min before the onset of ventricular fibrillation. Similar results were obtained in other baboons.

cAMP levels in the ischaemic zone there was a consistent increase in cAMP starting approximately 10 min before the onset of ventricular fibrillation. This increase occurred later than the increase in myocardial lactate. There was no accumulation of cAMP or lactate in non-ischaemic tissue. Depletion of creatine phosphate in the ischaemic zone was complete within 10 min after ligation followed by a slower decrease of ATP. ATP and creatine phosphate levels in non-ischaemic myocardium remained constant. After the onset of global ischaemia produced by ventricular fibrillation, creatine phosphate in previously non-ischaemic myocardium decreased within seconds.

The relationship between cAMP levels in ischaemic heart tissue of six baboons and the onset of ventricular fibrillation is illustrated in figure 11.4. There was again

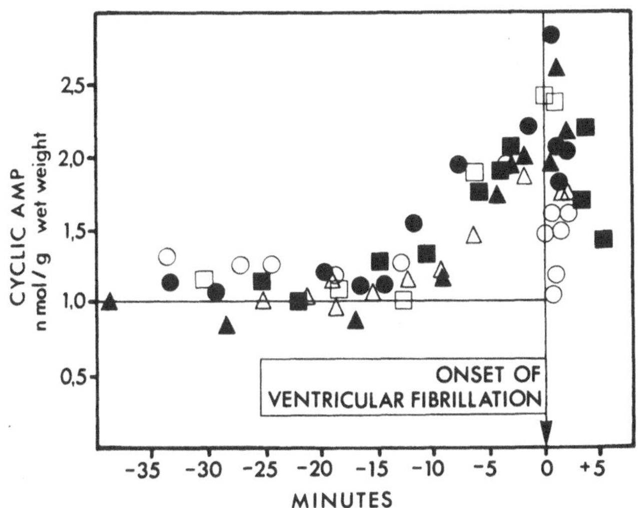

Figure 11.4 cAMP levels in the ischaemic myocardium of six baboons, developing ventricular fibrillation within 1 h of ligation of the anterior descending coronary artery two-thirds of the way from its origin. Data are plotted in relation to the onset of ventricular fibrillation (0 min). A specific symbol is assigned to each baboon. The horizontal line represents the mean cAMP level in non-ischaemic myocardium (1.0 nmol g^{-1} wet weight). Note the consistent increase of myocardial cAMP in the ischaemic zone starting approximately 10 min before the onset of ventricular fibrillation

a consistent increase of cAMP in the ischaemic zone starting approximately 10 min before ventricular fibrillation. Statistical analyses revealed that this increase of cAMP was associated with the onset of ventricular fibrillation rather than the onset of ligation (Podzuweit *et al.*, 1978b). Three baboons survived the first hour after coronary artery ligation and showed no comparable increase of myocardial cAMP.

Myocardial ischaemia and ventricular arrhythmias in the pig

Additional evidence for an arrhythmogenic role of cAMP was obtained by using White Landrace Cross pigs. The advantage of using pigs was that ligation of the anterior descending coronary artery two-thirds of the way from its origin produced an increased frequency of ventricular arrhythmias rather than an all or nothing ventricular fibrillation.

Arrhythmia distribution

Ligation of the anterior descending coronary artery in the pig precipitated ventricular arrhythmias, starting approximately 20 min after ligation. This was observed in all pigs studied and is illustrated in figure 11.5. Seven pigs (30 per cent) deve-

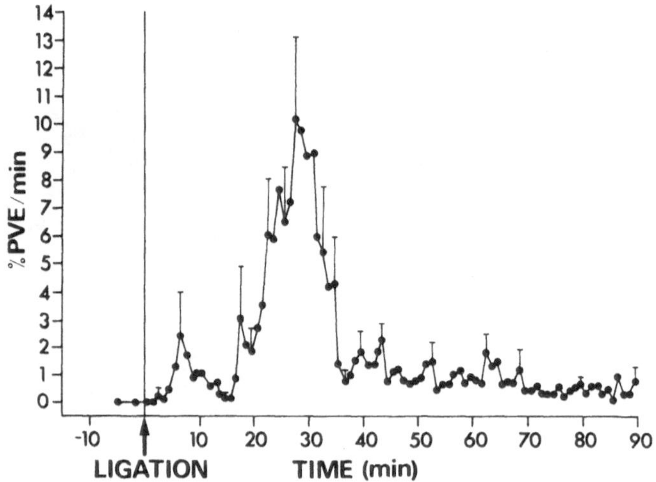

Figure 11.5 Frequency distribution of premature ventricular extrasystoles following ligation of the anterior descending coronary artery two-thirds of the way from its origin in the pig (n = 23 animals). The ordinate indicates the number of premature ventricular extrasystoles per minute as a percentage of the heart rate. Vertical bars represent standard errors of the mean.

loped ventricular fibrillation, while 16 pigs developed a cluster of ventricular arrhythmias lasting approximately 10–20 min. There were no arrhythmias immediately associated with coronary artery ligation. In the majority of experiments the heart rhythm was regular until 20 min post-ligation. In five pigs there was an early episode of premature ventricular extrasystoles between 3 and 12 min post-ligation and in two of these pigs this early arrhythmic episode included ventricular bigeminy. The major arrhythmias ceased between 35 and 45 min post-ligation. Ninety minutes post-ligation the heart rhythm was again normal.

The observed arrhythmias consisted of premature ventricular extrasystoles, bigeminal rhythm, repetitive extrasystoles in pairs, ventricular tachycardia and ventricular fibrillation. Supra-ventricular arrhythmias were not encountered. Five of the episodes of ventricular fibrillation occurred between 16 and 26 min post-ligation. One pig developed ventricular fibrillation 7 min after ligation and one pig 46 min after ligation.

Biochemical analysis of single biopsies

Biochemical analysis of epicardial to mid-myocardial mini-drill biopsies obtained from the left ventricular free wall of the beating pig heart showed a time-dependent variation of cAMP and lactate levels in the ischaemic zone after coronary artery ligation (Podzuweit and Lubbe, 1977; Podzuweit *et al.*, 1981). cAMP levels in the anticipated ischaemic region averaged 0.99 nmol g^{-1} wet weight prior to ligation (Table 11.1). At 20 min post-ligation, cAMP had increased by 63 per cent of its pre-ligation value. Duing the same period myocardial lactate levels increased approximately 10 times. These high levels of cAMP and lactate coincided with the

Table 11.1 Myocardial levels of cAMP and lactate within 90 min of ligation of the anterior descending coronary artery two-thirds of the way from its origin in the pig

Time of biopsy before (−) and after (+) ligation (min)	cAMP (nmol g^{-1} wet weight)	Lactate (μmol g^{-1} wet weight)
− 1	0.99 ± 0.05^1	3.2 ± 1.7^4 (4)
+ 20	1.62 ± 0.32^2	34.1 ± 4.0^5 (6)
+ 90	0.90 ± 0.24^3	45.8 ± 9.7^6 (5)

1 vs 2, $P < 0.01$; 2 vs 3, $P < 0.005$; 1 vs 3, n.s.; 4 vs 5, $P < 0.001$; 4 vs 6, $P < 0.001$; 5 vs 6, $P < 0.05$.

Epicardial biopsies were taken from the apical portion of the anterior free wall of the left ventricle of four pigs without coronary artery ligation. Additional biopsies were taken from the ischaemic zone of six pigs at 20 min post ligation and from the ischaemic zone of five other pigs at 90 min post ligation.

Values are means ± S.D. (number of pigs in parentheses). P values were calculated by comparing means according to the method of Scheffe (1959) following single classification analysis of variance.

onset of arrhythmias. At 90 min post-ligation cAMP levels in the ischaemic zone were decreased to pre-ligation levels. In contrast, lactate levels in the ischaemic zone had further increased from their 20 min post-ligation levels.

Myocardial mapping

A special biopsy technique was developed to pursue the above findings. This technique was based upon our observation that quick-freezing of pig hearts *in situ* with the aid of melting Freon 502 or liquid nitrogen is sufficiently rapid to preserve levels of labile metabolites such as cAMP, lactate and ATP within the outer 6 mm layer of the myocardium in a state close to that existing *in vivo*. This allowed us to obtain myocardial cAMP, lactate and ATP maps at different times after ligation.

The cAMP map of a quick-frozen control heart is shown in figure 11.6(a). The mean myocardial contents of cAMP was 1.09 nmol g^{-1} wet weight and was not different to values found with the dental drill technique. The highest cAMP value found in this map was 1.29 nmol g^{-1} wet weight.

Twenty minutes post-ligation, when the first arrhythmias ensued, there was an increase of cAMP in the ischaemic zone (figure 11.6(b)). For example, some of the values were 1.56, 1.60, 1.52 and 1.62 nmol g^{-1} wet weight. This increase of cAMP was non-uniform and some areas of slightly increased cAMP levels (for example, 1.39 and 1.35 nmol g^{-1} wet weight) were also found in non-ischaemic tissue, close to the visible edge of ischaemia.

By 90 min post-ligation the arrhythmias had stopped (figure 11.5) and cAMP levels in the ischaemic area were now below those found in the non-ischaemic zone (figure 11.6(c)). Values such as 0.80, 0.69 and 0.71 nmol g^{-1} wet weight were common. There was no difference in dry weight to wet weight ratio between the ischaemic and non-ischaemic myocardium.

ATP levels in the ischaemic zone had decreased by 20 min post-ligation to about 50 per cent of the mean pre-ligation value of 3.6 ± 0.4 mol g^{-1} wet weight ($n = 40$ biopsies; figure 11.7(a) and (b)). Ninety minutes post-ligation ATP stores were practically exhausted in the ischaemic region (figure 11.7(c)).

Twenty minutes after ligation myocardial lactate was increased in the ischaemic zone (figure 11.8(b)) and 90 min post-ligation this increase was even more marked (figure 11.8(c)). Relative to the increase of myocardial cAMP this increase of lactate was uniform and was confined to the ischaemic area. The mean myocardial lactate content in non-ischaemic tissue 20 min post-ligation was 1.1 ± 0.4 μmol g^{-1} wet weight ($n = 26$ biopsies) and 90 min post-ligation was 2.5 ± 1.4 μmol g^{-1} wet weight ($n = 25$ biopsies). The respective mean values in ischaemic tissue were 25.6 ± 2.5 μmol g^{-1} wet weight ($n = 11$ biopsies) and 36.5 ± 2.3 μmol g^{-1} wet weight ($n = 15$ biopsies; mean ± S.D.)

Chemical induction of arrhythmias

Arrhythmias were induced in the ischaemic pig heart 90 min after coronary artery ligation (at a time when myocardial cAMP levels were low) by infusing various agents which increase myocardial cAMP subepicardially close to the visible edge of ischaemia (figure 11.1). Ventricular tachycardia was the most commonly induced arrhythmia. In some experiments, however, premature ventricular extrasystoles prevailed (Podzuweit *et al.*, 1981).

A typical arrhythmia induction experiment is shown in figure 11.9. Approximately 60 s after commencing the subepicardial infusion of 10^{-5} M noradrenaline VT ensued, precipitating a fall in blood pressure. This tachycardia could be maintained for several minutes, it was reversed to sinus rhythm within 1-5 min after

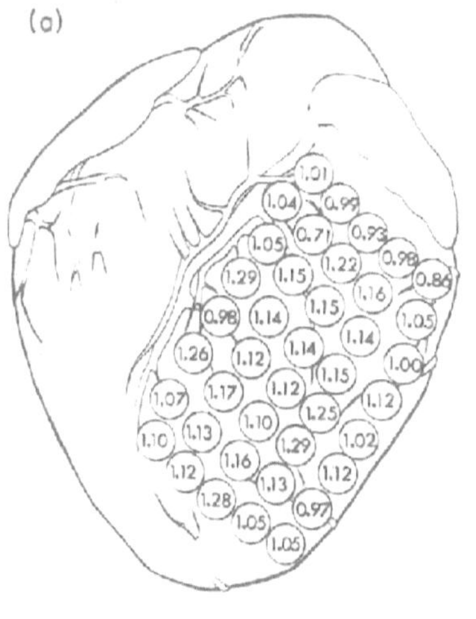

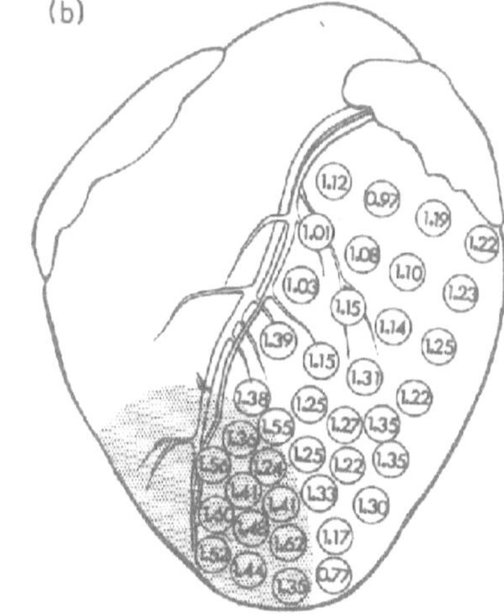

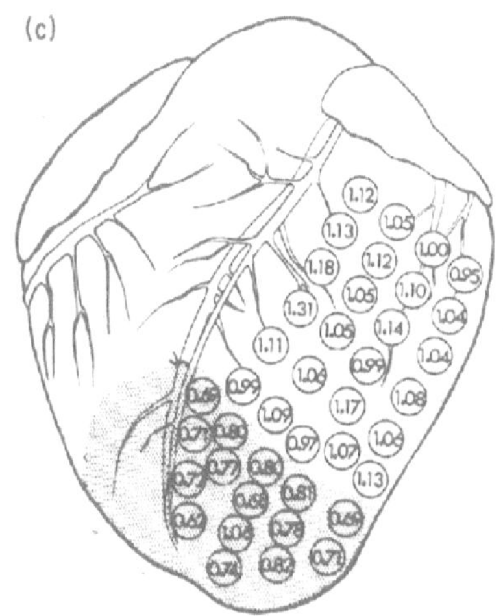

Figure 11.6 Myocardial maps of cAMP of pig hearts frozen *in situ* by immersion in liquid nitrogen (cf. figure 11.2(b)). The hearts were frozen prior to ligation (a), 20 min post-ligation (b) and 90 min post-ligation (c).

terminating the infusion. These experiments were readily reproducible. Ventricular arrhythmias could be induced repeatedly without changing the infusion site.

It was next demonstrated that catecholamines also induce ventricular tachycardia when infused subepicardially into the non-ischaemic pig heart (Podzuweit, 1980; Podzuweit *et al.*, 1980). This arrhythmogenic effect of noradrenaline, which was enhanced by increasing $[Ca^{2+}]_o$, could thus be ascribed to a local effect of the catecholamine.

The effect of the infusion of noradrenaline/calcium solutions on myocardial levels of cAMP and of cGMP was then examined (table 11.2). At the onset of ventricular tachycardia, myocardial cAMP at the infusion sites had increased by approximately 45 per cent relative to the adjacent control tissue ($P < 0.001$). These

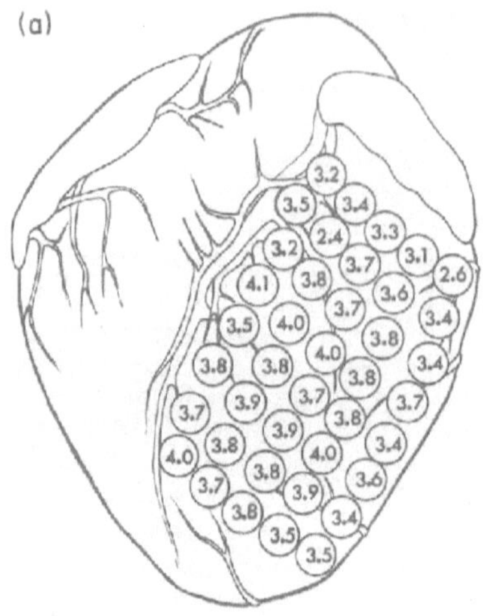

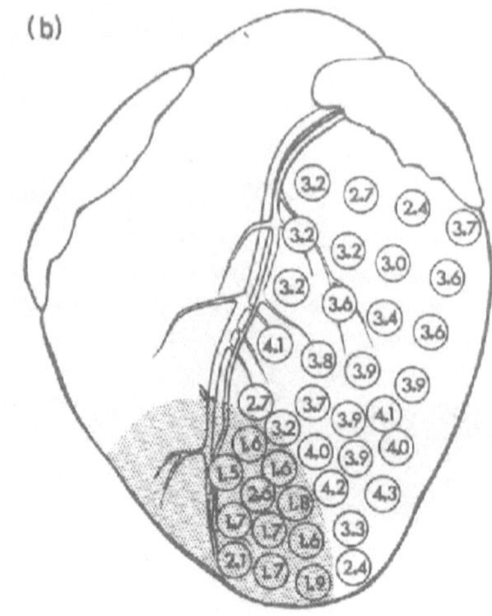

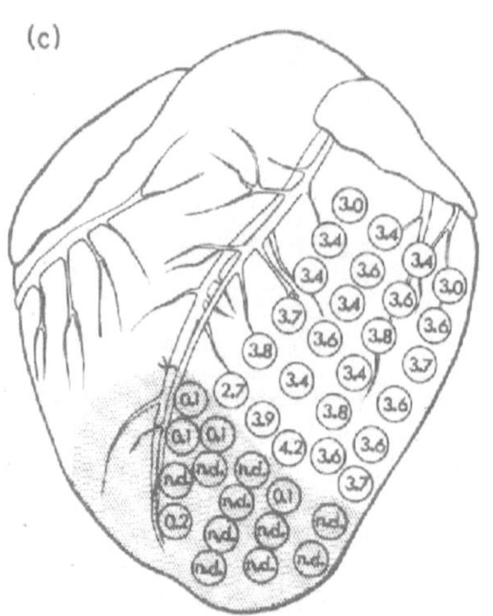

Figure 11.7 Myocardial maps of ATP of pig hearts frozen *in situ* by immersion in liquid nitrogen (cf. figure 11.2(b)). The hearts were frozen prior to ligation (a), 20 min post-ligation (b) and 90 min post-ligation (c).

increased cAMP levels were confined to 4 mm diameter cores around the infusion sites; there was no effect on myocardial cGMP levels. Previous investigations had shown that ATP levels at the infusion site remained constant during the arrhythmia induction period of 60 s (Podzuweit *et al.*, 1980).

We then began to examine the effects on cardiac rhythm in the normal heart of other agents related to cAMP. Some of these agents were found to be active only in the ischaemic heart. The results of these experiments are summarised in figure 11.10. The centre position in this scheme is taken by cAMP. Grouped around it are agents which were found to be either arrhythmogenic or antiarrhythmic. Adrenaline, noradrenaline (10^{-5} M each) and isoprenaline (10^{-6} M) were found to be potent arrhythmogenic agents. Dopamine (10^{-3} M) was effective only in the

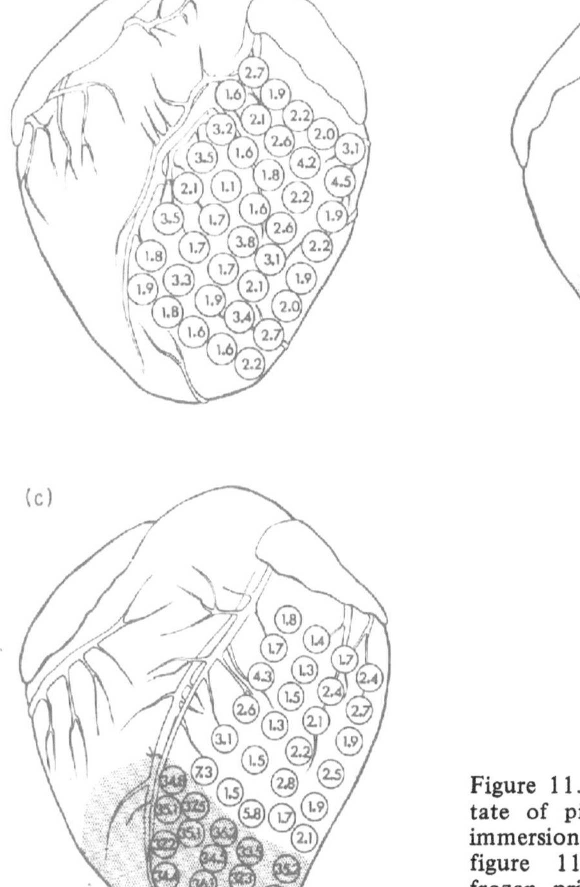

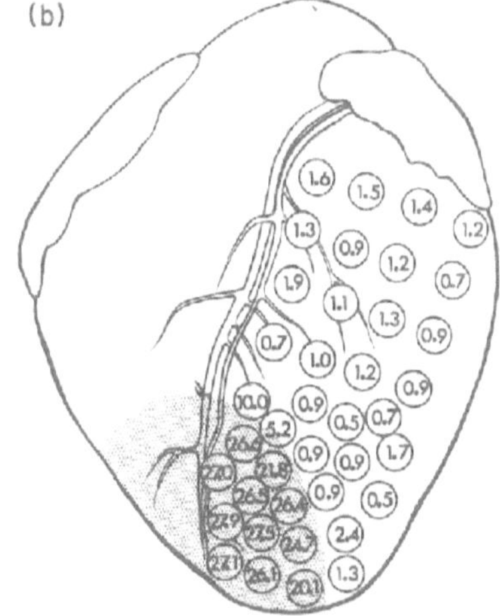

Figure 11.8 Myocardial maps of lactate of pig hearts frozen *in situ* by immersion in liquid nitrogen (cf. figure 11.2(b)). The hearts were frozen prior to ligation (a), 20 min post-ligation (b) and 90 min post-ligation (c).

ischaemic heart. We have presented evidence that noradrenaline increases myocardial cAMP at the infusion site and that this coincides with the onset of arrhythmias (table 11.2). The butyryl analogues of cAMP, N^6-monobutyryl-cAMP and $N^6,O^{2'}$-dibutyryl-cAMP (5×10^{-2} M each) produced severe and persistent arrhythmias (see also Podzuweit, 1980). In contrast, neither infusion of sodium butyrate (100 mM) nor N^6-monobutyryl-2′-deoxy-cAMP (5×10^{-2} M) precipitated arrhythmias, nor did infusion of another butyryl analogue of cAMP, $O^{2'}$-monobutyryl-cAMP. The catecholamine arrhythmias were abolished by β-adrenoceptor blockade. The order of potencies of such agents in abolishing VT induced by subepicardial infusion of a solution containing 10^{-5} M noradrenaline and 2.5 mM $CaCl_2$ in 150 mM NaCl was pindolol (10^{-6} M) > D,L-propranolol (10^{-4} M) > di-

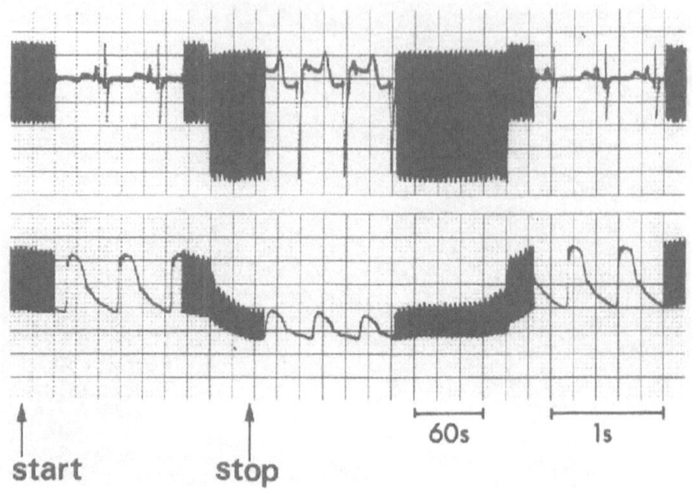

Figure 11.9 Induction of ventricular tachycardia in the infarcting pig heart by the subepicardial infusion, close to the visible edge of ischaemia of 10^{-5} M noradrenaline dissolved in 150 mM NaCl. The infusion rate was 10 μl min^{-1}. The ECG (lead II) (upper trace) and aortic blood pressure (lower trace) are shown. The recording speeds were 0.25 mm s^{-1} and 25 mm s^{-1}. The blood pressure calibration was 20 mmHg per division.

Table 11.2 Levels of myocardial cyclic nucleotides at the onset of ventricular tachycardia, induced by a 60 s infusion of a mixture of 10^{-5} M noradrenaline and 2.5 mM $CaCl_2$ in 150 mM NaCl

Biopsy site	cAMP (nmol g^{-1} wet weight)	cGMP (nmol g^{-1} wet weight)
Control	1.04 ± 0.04[1] (6)	0.042 ± 0.003[2] (6)
Infusion site	1.49 ± 0.08[1] (6)	0.041 ± 0.010[2] (6)

1, $P < 0.001$; 2, n.s. P calculated using Student's t test for unpaired observations.

Noradrenaline (10^{-5} M) and 2.5 mM $CaCl_2$ in 150 mM NaCl was infused at six subepicardial sites of the left ventricle. The infusion depth was 5 mm and the infusion rate 10 μl min^{-1}. The heart was contained in a plastic cradle made of surgical drapes. As soon as tachycardia commenced the heart was immersed in liquid nitrogen. The frozen heart was then transferred to a liquid nitrogen bath and subjected to core-drilling after the infusion needles had been removed. The retrieved tissue cores (approximately 6 mm length, 4 mm diameter) were analysed for cAMP and cGMP. Values are means ± S.D. (number of biopsies in parentheses).

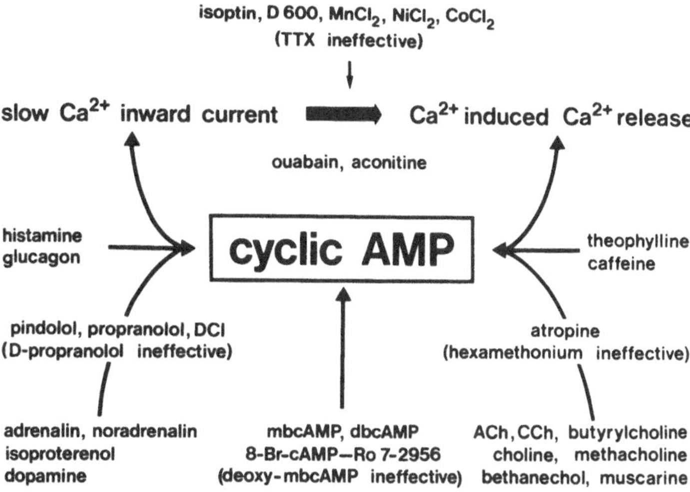

Figure 11.10 Hypothetical scheme for the induction of ventricular arrhythmias by cAMP. This scheme was derived from subepicardial infusion experiments in the pig. For details see text.

chloroisoproterenol (10^{-3} M). Relative to D,L-propranolol, D-propranolol was ineffective. Administration of β-adrenoceptor blocking drugs in the above concentrations did not inhibit arrhythmias induced by butyryl analogues of cAMP (5×10^{-2} M). The induction of arrhythmias was facilitated by inhibitors of cyclic nucleotide phosphodiesterase. For example, tachycardia could be induced by infusing a mixture of 8-Br-cAMP (5×10^{-2} M) and Ro 7-2956 (5×10^{-4} M): neither agent alone had such an effect. Theophylline and caffeine (5×10^{-2} M each) precipitated ventricular arrhythmias when infused into the ischaemic myocardium. The same was true for histamine and glucagon (10^{-3} M each).

Calcium (2.5 mM $CaCl_2$) facilitated the induction of arrhythmias without itself producing arrhythmias. Arrhythmias induced by either 10^{-5} M noradrenaline or by 5×10^{-2} M N^6-butyryl-cAMP were inhibited by calcium antagonists such as isoptin. D 600 (10^{-4} M each) and $MnCl_2$ (5×10^{-4} M). In addition, $NiCl_2$ and $CoCl_2$ (2.5×10^{-3} M each) were found to be effective in preventing arrhythmias induced by the infusion of noradrenaline and $CaCl_2$. These agents inhibit the transsarcolemmal slow inward current, primarily carried by calcium ions (Kohlhardt *et al.*, 1972). Tetrodotoxin (up to 10^{-5} M), which blocks the fast inward sodium current, did not protect against noradrenaline/calcium arrhythmias.

Acetylcholine is known to antagonise some effects of catecholamines by decreasing sarcolemmal calcium inflow (Ten Eick *et al.*, 1976). In our experiments choline esters (for example, acetylcholine (10^{-4} M), carbamylcholine (10^{-6} M), butyrylcholine (10^{-4} M)), β-methylcholine esters (for example, methacholine (10^{-6} M) and bethanechol (10^{-5} M)) and muscarine (10^{-6} M) proved to be potent antiarrhythmic agents. Choline abolished VT induced by noradrenaline/calcium at higher concentrations (10^{-2} M). This effect was blocked by atropine (10^{-6} M) but not by hexamethonium (up to 10^{-4} M). Biochemical analysis revealed that choline esters in the absence of atropine attenuate the accumulation of myocardial cAMP during noradrenaline/calcium infusions (Podzuweit, 1982).

Ouabain (10^{-5} M) and aconitine (10^{-6} M) were two other agents which precipitated ventricular arrhythmias in the intact heart. There is no evidence which linked this action with cAMP accumulation. It is, however, possible that these agents increase cellular calcium uptake by a cAMP-independent mechanism. This supposition is supported by the finding that ouabain arrhythmias are abolished by calcium antagonists (verapamil, $MnCl_2$). In addition, recent electrophysiological studies have shown that strophanthidin increases the slow calcium inward current (Weingart *et al.*, 1978).

Myocardial ischaemia in the dog

In contrast to the pig and baboon experiments ventricular fibrillation did not occur in dogs after ligation of the anterior descending coronary artery two-thirds of the way from its origin. There was also no accumulation of myocardial cAMP within the 60 min period studied (Podzuweit *et al.*, 1978b). This absence of cAMP accumulation seemed to be related to the less severe ischaemia in the epicardial to midmyocardial region in this species in comparison with pigs and baboons. This was judged from the less severe depletion of myocardial ATP and creatine phosphate (Podzuweit *et al.*, 1978b). In contrast, proximal ligation of the anterior descending coronary artery precipitated ventricular fibrillation within 1-3 min in seven out of eight dogs. In four of these dogs ventricular fibrillation was preceded by accumulation of myocardial cAMP. In one dog in which an increase in cAMP did not occur, the last biopsy was taken 1 min before the onset of fibrillation; a later increase in cAMP cannot thus be excluded. In two other dogs with low levels of cAMP 30-64 s before ventricular fibrillation, fibrillation appeared to be precipitated by an unsuccessful biopsy.

Arrhythmias resulting from global ischaemia in the isolated perfused rat heart

Global ischaemia produced by decreasing the perfusion pressure in rat hearts retrogradely perfused, according to the Langendorff technique, with non-glucose substrates, led to marked accumulation of myocardial cAMP within 30-45 min of ischaemia (tables 11.3 and 11.4). This increase was pronounced in hearts perfused with 5 mM pyruvate, 5 mM acetate, 0.5 mM octanoate, 0.5 mM palmitate-0.1 mM albumin or 0.9 mM palmitate-0.25 mM albumin and did not occur in hearts perfused with 11 mM glucose. Upon re-establishing the normal perfusion pressure (100 cm H_2O) ventricular arrhythmias ensued (see also Bricknell and Opie, 1978). These were most severe in hearts with increased myocardial cAMP. The arrhythmogenic effect of ischaemic perfusion with palmitate conjugated to albumin was

Table 11.3 Effects of substrates and perfusion pressure on myocardial levels of cAMP, ATP and creatine phosphate in isolated perfused rat hearts

Substrate	cAMP (nmol g^{-1} fresh weight)		ATP (μmol g^{-1} fresh weight)		Creatine phosphate (μmol g^{-1} fresh weight)	
	100 cm	20 cm	100 cm	20 cm	100 cm	20 cm
11 mM glucose	0.42 ± 0.10[1] (6)	0.48 ± 0.06[6] (6)	4.2 ± 0.4[11] (6)	4.2 ± 0.1[16] (6)	3.6 ± 0.5[21] (6)	4.7 ± 0.5[26] (6)
5 mM pyruvate	0.51 ± 0.08[2] (6)	0.68 ± 0.17[7] (11)	4.5 ± 0.4[12] (6)	3.8 ± 0.6[17] (11)	7.8 ± 1.2[22] (6)	6.3 ± 1.5[27] (11)
5 mM acetate	0.53 ± 0.06[3] (6)	0.78 ± 0.13[8] (6)	4.1 ± 0.5[13] (6)	1.7 ± 0.8[18] (6)	6.6 ± 0.9[23] (6)	3.9 ± 1.6[28] (6)
0.5 mM octanoate	0.47 ± 0.05[4] (5)	0.87 ± 0.16[9] (6)	4.2 ± 0.1[14] (5)	1.7 ± 1.1[19] (6)	4.9 ± 0.4[24] (5)	3.2 ± 2.1[29] (6)
0.5 mM palmitate–0.1 mM albumin	0.57 ± 0.08[5] (4)	0.73 ± 0.14[10] (12)	3.3 ± 1.4[15] (4)	2.3 ± 1.1[20] (12)	4.7 ± 1.0[25] (4)	3.4 ± 1.6[30] (12)

Student's t *test*: 1 vs 6, 11 vs 16, 16 vs 20, 24 vs 29, 25 vs 30, n.s.; 2 vs 7, 5 vs 10, 12 vs 17, 22 vs 27, $P < 0.05$; 21 vs 26, 23 vs 28, $P < 0.01$; 3 vs 8, $P < 0.02$; 4 vs 9, 13 vs 18, 14 vs 19, $P < 0.001$.

Scheffe test (comparison data 1–5, 6–10, 11–15, 16–20, 21–25, 26–30): 6 vs 10, $P < 0.05$; 6 vs 8, 27 vs 29, $P < 0.025$; 6 vs 9, 16 vs 20, 17 vs 18, 17 vs 19, 17 vs 20, 27 vs 30, $P < 0.005$; 16 vs 18, 16 vs 19, $P < 0.001$; others, n.s.

Rat hearts were perfused for a 15 min pre-perfusion period at 100 cm H_2O perfusion pressure by the method of Langendorff with a Krebs–Henseleit buffer plus substrate, gassed with 95 per cent O_2 and 5 per cent CO_2 (pH = 7.4). This was followed by 30 min perfusion at 20 or 100 cm H_2O. Hearts were freeze-clamped at the end of the perfusion period using an automated freeze-clamp (see figure 11.2(c)). Values are means ± S.D. (number of hearts in parentheses).

Table 11.4 Effects of substrates and low perfusion pressure on myocardial levels of cAMP, ATP and creatine phosphate in isolated perfused rat hearts

Substrate	cAMP (nmol g^{-1} fresh weight)	ATP (μmol g^{-1} fresh weight)	Creatine phosphate (μmol g^{-1} fresh weight)
11 mM glucose	0.58 ± 0.06^{1} (5)	4.6 ± 0.2^{5} (5)	4.7 ± 0.4^{9} (5)
0.9 mM palmitate–0.25 mM albumin	0.77 ± 0.14^{2} (6)	2.0 ± 1.0^{6} (6)	2.3 ± 1.1^{10} (6)
0.9 mM palmitate–0.25 mM albumin–11 mM glucose	0.65 ± 0.10^{3} (7)	3.5 ± 0.4^{7} (7)	2.9 ± 1.2^{11} (7)
0.9 mM palmitate–0.25 mM albumin–22 mM glucose	0.56 ± 0.10^{4} (6)	4.4 ± 0.4^{8} (6)	4.6 ± 0.4^{12} (6)

Scheffe test: 1 vs 2, $P < 0.05$; 2 vs 4, $P < 0.05$; 5 vs 6 and 6 vs 8, $P < 0.001$; 5 vs 7, $P < 0.05$; 6 vs 7, $P < 0.005$; 9 vs 10 and 10 vs 12, $P < 0.005$; 9 vs 11 and 11 vs 12, $P < 0.025$; others, n.s.

Rat hearts were perfused for a 15 min pre-perfusion period at 100 cm H_2O perfusion pressure by the method of Langendorff with Krebs–Henseleit buffer, containing 11 mM glucose, gassed with 95 per cent O_2 and 5 per cent CO_2 (pH = 7.4). This was followed by 45 min low pressure perfusion (20 cm H_2O) with the respective substrate. Hearts were freeze-clamped at the end of the perfusion period using an automated freeze-clamp (see figure 11.2(c)). Values are means ± S.D. (number of hearts in parentheses).

markedly reduced by adding glucose (11 mM). The increase of myocardial cAMP in hearts perfused with non-glucose substrates was associated with a concomitant decrease of myocardial ATP (Tables 11.3 and 11.4). Addition of glucose attenuated cAMP accumulation and also the decrease of myocardial ATP in hearts perfused with palmitate-albumin (table 11.4).

11.4 DISCUSSION

These data imply that accumulation of cAMP in the ventricular myocardium may be a critical event in the genesis of ventricular arrhythmias such as fibrillation. Such a dependence of arrhythmias upon cAMP is suggested by the following observations:

(1) cAMP levels increase in the ischaemic zone of the infarcting baboon heart prior to the onset of ventricular fibrillation (Podzuweit *et al.*, 1978b; figures 11.3 and 11.4).

(2) A relationship exists in the pig between post-ligation ventricular arrhythmias (figure 11.5) and the accumulation of myocardial cAMP (Podzuweit and Lubbe, 1977, and table 11.1).

(3) Perfusion, under reduced perfusion pressure, of isolated rat hearts with non-glucose substrates (palmitate-albumin, octanoate, pyruvate, acetate) increases myocardial cAMP levels and precipitates arrhythmias upon re-establishment of normal perfusion pressure (tables 11.3 and 11.4).

(4) Ventricular arrhythmias can be induced in the pig heart by the subepicardial infusion of agents increasing myocardial cAMP (Podzuweit, 1980; Podzuweit *et al.*, 1980, 1981; figures 11.9 and 11.10).

From these observations a mechanism for arrhythmogenesis can be suggested and is depicted in figure 11.10. Arrhythmias are thought to result from extreme overactivation by cAMP of trans-sarcolemmal calcium inflow (Podzuweit, 1980; Podzuweit *et al.*, 1980). It follows that agents may induce arrhythmias by by-passing cAMP if they either increase the calcium inward current directly or if they effect calcium uptake by other means, for example, via electrogenic Na/Ca-exchange. Such mechanisms may contribute to arrhythmias induced by cardiac glycosides (Weingart *et al.*, 1978; Fischmeister and Vassort, 1981).

This concept of cAMP inducing arrhythmias by augmenting the slow calcium inward current rests on the following findings. First, the induction of ventricular arrhythmias in the intact pig heart by subepicardial infusion of noradrenaline is facilitated by increasing $[Ca^{2+}]_o$ (Podzuweit, 1980; Podzuweit *et al.*, 1980). Secondly, infusion of calcium ions (up to 5×10^{-2} M) in the absence of β-adrenoceptor stimulation does not precipitate arrhythmias. Thirdly, arrhythmias induced by the infusion of a combination of noradrenaline and Ca^{2+} can either be inhibited by preventing the cAMP elevating effect of catecholamines (β-adrenoceptor blockade) or by using slow channel blockers to impede the calcium influx across the sarcolemma. This postulated effect of cAMP on the calcium inward current in arrhythmogenesis is consistent with the finding that cAMP increases the sarcolemmal conductance of myocardial fibres to Ca^{2+} (Reuter, 1974). However, it depends in part on the assumption that calcium antagonists inhibit the slow calcium inward current (Kolhardt *et al.*, 1972; Watanabe and Besch, 1974) yet do not attenuate the generation of cAMP. The possible role of calcium in the genesis of early post-ischaemia ventricular arrhythmias is discussed by Parratt in chapter 18.

Evidence from other laboratories for an arrhythmogenic role of cAMP has also been increasing during recent years. The cAMP hypothesis is, for instance, supported by the demonstration in cats with regional myocardial ischaemia that ventricular arrhythmias were accompanied by increased myocardial cAMP levels (Corr *et al.*, 1978). Dibutyryl-cAMP has also been shown to lower the ventricular fibrillation threshold and to increase the duration of the vulnerable period in the isolated perfused rat heart (Lubbe *et al.*, 1976, 1978). Ventricular fibrillation induced by aminophylline in dogs has been associated with increased left ventricular cAMP concentrations (Sugiura *et al.*, 1979). Prostacyclin prevents cAMP accumulation following coronary artery ligation in the pig (Rösen *et al.*, 1981) and decreases the incidence of post-ligation arrhythmias (Zylka *et al.*, 1981, and chapter 13).

The electrophysiological mechanism(s) of cAMP-mediated arrhythmias are as yet undefined. A particularly unresolved question is whether or not cAMP-mediated arrhythmias in the intact non-ischaemic heart (Podzuweit, 1980) and in the ischaemic heart (Podzuweit *et al.*, 1981) depend upon the same mechanism.

The following evidence suggests a role for cAMP in inducing spontaneous automaticity in the myocardium. Adrenaline has an acceleratory effect on cardiac pacemaker fibres as a result of increasing phase 4 diastolic depolarisation (Otsuka, 1958). This effect of adrenaline is mimicked by iontophoretically injecting cAMP into spontaneously active Purkinje fibres (Tsien, 1973) or sinus node cells (Yamasaki *et al.*, 1974). Exogenous cAMP analogues increase the rate of beating of isolated perfused atria (Drummond and Hemmings, 1972) and of heart cells in culture (Goshima, 1976). Moreover, catecholamines are known to induce automaticity in Purkinje fibres (Otsuka, 1958), heart cells in culture (Goshima, 1974) and isolated ventricular muscle fibres (Tritthart, 1974). In the latter experiments automaticity was also obtained by superfusing fibres with cAMP analogues. These findings show that automaticity is not a unique property of specialised conducting fibres, but can also be demonstrated in working muscle cells (Tritthart, 1974), implying that any part of the ventricular myocardium may take on an additional pacemaker role.

Slow diastolic depolarisation may not be the only cause of automaticity. In partially depolarised cells automaticity may arise from slow response formation (Cranefield, 1975; Sano *et al.*, 1977). In canine ventricular preparations superfused with β-adrenoceptor agonists automaticity is due to transient after-depolarisations. Slow diastolic depolarisation is only observed at higher agonist concentrations and especially in partially depolarised cells (Lazzara *et al.*, 1978).

cAMP could also be involved in triggered automaticity, which has been demonstrated in ventricular conducting tissue (Vassalle and Carpentier, 1972; Cranefield and Aronson, 1974), and more recently in canine ventricular preparations superfused with noradrenaline (Lazzara *et al.*, 1978). The importance of adrenergic enhancement in overdrive excitation is emphasised by the demonstration that ventricular rhythms can be induced by pacing in dogs with AV block during stimulation of the left stellate ganglion (Vassalle *et al.*, 1976). Although automaticity and triggered automaticity may have fundamentally different causes, both phenomena may be related to diastolic calcium inward current, mediated by cAMP (Tritthart, 1974; Lazzara *et al.*, 1978).

The available evidence favours re-entrant excitation within the ischaemic myocardium as the cause of early malignant ventricular arrhythmias (see chapters 3 and 4). The ischaemic action potential is thought to consist of slow response action potentials (Cranefield *et al.*, 1972; Wit and Bigger, 1975) and/or depressed fast response action potentials (El-Sherif and Lazzara, 1979). Slow responses and abnormal fast responses are both markedly reduced in amplitude and upstroke velocity relative to the normal action potential (range for the occurrence of fast responses −90 to −55 mV; range for slow responses −60 to −40 mV). A vital difference between these two types of action potentials is that the upstroke of the fast response depends on the fast Na^+ channel and that of the slow response on the slow Ca^{2+} channel.

The slow response is promoted by catecholamine-cAMP (Schneider and Sperelakis, 1975). The formation of cAMP due to a given stimulus is rapid, occurring within seconds (Cheung and Williamson, 1965) or even within milliseconds (Brooker, 1973; Wollenberger *et al.*, 1973). In myocardium previously rendered inexcitable by ischaemic depolarisation, cAMP accumulation may induce short-lived slow responses. These could initiate slow conduction, intermittency of conduction and unidirectional conduction block, thereby satisfying the requisite for the occurrence of re-entrant ventricular arrhythmias (Cranefield *et al.*, 1972). Evidence for an involvement of the slow response in ischaemic arrhythmogenesis is growing (Wit and Bigger, 1975), although recordings of intracellular action potentials *in vivo* have as yet failed to demonstrate slow response action potentials in the ischaemic subepicardium (see chapter 4). Likewise, these studies have so far failed to show that spontaneous or triggered abnormal automaticity occurs in the ischaemic region. The possibility that automaticity is a cause of early post-ischaemia arrhythmias is not supported by the finding that arrhythmias in dogs with AV block can be interrupted by cessation of pacing (Horacek *et al.*, 1981).

The mechanisms by which cAMP increases in the acutely ischaemic myocardium still require clarification. Conceivably, accumulation of myocardial cAMP during the early arrhythmogenic phase may be caused by liberation of endogenous catecholamines from the myocardium, a possibility discussed in detail in chapters 8-10 and 16. Early release of catecholamines from the ischaemic heart is also suggested by the protective effects of chronic cardiac denervation, of reserpine pretreatment and of α- and β-adrenoceptor blocking agents.

Ventricular arrhythmias and fibrillation during the Harris phase 1 arrhythmias show a biphasic distribution in time (phases 1a and 1b; chapter 6). This biphasic distribution of arrhythmias was also evident in our own pig experiments (figure 11.5). However, phase 1a arrhythmias were observed rather infrequently and seemed to be associated with a slightly larger than normal mass of ischaemic myocardium. Our dog experiments showed that proximal ligation of the anterior descending coronary artery increased myocardial cAMP within 1-3 min preceding the onset of ventricular fibrillation. These observations suggest that the early 1a phase of arrhythmias may also be related to myocardial cAMP. Accumulation of myocardial cAMP in our pig experiments occurs during phase 1b (20 min post-ligation) predominantly in the ischaemic zone. The data of Krause *et al.* (1978) suggest a biphasic increase of myocardial cAMP in ischaemic and non-ischaemic regions of the myocardium following coronary artery ligation. The early increase of myocardial cAMP during ischaemia was suggested by Krause and Wollenberger (1980) to result from catecholamine liberation from efferent cardiac sympathetic nerves. The secondary and more protracted post-occlusion rise of myocardial cAMP was assumed to be largely due to catecholamine release from the adrenal medulla.

Our experiments with isolated underperfused rat hearts show that cAMP levels in the ischaemic myocardium may be substrate dependent. Low pressure perfusion (20 cm H_2O) for 30-45 min with non-esterified fatty acid (0.5-0.9 mM palmitate) bound to albumin (0.1-0.25 mM) increased myocardial cAMP by 30-50 per cent compared to low pressure perfusion for the same period with 11 mM glucose (tables 11.3 and 11.4). Similar observations were made when using octanoate, pyruvate or acetate as the sole exogenous substrate. During subsequent perfusion under normal (100 cm H_2O) perfusion pressure such hearts exhibited an increased frequency of arrhythmias and fibrillation. Addition of glucose to the palmitate-albumin perfusate prevented cAMP accumulation and arrhythmias. Besides increasing myocardial cAMP, ischaemic perfusion with non-glucose substrates consistently decreased ATP. This effect was prevented by adding glucose (table 11.4). These findings suggest that myocardial cAMP levels during ischaemia may be related in some way to glycolytic ATP.

Inhibition of cyclic nucleotide phosphodiesterase, the enzyme which hydrolyses cAMP to 5'-AMP, could contribute to cAMP-mediated arrhythmogenesis in the ischaemic myocardium. Subepicardial infusion of methylxanthines precipitated arrhythmias in the ischaemic heart (figure 11.10). Arrhythmias could also be induced in the intact non-ischaemic heart by 8-Br-cAMP in the presence of the phosphodiesterase inhibitor Ro 7-2956 (figure 11.10).

It is conceivable that liberation of cardioactive compounds other than catecholamines may contribute to the genesis of early arrhythmias and to the accumulation of myocardial cAMP in the ischaemic heart. One such compound may be histamine, which produces severe arrhythmias when infused into the ischaemic myocardium (Podzuweit *et al.*, 1979).

Our data also suggest a potentially important role for post-synaptic muscarinic inhibition in cAMP-mediated arrhythmogenesis. Choline esters, β-methylcholine esters and the fly-mushroom poison muscarine were found to exert a strong anti-arrhythmic effect in a system in which arrhythmias were produced by adrenergic overstimulation (Podzuweit, 1982). This antiarrhythmic effect of choline esters was blocked by atropine. In the absence of atropine, choline esters attenuated the accumulation of cAMP by catecholamines. These findings suggest, firstly, that atropine competes with choline esters for binding sites on muscarinic receptors and, secondly, that these receptors are linked to the cAMP system. Cholinergic interventions have no effect on cGMP levels. Although the degree of cholinergic innervation of the ventricular myocardium is controversial (Rosen and Hoffman, 1978), in our experiments this muscarinic inhibition could be demonstrated anywhere in ventricular myocardium.

ACKNOWLEDGEMENTS

This work was supported between 1973 and 1980 by the South African Medical Research Council, the Chris Barnard Fund and the Cape Provincial Administration. I thank Professors B. C. Shanley, J. J. F. Taljaard and L. H. Opie for support, J. McCarthy, M. Phillips, D. J. Els and G. C. J. Louw for technical assistance, Professor W. F. Lubbe for co-operation and Professor W. Schaper for commenting on the manuscript.

REFERENCES

Breckenridge, B. McL. (1964). The measurement of cyclic adenylate in tissues. *Proc. natn. Acad. Sci. U.S.A.*, **52**, 1580-6

Bricknell, O. L. and Opie, L. H. (1978). Effects of substrates on tissue metabolic changes in the isolated rat heart during underperfusion and on release of lactate dehydrogenase and arrhythmias during reperfusion. *Circulation Res.*, **43**, 102-15

Brooker, G. (1973). Oscillation of cyclic adenosine monophosphate concentration during the myocardial contraction cycle. *Science, N.Y.*, **182**, 933-4

Cheung, W. Y. and Williamson, J. R. (1965). Kinetics of cyclic adenosine monophosphate changes in rat heart following epinephrine administration. *Nature, Lond.*, **207**, 979-81

Clark, B. B. and Cummings, J. R. (1956). Arrhythmias following experimental coronary occlusion and their response to drugs. *Ann. N.Y. Acad. Sci.*, **64**, 543-51

Corr, P. B., Witkowski, F. X. and Sobel, B. E. (1978). Mechanisms contributing to malignant dysrhythmias induced by ischemia in the cat. *J. clin. Invest.*, **61**, 109-19

Cranefield, P. F. (1975). *The Conduction of the Cardiac Impulse. The Slow Response and Cardiac Arrhythmias*, Futura Publishing Company, Mount Kisko, N.Y.

Cranefield, P. F. and Aronson, R. S. (1974). Initiation of sustained rhythmic activity by single propagated action potentials in canine Purkinje fibers exposed to sodium-free solution or to ouabain. *Circulation Res.*, **34**, 477-81

Cranefield, P. F., Wit, A. L. and Hoffman, B. F. (1972). Conduction of the cardiac impulse. III. Characteristics of very slow conduction. *J. gen. Physiol.*, **59**, 227-46

Drummond, G. I. and Hemmings, S. J. (1972). Inotropic and chronotropic effects of dibutyryl cyclic AMP. *Adv. cyclic Nucleotide Res.*, **1**, 307-16

Ebert, P. A., Vanderbeek, R. B., Allgood, R. J. and Sabiston, D. C. (1970). Effect of chronic cardiac denervation on arrhythmias after coronary artery ligation. *Cardiovasc. Res.*, **4**, 141-7

El-Sherif, N. and Lazzara, R. (1979). Re-entrant ventricular arrhythmias in the late myocardial infarction period. 7. Effect of verapamil and D-600 and the role of the 'slow channel'. *Circulation*, **60**, 605-15

Fischmeister, R. and Vassort, G. (1981). The role of an electrogenic Na-Ca exchange in the regulation of cardiac rhythmic activity. Poster Session, Abstract, Meeting of the International Society for Heart Research, Burlington, Vermont, USA, 18-20 June

Goshima, K. (1974). Initiation of beating in quiescent myocardial cells by norepinephrine, by contact with beating cells and by electrical stimulation of adjacent FL cells. *Exp. Cell Res.*, **84**, 223-34

Goshima, K. (1976). Antagonistic influences of dibutyryl cyclic AMP and dibutyryl cyclic GMP on the beating rate of cultured mouse myocardial cells. *J. molec. cell. Cardiol.*, **8**, 713-25

Harris, A. S., Bisteni, A., Russell, R. A., Brigham, J. C. and Firestone, J. E. (1954). Excitatory factors in ventricular tachycardia resulting from myocardial ischemia. Potassium a major excitant. *Science, N.Y.*, **119**, 200-3

Hohorst, H. J., Kreutz, F. H. and Bücher, T. (1959). Über Metabolitgehalte und Metabolitkonzentrationen in der Leber der Ratte. *Biochem. Z.*, **332**, 18-46

Horacek, T., Neumann, M. and Meesmann, W. (1981). Dispersion of effective refractory periods, dispersion of excitability, and conduction velocity in relation to the early ventricular arrhythmias after acute coronary artery ligation and reperfusion in dogs. *Pflügers Arch. ges. Physiol.*, **389**, Suppl. R5, abstr. 18

Kolhardt, M., Bauer, B., Krause, H. and Fleckenstein, A. (1972). Differentiation of the transmembrane Na and Ca channels in mammalian cardiac fibres by the use of specific inhibitors. *Pflügers Arch. ges. Physiol.*, **335**, 309-22

Krause, E.-G. and Wollenberger, A. (1980). Cyclic nucleotides in heart in acute myocardial ischaemia and hypoxia. *Adv. cyclic Nucleotide Res.*, **12**, 49-61

Krause, E.-G., Ziegelhöffer, A., Fedelsová, M., Styk, J., Kostolansky, S., Gabauer, I., Blasig, I. and Wollenberger, A. (1978). Myocardial cyclic nucleotide levels following coronary artery ligation. *Adv. Cardiol.*, **25**, 119-29

Kurien, V. A. and Oliver, M. F. (1970). A metabolic cause for arrhythmias during acute myocardial hypoxia. *Lancet*, **i**, 813-5

Lazzara, R., Hope, R. R. and Yeh, B. K. (1978). Implication of cAMP and calcium as mediators of automaticity induced in working myocardium. *Am. J. Cardiol.*, **41**, 417 (abstr.)

Liedtke, A. J., Nellis, S. and Neely, J. R. (1978). Effects of excess free fatty acids on mechanical and metabolic function in normal and ischemic myocardium in swine. *Circulation Res.*, **43**, 652-61

Lubbe, W. F., Bricknell, O. L., Podzuweit, T. and Opie, L. H. (1976). Cyclic AMP as a determinant of vulnerability to ventricular fibrillation in the isolated rat heart. *Cardiovasc. Res.*, **10**, 697-702

Lubbe, W. F., Podzuweit, T., Daries, P. S. and Opie, L. H. (1978). The role of cyclic adenosine monophosphate in adrenergic effects on ventricular vulnerability to fibrillation in the isolated perfused rat heart. *J. clin. Invest.*, **61**, 1260-9

Maling, H. M. and Moran, N. C. (1957). Ventricular arrhythmias induced by sympathomimetic amines in unanaesthetised dogs following coronary artery occlusion. *Circulation Res.*, **5**, 409-13

Otsuka, M. (1958). Die Wirkung von Adrenalin auf Purkinje-Fasern von Säugetierherzen. *Pflügers Arch. ges. Physiol.*, **266**, 512-7

Podzuweit, T. (1980). Catecholamine-cyclic AMP-Ca^{2+}-induced ventricular tachycardia in the intact pig heart. *Basic Res. Cardiol.*, **75**, 772-9

Podzuweit, T. (1981). Cyclic AMP arrhythmias. Inhibition by choline esters. *Adv. Myocardiol.*, **3**, 193-8

Podzuweit, T. and Lubbe, W. F. (1977). Relation between post-ligation arrhythmias and myocardial cyclic AMP levels in the pig. *J. molec. cell. Cardiol.*, **9**, Suppl., 40

Podzuweit, T., Lubbe, W. F. and Opie, L. H. (1976). Cyclic adenosine monophosphate, ventricular fibrillation and antiarrhythmic drugs. *Lancet*, *i*, 341-2

Podzuweit, T., van der Werff, T. J., Bricknell, O. and Kay, A. (1978a). An automatic device for freeze-clamping of cardiac tissue within a fraction of the contraction cycle. *Cardiovasc. Res.*, **12**, 322-6

Podzuweit, T., Dalby, A. J., Cherry, G. W. and Opie, L. H. (1978b). Cyclic AMP levels in ischaemic and non-ischaemic myocardium following coronary artery ligation: relation to ventricular fibrillation. *J. molec. cell. Cardiol.*, **10**, 81-94

Podzuweit, T., Els, D. J. and Taljaard, J. J. F. (1979). Cyclic AMP-arrhythmias. Myocardial maps and infusion. *J. molec. cell. Cardiol.*, **11**, Suppl 2, 45 (abstr.)

Podzuweit, T., Louw, G. C. J. and Shanley, B. C. (1980). Catecholamine-cyclic AMP-Ca^{2+} induces arrhythmias in the healthy pig heart. *Adv. Myocardiol.*, 2, 133-43

Podzuweit, T., Els, D. J. and McCarthy, J. (1981). Cyclic AMP mediated arrhythmias induced in the ischaemic pig heart. *Basic Res. Cardiol.*, **76**, 443-8

Pool, P. E., Norris, G. F., Lewis, R. M. and Covell, J. W. (1968). A biopsy drill permitting rapid freezing. *J. appl. Physiol.*, **24**, 832-3

Reuter, H. (1974). Localization of beta adrenergic receptors, and effects of noradrenaline and cyclic nucleotides on action potentials, ionic currents and tension in mammalian cardiac muscle. *J. Physiol., Lond.*, **242**, 429-51

Rösen, M. R. and Hoffman, B. F. (1978). Editorial. The vagus and the ventricles. *Circulation Res.*, **42**, 1

Rösen, R., Rösen, P., Ohlendorf, R. and Schrör, K. (1981). Prostacyclin prevents ischaemia-induced increase of lactate and cyclic-AMP in ischaemic myocardium. *Eur. J. Pharmac.*, **69**, 489-91

Sano, T., Sawanobori, T. and Hiraoka, M. (1977). Re-evaluation of arrhythmogenetic role of slow responses. *J. molec. cell. Cardiol.*, **9**, Suppl, 18 (abstr.)

Scheffe, H. (1959). *The Analysis of Variance*, John Wiley, New York

Schneider, J. A. and Sperelakis, N. (1975). Slow Ca^{2+} and Na^{+} responses induced by isoproterenol and methylxanthines in isolated perfused guinea pig hearts exposed to elevated K^{+}. *J. molec. cell. Cardiol.*, 7, 249-73

Stanley, P. E. and Williams, S. G. (1969). Use of the liquid scintillation spectrometer for determining adenosine triphosphate by the luciferase enzyme. *Analyt. Biochem.*, **29**, 381-92

Sugiura, M., Ogawa, K. and Yamazaki, N. (1979). Concentration of myocardial cyclic AMP and ventricular fibrillation induced by aminophylline. *Jap. Heart J.*, **20**, 177-82

Ten Eick, R., Nawrath, H., McDonald, T. F. and Trautwein, W. (1976). On the mechanisms of the negative inotropic effect of acetylcholine. *Pflügers Arch. ges. Physiol.*, **361**, 207-13

Tritthart, H. (1974). The comparison of cAMP and β-adrenergic effects on Ca-mediated action potentials of cat ventricular myocardium. *Naunyn-Schmiedebergs Arch. Pharmac.*, **285**, Suppl., R85

Tsien, R. W. (1973). Adrenaline-like effects of intracellular iontophoresis of cyclic AMP in cardiac Purkinje fibres. *Nature, Lond.*, **245**, 120-2

Vassalle, M. and Carpentier, R. (1972). Overdrive excitation: onset of activity following fast drive in cardiac Purkinje fibers exposed to norepinephrine. *Pflügers Arch. ges. Physiol.*, **332**, 198-205

Vassalle, M., Knob, R. E., Lara, G. A. and Stuckey, J. H. (1976). The effect of adrenergic enhancement on overdrive excitation. *J. Electrocardiol.*, **9**, 335-43

Watanabe, A. M. and Besch, H. R. (1974). Subcellular myocardial effects of verapamil and D 600: comparison with propranolol. *J. Pharmac. exp. Ther.*, **191**, 241-51

Weingart, R., Kass, R. S. and Tsien, R. W. (1978). Is digitalis inotropy associated with enhanced slow inward calcium current? *Nature, Lond.*, **273**, 389-92

Wissner, S. B. (1974). The effect of excess lactate upon the excitability of the sheep Purkinje fibre. *J. Electrocardiol.*, 7, 17-26

Wit, A. L. and Bigger, J. T., Jr (1975). Possible electrophysiological mechanisms for lethal arrhythmias accompanying myocardial ischemia and infarction. *Circulation*, **51/52**, Suppl. III, 96-115

Wollenberger, A., Krause, E.-G. and Heier, G. (1969). Stimulation of 3′,5′-cyclic AMP formation in dog myocardium following arrest of blood flow. *Biochem. biophys. Res. Commun.*, **36**, 664-70

Wollenberger, A., Babskii, E. B., Krause, E.-G., Genz, S., Blohm, D. and Bogdanova, E. V. (1973). Cyclic changes in levels of cyclic AMP and cyclic GMP in frog myocardium during the cardiac cycle. *Biochem. biophys. Res. Commun.*, **55**, 446-52

Yamasaki, Y., Fujiwara, M. and Toda, N. (1974). Effects of intracellularly applied cyclic 3′,5′-adenosine monophosphate and dibutyryl cyclic 3′,5′-adenosine monophosphate on the electrical activity of sino-atrial nodal cells of the rabbit. *J. Pharmac. exp. Ther.*, **190**, 15-20

Zylka, V., Addicks, K., Deutsch, H.-J., Friedrich, R., Griebenow, R. and Hirch, Hj. (1981). Die antiarrhythmische Wirkung von Prostazyklin (PGI_2) am Schweineherzen. *Z. Kardiol.*, **70**, 308, abstr. 200

12

Amphiphilic Lipid Metabolism and Ventricular Arrhythmias

Peter B. Corr and Burton E. Sobel

12.1 INTRODUCTION

Sudden death associated with coronary artery disease results primarily from disturbances in cardiac rhythm culminating in ventricular fibrillation (Armstrong *et al.*, 1972). During the past decade, the electrophysiological derangements induced by ischaemia have been characterised and several arrhythmogenic mechanisms proposed to explain the high incidence of ventricular fibrillation coincident with an ischaemic insult.

12.2 THE ELECTROPHYSIOLOGICAL DERANGEMENTS CHARACTERISTIC OF EARLY ISCHAEMIA

Ventricular dysrhythmias after coronary occlusion in experimental animals occur during three distinct phases. The earliest (phase 1), which begins within minutes and persists for approximately 30 min, may be analogous to the malignant, prehospital phase of acute myocardial infarction. Arrhythmias appearing 12-24 h later (phase 2) or days to weeks after acute myocardial infarction (phase 3) appear to depend upon different electrophysiological alterations and hence different arrhythmogenic mechanisms (Corr and Sobel, 1979). The primary focus of this discussion will be those derangements responsible for the early phase 1 ventricular arrhythmias.

Early phase 1 malignant arrhythmias appear to result from sustained re-entry within ventricular muscle. Thus, extracellular electrograms recorded from ischaemic segments *in vivo* demonstrate delays in excitation, prolonged electrical activity, fractionation of the waveform and significant reduction of waveform amplitude (Scherlag *et al.*, 1974; Bigger *et al.*, 1977; Penkoske *et al.*, 1978). In addition, intracellular transmembrane potentials recorded *in vivo* from ischaemic regions manifest prompt reduction of resting membrane potential, amplitude, $\dot{V}_{max}$ of phase 0 and action potential duration (Downar *et al.*, 1977a; Russell *et al.*, 1977; Akiyama, 1981). Fractionation of the action potential and also shortening of refractory period and post-repolarisation refractoriness occur as well, resulting in increased disparity of refractoriness (see chapter 4). The appearance of ventricular fibrillation during the interval soon after the onset of ischaemia has been correlated not only with a delay in activation of the epicardial ischaemic zone persisting beyond the duration of inscription of the T-wave on the surface electrocardiogram (Williams *et al.*, 1974) but also with the appearance of electrical alternans in the intracellular action potentials, probably reflecting intermittent variation of regional refractoriness. Other evidence (Scherlag *et al.*, 1974) implicating re-entry as opposed to enhanced ventricular automaticity as a probable mechanism underlying phase 1 ventricular dysrhythmias includes the following: (1) exacerbation by high right atrial electrical pacing; (2) a slow idioventricular escape rate; (3) inhibition of arrhythmia by efferent vagal nerve stimulation; and (4) absence of enhanced automaticity *in vitro* in Purkinje cells isolated from ischaemic regions.

Despite each of these findings, specific re-entrant pathways responsible for early phase 1 arrhythmias have not been delineated.

Recently, data implicating two different types of arrhythmogenic mechanisms during phase 1 ventricular arrhythmias have been obtained (Janse *et al.*, 1980, and chapter 4). Findings suggesting that ventricular ectopic activity which initiates ventricular tachycardia or fibrillation is not due to a re-entrant mechanism include the observations that the earliest activation occurs in the normal zone adjacent to the ischaemic border zone and that activation of Purkinje fibres precedes activation in myocardial segments. However, the maintenance of ventricular tachycardia or ventricular fibrillation appears to depend upon both macro and micro re-entrant circuits through the ischaemic regions (Janse *et al.*, 1980, and chapter 4).

Possible electrophysiological mechanisms responsible for initiation of earliest activation in the normal region include current flow from ischaemic to normal regions due to delayed activation of ischaemic regions and hence earlier repolarisation in normal zones. Others include enhancement of phase 4 diastolic depolarisation in Purkinje fibres by depolarising electrotonic current or induction of abnormal types of automaticity, including oscillatory activity at reduced resting membrane potentials due to disparities in the magnitude of depolarisation in ischaemic compared to non-ischaemic regions. Thus, the early phase 1 ventricular arrhythmias may be initiated by alterations in current flow across the ischaemic border sufficient to prematurely excite normal regions. Maintenance of ventricular tachycardia or fibrillation may involve a perpetuation of this early excitation through re-entrant circuits involving slowed conduction and variable refractoriness in ischaemic regions.

In addition to induction of ventricular arrhythmias by sustained occlusion, a rapid onset-ventricular arrhythmia occurs after reperfusion of ischaemic regions and is associated with a high incidence of ventricular fibrillation. Arrhythmias induced by reperfusion may play an important role in the aetiology of sudden cardiac death since relief of coronary spasm may occur spontaneously (Oliva and

Breckenridge, 1977), platelet aggregation and lysis may occur *in vivo* with phasic alterations in flow, and variations in collateral flow may lead to some increased perfusion in ischaemic regions (Marcus *et al.*, 1976). Recent evidence indicates that reperfusion-induced malignant arrhythmias are distinctly different from arrhythmias due to occlusion alone. In contrast to arrhythmias induced by sustained occlusion, those induced by reperfusion are associated with significant improvement in mid-myocardial conduction, synchronous depolarisation in the ischaemic region and an elevated idioventricular rate (Penkoske *et al.*, 1978). Since different arrhythmogenic mechanisms may underlie arrhythmias due to occlusion alone in contrast to those due to reperfusion, effective prophylactic or therapeutic interventions required for each may differ.

The electrophysiological alterations responsible for ventricular arrhythmias accompanying ischaemia are likely to depend ultimately on changes in membrane structure. Prior to considering several biochemical events which may be responsible for such sarcolemmal alterations, a brief review of membrane chemistry and its relationship to electrical events may be helpful.

12.3 SARCOLEMMAL STRUCTURE: RELATIONSHIP TO ELECTRICAL EVENTS

Modern membrane biochemistry began with the findings of Gorter and Grendel (1925) which suggested that membranes were composed of a bilayer of lipids. Subsequent observations of Danielli and colleagues (Danielli and Davson, 1935; Danielli and Harvey, 1935; Stein and Danielli, 1956) indicated that protein played an integral role in membrane structure, possibly providing a structural basis for the functional pores through the lipid bilayer. Subsequently, Robertson (1959) proposed the unit membrane model in which it was assumed that all membranes have an identical subunit molecular structure consisting of a bilayer of mixed polar lipids (phospholipids with hydrocarbon chains (hydrophobic) oriented toward the centre of the membrane forming a continuous hydrophobic phase). The hydrophilic moieties of the lipids orient toward the cytoplasm in one direction and toward the cell exterior in the other direction, with each surface of the membrane covered by a layer of protein (figure 12.1). More recent evidence indicates, however, that membranes vary in thickness, lipid composition, enzymatic activity, transport and electrical excitability. Thus, structural differences between different types of membranes confer specificity. It has become clear that, as the ratios change among different phospholipids containing polar head-groups with different geometry, electrical charge and polarity, the functional specificity of the membrane is altered (Korn, 1966). Likewise, differences in membrane proteins confer functional specificity. The predominant phospholipids in human heart muscle are phosphatidylcholine (PC) (39 per cent) and phosphatidylethanolamine (PE) (26 per cent). Smaller quantities of phosphatidylserine (2 per cent) and phosphatidylinositol (6 per cent) are present as well.

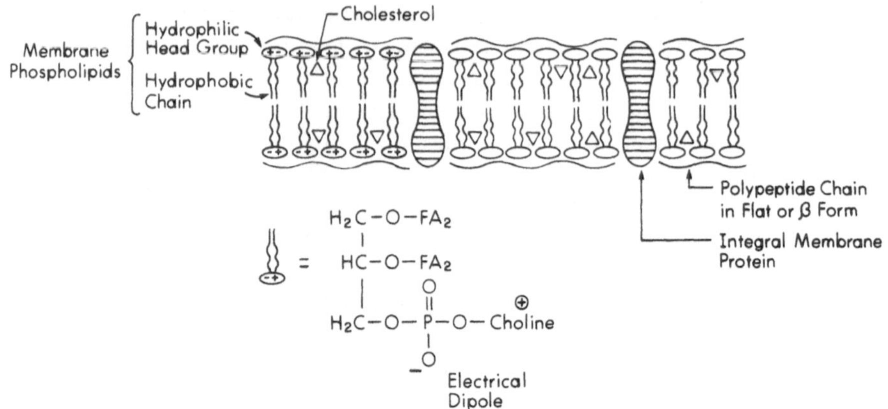

Figure 12.1 Diagramatic representation of a membrane illustrating the orientation of phospholipids, cholesterol and intrinsic and extrinsic proteins. The hydrophilic head-group of the phospholipid forms a dipole, as illustrated, which appears to mediate at least in part the ionic currents in excitable tissue. See text for details.

The organisation of membrane phospholipids appears to determine the relative membrane permeability to ions, maintenance of membrane resistance, resting membrane potential, and generation of the cardiac action potential (Goldman, 1964; Tobias, 1964; Blaustein and Goldman, 1966; Baker, 1968). However, structure-function relationships have not yet been elucidated definitively. Alterations in permeability may depend on membrane potential because of the effect of the electrical field (voltage) on the orientation of charged molecules, which in turn may modify the functional channels through the membrane. The transient nature of specific currents may be explained by the time- and voltage-dependent orientation of the charged particles, which under some conditions may result in blockade of the channel (Goldman, 1964). Presumably a separate channel exists for each ion, since the kinetics of activation and deactivation for each current differ so dramatically (Baker, 1968). Tobias (1964) has suggested that the hydrophilic head group of membrane phospholipids (choline, ethanolamine) are ion exchange sites involved in the control of ionic permeability (figure 12.1). Phospholipids contain dipoles in some head groups involving phosphate, oxygen and ionised nitrogen; rotation of such dipoles in the presence of an applied electrical field may alter the membrane permeability for specific ions.

Tobias hypothesised that in nerve, calcium ions associated with the polar head-groups of membrane phospholipids are displaced by K^+ ions during depolarisation, resulting in a deformation of membrane proteins with a consequent alteration of membrane resistance. The experiments of DeMello (1972) support the hypothesis that the polar head-groups of membrane phospholipids are important determinants of the electrophysiological properties of membranes. Treatment of excitable tissue with phospholipase C, which hydrolyses the ester bond between glycerol and the phosphate group, and removes the polar group of the phospholipid, abolishes membrane potentials in nerve and skeletal muscle. This response is preceded by a loss of excitability and depression of conduction velocity. A similar effect is seen in cardiac tissue (DeMello, 1972). In pacemaker tissue from the heart, phospholipase C treatment does not exert marked electrophysiological effects, suggesting that different mechanisms are responsible for pacemaker cell action potentials, that penetration of phospholipase C into membranes of pacemaker tissue is in some way inhibited, or that phospholipid composition of pacemaker tissue is unique (DeMello, 1972).

The role of membrane proteins in the maintenance of the membrane potential seems less important than that of phospholipids since treatment of nerve, skeletal muscle and cardiac muscle with trypsin or chymotrypsin fails to alter membrane polarisation or excitability (DeMello, 1972). However, the importance of membrane-bound enzymes, including Na^+, K^+ ATPase, should not be underestimated. The negative results with proteases such as trypsin may be secondary to a lack of access of the enzyme to the membrane proteins. Some proteins (peripheral or extrinsic proteins) can be dissociated easily from the membrane without alteration in its structural integrity but others, including some enzymes, can be removed from the membrane only with concomitant destruction of the membrane (integral or intrinsic proteins) or profound alterations of the membrane's physiological properties (Coleman, 1973). Thus, membrane phospholipids appear to be intimately associated with the changes in ionic conductances which occur across the sarcolemma. Changes in the relative conformation of membrane phospholipids may alter the electrical characteristics of the membrane.

12.4 MEDIATION OF ISCHAEMIA-INDUCED ELECTROPHYSIOLOGICAL DISTURBANCES BY METABOLITES

Since the electrophysiological derangements characteristic of ischaemic tissue *in vivo* appear to reflect alterations in the integrity of the membrane and consequent changes in ionic conductances, it is not surprising that ischaemia induces electrophysiological alterations which differ in several important respects from those due to hypoxia *per se*. The ischaemic heart is far more vulnerable to ventricular fibrillation than the heart made hypoxic without reduction of flow (Bagdonas *et al.*, 1961). In contrast to hypoxia alone, ischaemia results in (1) retention of metabolites; (2) accumulation of intra- or extracellular ions; and (3) regional acidosis. Thus it is not surprising that (1) perfusion of ischaemic regions *in vivo* with saline gassed with nitrogen restores normal subepicardial action potentials within 20 s (Downar *et al.*, 1977a) suggesting that washout of a noxious metabolite has occurred despite the persistence of hypoxia; (2) venular blood from ischaemic regions elicits electrophysiological changes in isolated myocardial tissue resembling those characteristic of ischaemic myocardium *in vivo* (Downar *et al.*, 1977b); and (3) electrophysiological alterations occurring within the first 20 min after the onset of myocardial ischaemia *in vivo* do not persist when the tissue is superfused *in vitro* (Lazzara *et al.*, 1973).

In concert, these findings suggest that soon after myocardial ischaemia accumulation of metabolites may be of primary importance in the genesis of electrophysiological alterations underlying malignant ventricular dysrhythmias. Potentially arrhythmogenic biochemical factors that do not induce electrophysiological alterations directly may result in secondary or tertiary arrhythmogenic phenomena. Furthermore, one metabolite may 'sensitise' the membrane to adverse influences of others or enhance the synthesis or inhibit degradation of other noxious agents. In addition, alterations of membrane structure may alter the density or affinity of receptors which may in turn mediate adverse electrophysiological responses.

One class of metabolites which has been implicated strongly in the mediation of arrhythmias induced by ischaemia includes lysophosphoglycerides and long chain acyl carnitines. Both types of compound are amphiphiles, that is, endowed with both hydrophilic and hydrophobic constituents - a structural conformation facilitating induction of potentially deleterious effects on membranes (figure 12.2).

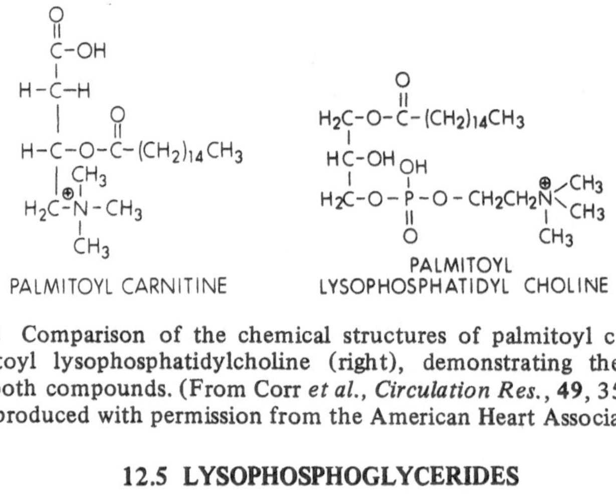

PALMITOYL CARNITINE

PALMITOYL LYSOPHOSPHATIDYL CHOLINE

Figure 12.2 Comparison of the chemical structures of palmitoyl carnitine (left) and palmitoyl lysophosphatidylcholine (right), demonstrating the amphiphilic nature of both compounds. (From Corr *et al.*, *Circulation Res.*, **49**, 354–63 (1981). Reproduced with permission from the American Heart Association.)

12.5 LYSOPHOSPHOGLYCERIDES

In 1977, we presented evidence that lysophosphoglycerides (LPG), including lysophosphatidylcholine (LPC) and lysophosphatidylethanolamine (LPE), accumulate in ischaemic myocardium with lower, but still large, concentrations in normal myocardium (Sobel *et al.*, 1978). In these initial studies, tissue samples were extracted with acidified media to improve recovery of the LPGs, as described by Bjerve *et al.* (1974). Subsequently, with the use of ^{31}P-NMR, we demonstrated that the conventionally employed acidification of the extraction media used to enhance recovery of extracted lipids led to substantial intrapreparative conversion of plasmalogens to LPGs, thereby falsely elevating the tissue LPG levels (Mogelson *et al.*, 1980). Plasmalogens are diacyl phospholipid moieties with a vinyl ether linkage in the 1-position. They comprise approximately 40 per cent of myocardial phospholipid. Thus, an artefact of this type is likely to be a particularly serious problem with cardiac tissue. Despite the elevated baseline values of LPG under such conditions, however, a substantial increase of LPG was found in ischaemic compared to control myocardium (Sobel *et al.*, 1978). A comparable percentage increase in ischaemic tissue was reported subsequently by others when non-acidified extraction media were utilised (Shaikh and Downar, 1981). Lower concentrations of LPC bound to albumin induced marked electrophysiological derangements in isolated tissue *in vitro* (Corr *et al.*, 1979), analogous to those alterations characteristic of ischaemic myocardium *in vivo*, as well as those changes induced by venous effluents from ischaemic zones (Downar *et al.*, 1977b). Neither glycerophosphorylcholine (GPC) nor free fatty acids (FFA), both catabolites of LPC, induced significant alterations of the transmembrane action potential resembling those elicited by LPC (Corr *et al.*, 1979). Thus, it appeared that the accumulation of LPGs within ischaemic myocardium may contribute to the electrical instability of the ischaemic heart.

More recently we have employed non-acidified extraction media (chloroform-methanol) with separation and assay of phospholipids by isocratic HPLC and found that LPGs increase by 53 per cent in ischaemic compared to control myocardium within 10 min after the onset of coronary occlusion in the cat (LPC, 2.76 ± 0.2 to 4.5 ± 0.4 nmol (mg protein)$^{-1}$, $P < 0.001$; lysophosphatidylethanolamine (LPE), 2.1 ± 0.1 to 3.0 ± 0.6, $P < 0.05$; and LPC plus LPE, 4.9 ± 0.27 to 7.5 ± 0.33, $P < 0.001$). Although others (Chien *et al.*, 1981) have demonstrated degradation of the diacyl phospholipids (PC and PE) after 1 h or more of ischaemia, in our studies with 10 min of ischaemia no significant changes in the concentration of those diacyl phospholipids were found. Since the mean value of LPC plus LPE in ischaemic tissue was found to be 7.5 nmol (mg protein)$^{-1}$, based on an assumed 220 mg protein (g wet weight)$^{-1}$ their overall cellular concentration would be 1650 nmol mg^{-1} or 1.65 mM. This is a conservative estimate since the LPGs are not distributed homogenously. Thus, the sarcolemmal LPG concentrations are likely to exceed this overall cellular concentration of 1.6 mM. In the presence of albumin (0.4 mM) a concentration of 1.6 mM LPG induced marked electrophysiological derangements in isolated tissue (Corr *et al.*, 1979) closely analogous to those changes seen in ischaemic tissue *in vivo*, including (1) reduction of maximum diastolic potential, $\dot{V}_{max}$ of phase 0, amplitude, over-shoot of phase 0 and action potential duration; (2) fractionation of the upstroke of phase 0 depolarisation and unresponsiveness to external stimulation; (3) enhanced automaticity at normal and reduced membrane potentials; (4) a rightward and downward shift in the membrane response curve with a prolongation of conduction time; and (5) an increase in the ratio of effective refractory period to action potential duration (APD) such that the effective refractory period persists beyond the APD, resulting in post-repolarisation refractoriness. Effects of free LPG in the absence of albumin are seen at 10-fold lower concentrations. Even lower concentrations of LPC increase membrane resistance, length, and time constants and elicit biphasic effects on excitability with an increase in excitability due to alteration of passive membrane properties and a decrease due to changes in active membrane properties (Arnsdorf and Sawicki, 1981).

Recently we have found that the concentration of LPC increases twofold in effluents from ischaemic regions *in vivo* within 10 min of coronary occlusion. The increase in the concentration of LPC together with a concomitant decrease in pH (to 6.7) is sufficient to induce marked electrophysiological alterations in the intracellular action potentials of normoxic ventricular tissue, typical of ischaemic tissue *in vivo*. Thus, LPC may account in part for the arrhythmogenic properties of venous effluents from ischaemic zones, particularly since the arrhythmogenic properties of LPC are intensified markedly in the presence of concomitant acidosis, characteristic of ischaemic myocardium *in vivo*. The apparent increase in sensitivity to LPC under conditions of acidosis results in a threefold shift to the left of the concentration response curve for LPC, even in the absence of albumin. Together, these observations support the hypothesis that lysophosphoglycerides may be important contributors to electrophysiological deterioration of the ischaemic heart and to the evolution of malignant ventricular arrhythmias.

The toxicity of amphiphiles such as LPC has been demonstrated in several other systems as well. For example, low concentrations of LPC induce alterations in the conformation of the red blood cell membrane, causing formation of echinocytes and in isolated perfused hearts, LPC induces tetanic contracture, elevating LVEDP profoundly (Bergmann *et al.*, 1981). LPC alters the activities of membrane-bound enzymes such as Na^+, K^+ ATPase (Karli *et al.*, 1979) and adenylate cyclase (Ahumada *et al.*, 1979). Thus, its accumulation may contribute to the augmentation of myocardial cyclic AMP in ischaemic heart muscle, which has been associated with arrhythmias (Corr *et al.*, 1978; Podzuweit *et al.*, 1978, and reviewed in chapter 10). LPC also increases release of K^+ from erythrocytes prior to lysis and loss of haemoglobin (Lawrence *et al.*, 1974). Thus, potentially detrimental effects of LPG during ischaemia may be related in part to a loss of cellular K^+ contributing to the observed increase in extracellular K^+ (chapter 6).

LPC also alters the structure and function of cardiac mitochondria. Organelles isolated from myocardium rendered ischaemic demonstrate depressed basal and state 3 respiration, lack of respiratory and substrate control, and ultrastructural alterations ranging from moderate swelling to complete disruption (Jennings and Ganote, 1974).

Albumin-bound LPC, in concentrations simulating those present in ischaemic myocardium, alters respiratory function, ATPase activity and ultrastructure of mitochondria isolated from normal guinea-pig hearts simulating changes seen in organelles isolated from ischaemic hearts. The deterioration of mitochondrial function elicited by LPC was associated with concentration-dependent alterations in mitochondrial structure, reflected by changes in turbidity of mitochondrial suspensions incubated with LPC and by ultrastructural changes characterised by electron microscopy. In ischaemic myocardium, cellular energetics would be impaired if only a fraction of the accumulating amphiphiles had immediate access to mitochondrial membranes with similar deleterious effects. Inhibition of oxidative phosphorylation and augmentation of ATPase activity by LPC might reduce the intracellular concentrations of ATP available for maintenance of cellular integrity. These observations may be particularly important since mitochondrial dysfunction is a hallmark of, and a possible aetiological factor in, the genesis of irreversible injury. Thus, amphiphiles may play a role not only in arrhythmogenesis but also in compromising cell viability by impairing mitochondrial functional integrity.

12.6 ACYL CARNITINE

Long chain acyl carnitines are amphiphiles which possess many structural similarities to LPC (figure 12.2). Like lysophosphoglycerides their concentrations increase in ischaemic tissue *in vivo* particularly when plasma FFA concentrations are elevated (Liedtke *et al.*, 1978). Acyl carnitines induce electrophysiological derangements analogous to those elicited by LPC with the arrhythmogenic effects significantly enhanced in the presence of concomitant acidosis. Furthermore, electrophysiological effects induced by long chain acyl carnitine are additive to those induced by LPC, suggesting that modest changes in tissue or plasma concentrations of several metabolites may elicit substantial electrophysiological consequences in combination, particularly in a milieu of reduced pH. The parallelism between increased tissue acyl carnitine and increased circulating FFA may help to explain the arrhythmogenicity of circulating FFA under some conditions.

12.7 POTENTIAL MECHANISMS UNDERLYING THE ELECTROPHYSIOLOGICAL EFFECTS OF AMPHIPHILES

The mechanisms whereby LPGs induce their effect on membranes are not known with certainty. Since LPGs are asymmetrical moieties with both hydrophobic and hydrophilic constituents, they can profoundly influence membrane integrity (figure 12.2). The functional integrity of membranes is dependent upon the physical characteristics of phospholipid constituents. Therefore, LPGs with both hydrophilic and hydrophobic properties readily incorporate into membranes and thereby induce marked alterations in membrane permeability. Since LPC will increase K^+ release from the erythrocyte prior to haemolysis, this mechanism may be applicable to ischaemic cardiac cells as well since increased extracellular K^+ is a characteristic finding *in vivo* (chapter 6). Recent evidence (Weltzien, 1979) suggests that the effect of LPC on the membrane is not due to incorporation of micelles into the membrane but rather due to 'wedging' of individual molecules of LPC into the membrane, thereby inducing their effect when two closely adjacent molecules are incorporated (figure 12.3). It is not known whether the LPC incorporated into the membrane during ischaemia is required in specific association with membrane proteins, lipids or both. Recent results in our laboratory obtained in studies of ventricular muscle demonstrate that less than 1 per cent of cellular phospholipid supplanted by additional LPC is sufficient to induce the electrophysiological

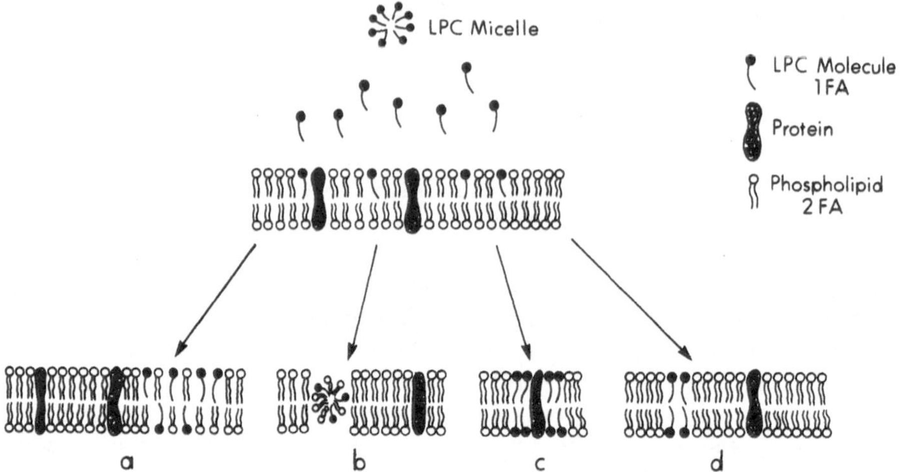

Figure 12.3 Schematic representation illustrating some of the possible mechanisms whereby LPC may be incorporated into membranes and thereby alter the symmetrical structure of the phospholipids and hence dipole–dipole interactions. These changes may explain the alteration in both active and passive membrane properties induced by LPC. In the top portion of the figure, LPC can exist in either the micelle or monomer form. Most evidence suggests incorporation of the monomer form initially into the outer bilayer. In the bottom portion of the figure, several examples (a–d) are given to represent subsequent orientation of the LPC which would thereby alter membrane properties and possibly ionic permeabilities. (Modified from Weltzien (1979).)

derangements characteristic of ischaemia and that, based on electron microscopic autoradiography with [^{14}C] LPC, selective sarcolemmal accumulation of LPG of less than 5 per cent is required to induce profound electrophysiological derangements. Thus, *in vivo*, only modest alterations in sarcolemmal LPGs synthesised endogenously would be required to exert the profound disturbances in membrane function characteristic within minutes of ischaemia.

Although the effects of LPC on specific ionic currents have not yet been delineated, depression in the rapid inward current carried by Na^+ appears likely since $\dot{V}_{max}$ of phase 0 is reduced (Corr *et al.*, 1979) and there is a downward and rightward shift in the membrane response curve. Thus, although $\dot{V}_{max}$ may be reduced in part as a consequence of the reduction in resting membrane potential (RMP), LPC appears to exert a direct depressant effect on gNa^+ independent of alterations in RMP (Corr *et al.*, 1979). The effects of LPC on refractoriness are complex and include a shortening of refractory period at lower concentrations with lengthening of refractoriness and induction of post-repolarisation refractoriness at higher concentrations. This inhomogeneity of refractoriness is a characteristic finding during ischaemia *in vivo* (Russell and Oliver, 1978) and may occur secondarily to differences in the accumulation of LPGs across the ischaemic region. This disparity of refractoriness may be of ultimate importance in the induction of unidirectional block and, together with the slowed conduction induced by LPC (Corr *et al.*,

1979), the maintenance of re-entrant pathways within ischaemic myocardium. Indeed, the occurrence of electrical alternans in subepicardial ischaemic zone action potentials (Downar *et al.*, 1977a; Russell *et al.*, 1977), a phenomenon also seen with LPC (Corr *et al.*, 1979), may be secondary to regional alterations in refractoriness. Changes in excitability during ischaemia *in vivo* including a transient increase for 1-3 min followed by a marked decrease in excitability (Elharrar *et al.*, 1977) may also be a reflection of accumulating LPGs. This is based on the observation that LPC elicits biphasic effects on excitability with an initial increase due to alteration of passive membrane properties and a decrease in excitability due to changes in active membrane properties (Arnsdorf and Sawicki, 1981). These alterations in excitability appear to differ across the ischaemic region and thereby may influence refractoriness as well as alterations in regional conduction time secondary to the inhomogenous accumulation of LPGs. Since LPC also increases membrane resistance (Arnsdorf and Sawicki, 1981), a phenomenon recently shown to occur during hypoxia *in vitro* (Wojtczak, 1979), block of conduction secondary to increases in membrane resistance with cell to cell uncoupling may also be mediated by LPGs.

Recent evidence suggests that two arrhythmogenic mechanisms may be responsible for arrhythmias associated with ischaemia (Janse *et al.*, 1980). These findings indicate that ventricular ectopic activity which initiates ventricular tachycardia or fibrillation is due to a mechanism which initiates earliest activation in the Purkinje fibres of the normal zone immediately adjacent to the ischaemic zone. Since elevated concentrations of LPGs increase automaticity of isolated Purkinje fibres at a normal and a reduced RMP (Corr *et al.*, 1979), the accumulation of these amphiphiles may influence the immediately adjacent normal zone. In addition, earliest activation in the normal zone may be secondary to current flow from the ischaemic to normal regions due to delayed activation of ischaemic regions and hence earlier repolarisation in normal regions. Thus, although LPGs shorten action potential duration, a finding characteristic of ischaemic myocardium *in vivo*, the delay in excitation through the ischaemic zone due to slowing in conduction velocity and regional conduction block would allow earlier excitation and hence repolarisation in normal regions. This may then result in a current flow from ischaemic to normal regions with earlier excitation in the normal region with subsequent excitation back through the ischaemic zone (Janse *et al.*, 1980). The increased idioventricular rate (IVR) characteristic of reperfused myocardium (Penkoske *et al.*, 1978), possibly a reflection of enhanced ventricular automaticity, may also be secondary to the accumulation of LPGs with associated increases in automaticity. It is possible that the reason why IVR is not elevated despite increased levels of LPGs during sustained occlusion is because of the concomitant accumulation of extracellular K^+, a phenomenon known to suppress ventricular automaticity (Vassalle *et al.*, 1964). However, with reperfusion, the extracellular K^+ falls rapidly, thus allowing LPGs to elicit the increase in IVR.

During myocardial ischaemia the importance of depolarisation dependent exclusively on the slow inward current (I_{si}) remains controversial. Several studies suggest that acidosis may inhibit I_{si}, thereby precluding a role of I_{si} during early myocardial ischaemia (Chesnais *et al.*, 1975; Davis *et al.*, 1976; Vogel and Sperelakis, 1977). Since I_{si} appears to depend upon cyclic AMP (Watanabe and Besche, 1974) and since we have recently shown that LPC stimulates adenylate cyclase independent of catecholamines (Ahumada *et al.*, 1979), LPC may induce potentials exclusively dependent on I_{si} despite concomitant acidosis. Furthermore, LPC also stimulates ^{45}Ca uptake into isolated cardiac myocytes, possibly augmenting I_{si} (Ahumada *et al.*, 1980). In isolated canine Purkinje fibres, LPC (200 μM) at pH 7.4 induced potentials dependent exclusively on I_{si} as judged by abolition by Mn^{2+} or verapamil and unresponsiveness to tetrodotoxin. Likewise, after prolonged exposure to pH 6.5, LPC at lower concentrations (100 μM) also induced action potentials dependent on I_{si}. However, these responses were not unique to LPC-induced alterations since I_{si} potentials produced by elevated K^+ (27 mM) plus isoprenaline were also maintained with prolonged (30 min) acidosis in both canine Purkinje fibres and ventricular muscle. Thus, it appears that under conditions of acidic pH, comparable to that seen in early ischaemia *in vivo*, potentials dependent exclusively on I_{si} may mediate in part the slowed conduction and altered refractoriness. Later during ischaemia, when I_{si} is inhibited, slowed conduction may be mediated by depressed fast response action potentials. These conclusions are supported by recent findings that intracoronary infusion of Mn^{2+} during 10 min of ischaemia *in vivo* significantly delays conduction time and shortens the ERP in the ischaemic epicardium but not endocardium (Kupersmith and Cohen, 1980). In contrast, 1 h after coronary occlusion, Mn^{2+} has no effect on either conduction time or ERP of the ischaemic region. Likewise, verapamil or D-600 fails to alter subepicardial conduction time 3-7 days after coronary occlusion (El-Sherif and Lazzara, 1979). Thus, action potentials dependent exclusively on I_{si} and induced by LPGs may play an important role in arrhythmogenesis during early ischaemia, although other factors appear to be operative at later time periods.

12.8 MECHANISMS RESPONSIBLE FOR THE ACCUMULATION OF AMPHIPHILES

Long chain acyl carnitines

FFA taken up by the heart is rapidly esterified to FFA-CoA (coenzyme A) esters (acyl CoA) by acyl CoA synthetases at the outer mitochondrial membrane. Prior to β oxidation, the acyl group is transferred to carnitine and the acyl carnitine transported across the mitochondrial membrane. Total carnitine content on each side of the mitochondrial membranes remains relatively constant (Morgan *et al.*, 1978). Acyl carnitine within the mitochondria is reconverted to acyl CoA and the acyl group metabolised via β-oxidation. Since the cytoplasm of myocardial cells contains high concentrations of carnitine, the flux through β-oxidation predominates. β-Oxidation of fatty acid derivatives results in conversion of acyl CoA to two-carbon acetyl CoA moieties with simultaneous reduction of nicotinamide adenine nucleotide (NAD) and flavin adenine dinucleotide (FAD) to NADH and $FADH_2$, which are oxidised through mitochondrial electron transport with concomitant production of ATP. The acetyl CoA enters the citric acid cycle resulting in production of NADH, a substance oxidised via mitochondrial electron transport with consequent production of ATP. Under physiological conditions, oxygen availability is sufficient to oxidise the reduced nucleotides (NADH and $FADH_2$). However, in tissue rendered ischaemic the concentrations of $FADH_2$ and NADH increase and β-oxidation of fatty acid derivatives is inhibited, with a consequent reduction in the production of acetyl CoA and ATP. Under these conditions, concentrations of acyl CoA and acyl carnitine increase (Liedtke *et al.*, 1978). The increases are accentuated when plasma FFA levels are elevated, thereby providing a possible explanation of the arrhythmogenic influence of elevated circulating FFA evident in experimental animals (Kurien *et al.*, 1971) and patients (Simonsen and Kjekshus, 1978).

Lysophosphoglycerides

Sarcolemmal phospholipids undergo continuous turnover, but accumulation of their lysophospholipid catabolites is prevented under physiological conditions by either re-acylation to form diacyl phospholipids or hydrolysis of the lysophospholipids to form glycerophosphoryl choline (GPC, figure 12.4). Several potential mechanisms may be responsible for the accumulation of lysophosphoglycerides during ischaemia. One is enhanced phospholipase A_2 (PLA_2) activity (figure 12.4, pathway a). Accordingly, we recently evaluated activity of myocardial phospholipase A_2, an enzyme that cleaves the fatty acid from the 2-position of phospholipids resulting in synthesis of 2-deacyl LPC (Lee and Sobel, 1981). Radiolabelled

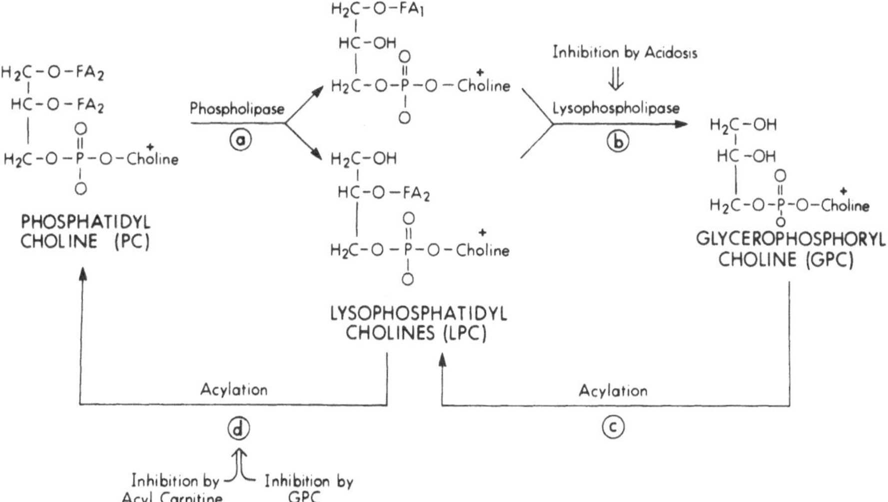

Figure 12.4 Pathways of synthesis of the major phospholipid moieties. FA = fatty acid. Phosphatidyl choline is a physiological constituent found in high concentrations in the sarcolemma.

phospholipid substrates ([^{14}C]linoleic acid in the 2-position of phosphatidylcholine or phosphatidylethanolamine) were employed to quantify phospholipase A_2 activity of rabbit heart mitochondria and microsomes, and to compare enzyme activities in fractions from normal and ischaemic tissue. The effects of substrate and pH on PLA_2 activity in fractions from rabbit hearts are shown in figure 12.5.

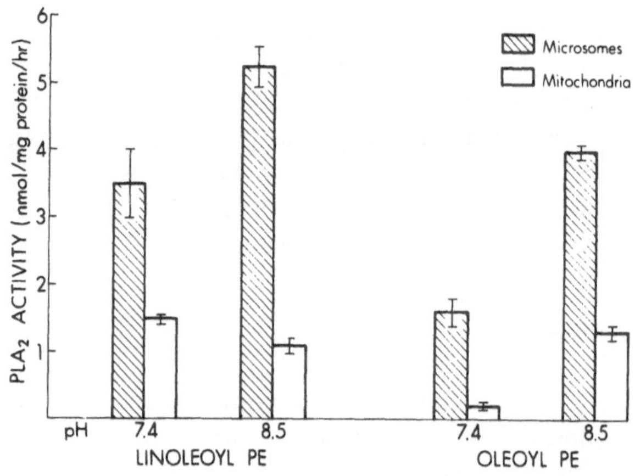

Figure 12.5 Effects of substrate and pH on PLA_2 activity. Incubations were performed for 1 h at 37 °C in the presence of 2 mM Ca^{2+}, 25 nmol substrate, and 0.1 mg microsomal or 0.2 mg mitochondrial protein.

With the single exception of mitochondria incubated at pH 8.5, linoleoyl phosphatidylethanolamine (PE) was a more effective substrate than oleoyl PE. Microsomal PLA_2 activity was higher at pH 8.5 compared to pH 7.4 with either oleoyl PE ($P < 0.001$) or linoleoyl PE ($P < 0.05$) as substrates. Mitochondria exhibited higher activity at pH 8.5 with oleoyl PE ($P < 0.001$), but activity was greater at pH 7.4 with linoleoyl PE ($P < 0.02$). PLA_2 activity was only moderately dependent on concentrations of Ca^{2+} between 0 and 2 mM (figure 12.6). To assess whether changes induced by ischaemia altered PLA_2 activity in isolated organelles, assays were performed in the microsomal and the mitochondrial fractions. Yields of each of the two types of organelles expressed as protein per gram of tissue were equivalent in extracts from ischaemic compared to control hearts. Microsomal PLA_2 activity was 14.8 ± 1.3 nmol (mg protein)$^{-1}$ h^{-1} in fractions from control hearts and 12.1 ± 1.5 nmol mg^{-1} h^{-1} in those from ischaemic hearts. Corresponding values for mitochondrial PLA_2 activity were 7.5 ± 1.2 and 4.9 ± 0.6 nmol mg^{-1} h^{-1}. These differences in PLA_2 activity were not significant. Thus, PLA_2 activity in mitochondria and microsomes did not increase in fractions from ischaemic compared to those from control rabbit hearts. Despite the sensitivity of the techniques employed, we could detect no significant change in the content of PC, PE or lysophosphatides when cells were stimulated with potential modulators of PLA_2 including bradykinin or with concentrations of noradrenaline and adrenaline which caused a 75-100 per cent increase in rate of beating of cultured cardiac myocytes. Because concomitant activity of a lysophospholipase (figure 12.4, pathway b)

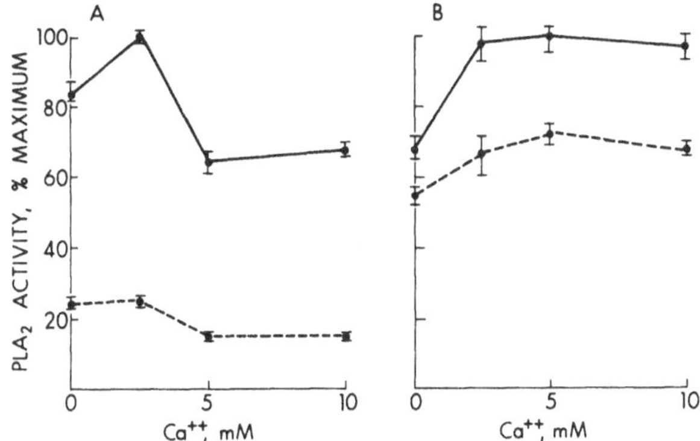

Figure 12.6 Effects of Ca^{2+} concentration on PLA_2 activity. Incubations were performed for 1 h at 37°C, pH 8.5, in the presence of 25 nmol substrate and 0.1 mg microsomal (●—●) or 0.2 mg mitochondrial (●---●) protein. A, substrate = linoleoyl PE; B, substrate = oleoyl PE. Results are expressed as a percentage of maximum activity obtained at optimum Ca^{2+} concentration with microsomes.

might have prevented accumulation of lysophosphoglycerides, we assayed selected samples for release of GPC, a product of lysophospholipase activity. There was no evidence of formation of either moiety. Thus, since PLA_2 activity is relatively low in fractions from rabbit heart compared to measured activity in corresponding liver fractions, since it does not increase in fractions isolated from ischaemic tissue, and since it fails to increase in intact cells in response to potential modulators, it is unlikely that PLA_2 activity plays a primary role in the mediation of membrane injury or augmentation of lysophosphoglyceride content observed in ischaemic myocardium *in situ*.

Because enhanced PLA_2 activity does not appear to be a major source of enhanced production of lysophosphoglycerides during ischaemia, several alternative pathways have recently been evaluated. For example, microsomal lysophospholipase (figure 12.4, pathway b) activity is inhibited 58 per cent by reduction in pH (Gross and Sobel, 1980a), which might thereby contribute to the accumulation of lysophosphoglycerides. Secondly, *de novo* synthesis of LPC by acylation of GPC to LPC (figure 12.4, pathway c) occurs in cardiac microsomal preparations (Gross and Sobel, 1980b), an effect which may be accentuated in ischaemic myocardium by the augmented concentrations of acyl CoA derivatives (Liedtke *et al.*, 1978). Thirdly, acyl CoA : LPC acyl transferase (figure 12.4, pathway d) is inhibited by increased GPC (Gross and Sobel, 1981a) and may thereby contribute to the accumulation of LPC in ischaemic myocardium. Fourthly, acyl carnitine, which increases in ischaemic tissue *in vivo*, inhibits cytosolic LPC transacylase (Gross and Sobel, 1981b; figure 12.4, pathway d) and may augment the accumulation of LPC in ischaemic tissue *in vivo*.

In plasma, concentrations of LPC may increase when cholesterol is elevated due to lecithin : cholesterol acyl transferase (LCAT) activity (Glomset *et al.*, 1962). In tissue, the LPC is converted to lecithin by acyl CoA : LPC acyl transferase. However, ischaemia may alter the rate or extent of local reconversion, leading to regional accumulation of LPC. Thus, although PLA_2 activity does not appear likely to account for the accumulation of lysophosphoglycerides with ischaemia, several mechanisms have been identified that may be responsible, alone or in combination.

12.8 THERAPEUTIC IMPLICATIONS

Presently, many commonly used antiarrhythmic agents are non-specific membrane depressants. In the milieu of myocardial ischaemia and the concomitant alterations of membrane function which result in early ventricular arrhythmias, many of these antiarrhythmic agents appear to be of only limited value. Delineation of the specific biochemical pathways responsible for the accumulation of arrhythmogenic metabolites and clarification of mechanisms involved in mediating their electrophysiological consequences should contribute to development of more specific and potentially more effective prophylactic and therapeutic measures. Such measures would be directed not only towards non-specific depression of membrane function but also towards inhibition of accumulation of metabolites potentially responsible for malignant ventricular arrhythmias.

ACKNOWLEDGEMENTS

Research from the authors' laboratory was supported by National Institutes of Health Grant HL17646, *SCOR* in Ischemic Heart Disease. Dr Corr is an Established Investigator of the American Heart Association.

REFERENCES

Ahumada, G. G., Bergmann, S. R., Carlson, E., Corr, P. B. and Sobel, B. E. (1979). Augmentation of cyclic AMP content induced by lysophosphatidyl choline in rabbit hearts. *Cardiovasc. Res.*, **13**, 377-82

Ahumada, G. G., Corr, P. B. and Sobel, B. E. (1980). Accelerated accumulation of calcium in cultured cardiac myocytes exposed to lysophosphatides. *Circulation*, **62**, Suppl. III, 113

Akiyama, T. (1981). Intracellular recording of *in situ* ventricular cells during ventricular fibrillation. *Am. J. Physiol.*, **9**, H465-71

Armstrong, A., Duncan, B., Oliver, M. F., Julian, D. G., Donald, K. W., Fulton, M., Lutz, W. and Morrison, S. L. (1972). Natural history of acute coronary heart attacks. A community study. *Br. Heart J.*, **34**, 67-80

Arnsdorf, M. F. and Sawicki, G. J. (1981). The effects of lysophatyl choline, a toxic metabolite of ischemia in the components of cardiac excitability in sheep Purkinje fibers. *Circulation Res.*, **49**, 16-30

Bagdonas, A. A., Stukey, J. H., Piera, J., Amer, N. S. and Hoffman, B. F. (1961). Effects of ischemia and hypoxia on the specialized conducting system of the canine heart. *Am. Heart J.*, **61**, 206-18

Baker, P. F. (1968). Nervous conduction. Some properties of the ion-selective channels which appear during the action potential. *Br. med. Bull.*, **24**, 179-82

Bergmann, S. R., Ferguson, T. B. and Sobel, B. E. (1981). Effects of amphiphiles on erythrocytes, coronary arteries and perfused hearts. *Am. J. Physiol.*, **9**, H229-37

Bigger, J. T., Dresdale, R. G., Heissenbuttel, R. H., Weld, F. M. and Wit, A. L. (1977). Ventricular arrhythmias in ischemic heart disease: mechanisms, prevalence, significance and management. *Progr. cardiovasc. Dis.*, **19**, 255-300

Bjerve, K. S., Daae, L. N. W. and Bremer, J. (1974). The selective loss of lysophospholipids in some commonly used lipid extraction procedures. *Analyt. Biochem.*, **58**, 238-45

Blaustein, M. P. and Goldman, D. E. (1966). Competitive action of calcium and procaine on lobster axon. *J. gen. Physiol.*, **49**, 1043-63

Chesnais, J. M., Coraboeuf, E., Sauviat, M. P. and Vassas, J. M. (1975). Sensitivity to H, and Li and Mg ions of the slow inward sodium current in frog atrial fibers. *J. molec. cell. Cardiol.*, **7**, 627-42

Chien, K. R., Reeves, J. P., Buja, L. M., Bonte, F., Parkey, R. W. and Willerson, J. T. (1981). Phospholipid alterations in canine ischemic myocardium. Temporal and topographical correlations with T_c-99m-PPi accumulation on an *in vitro* sarcolemmal Ca^{2+} permeability defect. *Circulation Res.*, **48**, 711-9

Coleman, R. (1973). Membrane-bound enzymes and membrane ultrastructure. *Biochim. biophys. Acta*, **300**, 1-30

Corr, P. B. and Sobel, B. E. (1979). The importance of metabolites in the genesis of ventricular dysrhythmia induced by ischemia. I. Electrophysiological considerations. *Mod. Concepts cardiovasc. Dis.*, **48**, 43-7

Corr, P. B., Witkowski, F. X. and Sobel, B. E. (1978). Mechanisms contributing to malignant dysrhythmias induced by ischemia in the cat. *J. clin. Invest.*, **61**, 109-19

Corr, P. B., Cain, M. E., Witkowski, F. X., Price, D. A. and Sobel, B. E. (1979). Potential arrhythmogenic electrophysiological derangements in canine Purkinje fibers induced by lysophosphoglycerides. *Circulation Res.*, **44**, 822-32

Danielli, J. F. and Davson, H. (1935). A contribution to the theory of permeability of thin films. *J. cell. comp. Physiol.*, **5**, 495-508

Danielli, J. F. and Harvey, E. N. (1935). The tension at the surface of mackeral egg oil, with remarks on the nature of the cell surface. *J. cell. comp. Physiol.*, **5**, 483-94

Davis, L. D., Helmer, P. R. and Ballantyne, F. (1976). Production of slow responses in canine cardiac Purkinje fibers exposed to reduced pH. *J. molec. cell. Cardiol.*, **8**, 61-76

DeMello, W. C. (1972). Membrane lipids and cardiac electrogenesis. In *Electrical*

Phenomena in the Heart (ed. W. C. DeMello), Academic Press, New York, pp. 89-110

Downar, E., Janse, M. J. and Durrer, D. (1977a). The effect of acute coronary artery occlusion on subepicardial transmembrane potentials in the intact porcine heart. *Circulation*, **56**, 217-24

Downar, E., Janse, M. J. and Durrer, D. (1977b). The effect of 'ischemic' blood on transmembrane potentials of normal porcine ventricular myocardium. *Circulation*, **55**, 455-62

Elharrar, V., Foster, P. R., Jirak, T. L., Gaum, W. E. and Zipes, D. P. (1977). Alterations in canine myocardial excitability during ischemia. *Circulation Res.*, **40**, 98-105

El-Sherif, N. and Lazzara, R. (1979). Reentrant ventricular arrhythmias in the late myocardial infarction period. 7. Effect of verapamil and D600 and the role of the 'slow channel'. *Circulation*, **60**, 605-15

Glomset, J. A., Parker, F., Tjaden, M. and Williams, R. H. (1962). Esterification *in vitro* of free cholesterol in human and rat plasma. *Biochim. biophys. Acta*, **58**, 398-406

Goldman, D. E. (1964). A molecular structural basis for the excitation properties of axons. *Biophys. J.*, **4**, 167-88

Gorter, E. and Grendel, F. (1925). On bimolecular layers of lipoids on the chromocytes of the blood. *J. exp. Med.*, **41**, 439-43

Gross, R. W. and Sobel, B. E. (1980a). Inhibition of rabbit myocardial lysophospholipase activity by acidosis: a potential cause of accumulation of lysophosphatides. *Circulation*, **62**, Suppl. III, 176

Gross, R. W. and Sobel, B. E. (1980b). Myocardial synthesis of phospho- and lysophosphoglycerides by acylation of glycerophosphorylcholine (GPC). *Clin. Res.*, **28**, 538A

Gross, R. W. and Sobel, B. E. (1981a). Inhibition of myocardial lysophosphatidyl choline (LPC) acyl transferase by glycerophosphoryl choline. *Clin. Res.*, **29**, 201A

Gross, R. W. and Sobel, B. E. (1981b). Inhibition of myocardial lysophosphatidyl choline (LPC) transcyclase by palmitoyl carnitine: implications for arrhythmogenesis. *Clin. Res.*, **29**, 562A

Janse, M. J., van Capelle, F. J. L., Morsink, H., Kleber, A. G., Wilms-Schopman, F., Cardinal, R., D'Alnoncourt, C. H. and Durrer, D. (1980). Flow of 'injury' current and patterns of excitation during early ventricular arrhythmias in acute regional myocardial ischemia in isolated porcine and canine hearts. Evidence for two different arrhythmogenic mechanisms. *Circulation Res.*, **47**, 151-65

Jennings, R. B. and Ganote, C. E. (1974). Structural changes in myocardium during acute ischemia. *Circulation Res.*, **34/35**, Suppl. III, 156-72

Jorgensen, L., Rowsell, H. C., Hovigt, T., Glynn, M. F. and Mustard, J. F. (1967). Adenosine diphosphate-induced platelet aggregation and myocardial infarction in swine. *Lab. Invest.*, **17**, 616-44

Karli, J. N., Karikas, G. A., Hatzipavlou, P. K., Levis, G. M. and Moulopoulos, S. N. (1979). The inhibition of Na^+ and K^+ stimulated ATPase activity of rabbit and dog heart sarcolemma by lysophosphatidyl choline. *Life Sci.*, **24**, 1869-76

Korn, E. D. (1966). Structure of biological membranes. *Science, N.Y.*, **153**, 1491-8

Kupersmith, J. and Cohen, R. (1980). Differing electrophysiological effects of slow response inhibiting agents manganese and verapamil on ischemic, infarcted and normal tissue *in situ*. *J. Pharmac. exp. Ther.*, **215**, 394-400

Kurien, A., Yates, P. A. and Oliver, M. F. (1971). The role of free fatty acids in the production of ventricular arrhythmias after acute coronary artery occlusion. *Eur. J. clin. Invest.*, **1**, 225-41

Lawrence, A. J., Morres, G. R. and Steele, J. (1974). A conductimetric study of erythrocyte lysis by lysolecithin and linoleic acid. *Eur. J. Biochem.*, **48**, 277-86

Lazzara, R., El-Sherif, N. and Scherlag, B. J. (1973). Electrophysiological properties of Purkinje cells in one-day-old myocardial infarction. *Circulation Res.*, **33**, 722-34

Lee, F. C. and Sobel, B. E. (1981). Phospholipid metabolism: myocardial phospholipase and acyltransferase. *Fedn Proc. Fedn Am. Socs. exp. Biol.*, **40**, 1631

Liedtke, A. J., Nellis, S. and Neely, J. R. (1978). Effects of excess free fatty acids on mechanical and metabolic function in normal and ischemic myocardium in swine. *Circulation Res.*, **43**, 652-61

Marcus, M. L., Kerber, R. E., Ehrhardt, J. and Abboud, F. M. (1976). Effects of time on volume and distribution of coronary collateral flow. *Am. J. Physiol.*, **230**, 279-85

Mogelson, S., Wilson, G. E. and Sobel, B. E. (1980). Characterization of rabbit myocardial phospholipids with ^{31}P nuclear magnetic resonance. *Biochem. biophys. Acta*, **619**, 680-8

Morgan, H. E., Neely, J. R. and LaNoue, K. F. (1978). Biochemical events in ischemic heart. In *Acute and Long-term Medical Management of Myocardial Ischemia* (ed. Å. Hjalmarson, L. Wilhelmsen, A. Lindren and A. B. Soner), Astra, Mölndal, pp. 10-22

Oliva, P. B. and Breckenridge, J. C. (1977). Arteriographic evidence of coronary arterial spasm in acute myocardial infarction. *Circulation*, **56**, 366-74

Penkoske, P. A., Sobel, B. E. and Corr, P. B. (1978). Disparate electrophysiological alterations accompanying dysrhythmia due to coronary occlusion and reperfusion in the cat. *Circulation*, **58**, 1023-35

Podzuweit, T., Dalby, A. J., Cherry, G. W. and Opie, L. H. (1978). Tissue levels of cyclic AMP in ischaemic and non-ischaemic myocardium following coronary artery ligation. *J. molec. cell. Cardiol.*, **10**, 81-94

Robertson, J. D. (1959). The ultrastructure of cell membranes and their derivatives. *Biochem. Soc. Symp.*, **16**, 3-43

Russell, D. C. and Oliver, M. F. (1978). Ventricular refractoriness during acute myocardial ischaemia and its relationship to ventricular fibrillation. *Cardiovasc. Res.*, **12**, 221-7

Russell, D. C., Oliver, M. F. and Wojtczak, J. (1977). Combined electrophysiological technique for assessment of the cellular basis of early ventricular arrhythmias. *Lancet*, *ii*, 686-88

Scherlag, B. J., El-Sherif, N., Hope, R. and Lazzara, R. (1974). Characterization and localization of ventricular arrhythmias resulting from myocardial ischemia and infarction. *Circulation Res.*, **35**, 372-83

Shaikh, N. A. and Downar, E. (1981). Time course of changes in porcine myocardial phospholipid levels during ischaemia. A reassessment of the lysolipid hypothesis. *Circulation Res.*, **49**, 316-25

Simonsen, S. and Kjekshus, J. K. (1978). The effect of free fatty acids on myocardial oxygen consumption during atrial pacing and catecholamine infusion in man. *Circulation*, **58**, 484-91

Sobel, B. E., Corr, P. B., Robison, A. K., Goldstein, R. A., Witkowski, F. X. and Klein, M. S. (1978). Accumulation of lysophosphoglycerides with arrhythmogenic properties in ischemic myocardium. *J. clin. Invest.*, **62**, 546-53

Stein, W. D. and Danielli, J. F. (1956). Structure and function in red cell permeability. *Discuss. Faraday Soc.*, **21**, 238-51

Tobias, J. M. (1964). A chemically specified molecular mechanism underlying excitation in nerve. A hypothesis. *Nature, Lond.*, **203**, 13-17

Vassalle, M., Greenspan, K., Jomain, S. and Hoffman, B. F. (1964). Effects of potassium on automaticity and conduction of canine hearts. *Am. J. Physiol.*, **207**, 334-40

Vogel, S. and Sperelakis, N. (1977). Blockage of myocardial slow inward current at low pH. *Am. J. Physiol.*, **233**, C99-103

Watanabe, A. M. and Besch, H. R. (1974). Cyclic adenosine monophosphate modulation of slow calcium influx channels in guinea pig hearts. *Circulation Res.*, **35**, 316-24

Weltzien, H. U. (1979). Cytolytic and membrane-perturbing properties of lysophosphatidyl choline. *Biochim. biophys. Acta*, **559**, 259-87

Williams, D. O., Scherlag, B. J., Hope, R. R., El-Sherif, N. and Lazzara, R. (1974). The pathophysiology of malignant ventricular arrhythmias during acute myocardial ischemia. *Circulation*, **50**, 1163-72

Wojtczak, J. (1979). Contractures and increase in internal longitudinal resistance of cow ventricular muscle induced by hypoxia. *Circulation Res.*, **44**, 88-95

NOTE ADDED IN PROOF

Some of the authors' most recent data has been published in the following reports:

Corr, P. B., Snyder, D. W., Cain, M. E., Crafford, W. A., Gross, R. W. and Sobel, B. E. (1981). Electrophysiological effects of amphiphiles on canine Purkinje fibers: implications for dysrhythmias secondary to ischemia. *Circulation Res.*, **49**, 354-63

Snyder, D. W., Crafford, W. A., Ginshow, J. L., Rankin, D., Sobel, B. E. and Corr, P. B. (1981). Lysophosphoglycerides in ischemic myocardial effluents and potentiation of their arrhythmogenic effects. *Am. J. Physiol.*, **241**, H700-7

13

Early Ventricular Arrhythmias Arising from Acute Myocardial Ischaemia; Possible Involvement of Prostaglandins and Thromboxanes

Susan J. Coker

13.1 INTRODUCTION

Prostaglandins are endogenous fatty acids which may influence cardiac arrhythmias in a number of different ways. Almost all the information about the effects of prostaglandins on arrhythmias has been derived from animal experiments using methods of inducing arrhythmias which bear little resemblance to those arising clinically as a result of an acute episode of myocardial ischaemia. There are only two groups who have reported on the clinical actions of prostaglandins on arrhythmias (Mann *et al.*, 1973; Mann, 1976; Mohr *et al.*, 1981). They have shown that prostaglandin (PG) $F_{2\alpha}$ and PGE_2 can exert antiarrhythmic effects against a variety of ventricular and supraventricular arrhythmias of mixed aetiology.

The question of the possible role of prostaglandins in early arrhythmias can be examined using three different experimental approaches. First, it is pertinent to examine the effects of exogenously administered prostaglandins on these arrhythmias. Secondly, the actions of drugs which either antagonise prostaglandins, or prevent their synthesis, can be investigated. Unfortunately there is a lack of specific antagonists but there are a number of compounds available which interfere with prostaglandin synthesis. This second approach will of course provide information on the role of endogenous prostaglandins. A third, and perhaps more useful approach is to attempt to detect and quantify prostaglandin release during acute myocardial ischaemia and look for a relationship with arrhythmias.

First of all, some aspects of the biosynthesis of prostaglandins and their pharmacological activity will be considered.

13.2 BIOSYNTHESIS OF PROSTAGLANDINS

The term 'prostaglandin' was first used by von Euler (1936) to describe the vasodepressor and smooth muscle stimulating substance which he found in accessory genital glands (von Euler, 1934, 1935). This 'substance' was also discovered independently by Goldblatt (1933) who detected its presence in human semen. Its activity was eventually found to be due to several different acidic lipids. In 1960 prostaglandin F was isolated from sheep prostate glands (Bergström and Sjövall, 1960) and since then a number of other prostaglandins have been isolated and their chemical structures elucidated.

It has been demonstrated that prostaglandins are synthesised from polyunsaturated fatty acids (Bergström *et al.*, 1964; Van Dorp *et al.*, 1964) such as dihomo-γ-linolenic acid, arachidonic acid and eicosapentaenoic acid. These three fatty acids give rise to the prostaglandins of the 1, 2 and 3 series respectively, the number indicating the number of double bonds in each. The most common of these prostaglandin precursors is arachidonic acid which is incorporated as a structural component of phospholipids in cell membranes. Arachidonic acid is derived directly from the diet or by metabolism from dietary linoleic acid and is present in all body tissues (Ramwell *et al.*, 1977).

Prostaglandins do not appear to be stored in tissues, indicating that release reflects *de novo* synthesis (see, for example, Ramwell *et al.*, 1966; Piper and Vane, 1971). The first step necessary for the synthesis of prostaglandins is the release of the precursor fatty acids from the membrane phospholipids. This is brought about by phospholipases which can be activated in a number of ways. Once the fatty acid is released prostaglandins are formed rapidly. The type and the proportions of the various prostaglandins that can be synthesised depends on the situation, the tissue and the conditions at the time.

Since arachidonic acid is the most common of the prostaglandin precursors and since there is little evidence that prostaglandins of the '1' series occur naturally in the cardiovascular system of mammals (Moncada and Vane, 1978; Lands, 1979), only the metabolism of arachidonic acid is detailed below. This particular fatty acid is initially metabolised by two types of enzyme. Figure 13.1 illustrates the two pathways and shows the chemical structures of the various substances that can be formed. One of these enzymes is a series of lipoxygenases (point 1, figure 13.1) which are responsible for the formation of the leukotrienes.

The other enzyme is a cyclo-oxygenase (point 2, figure 13.1) which converts arachidonic acid to the cyclic endoperoxide prostaglandin G_2 (PGG_2). This step involves the incorporation of oxygen (Samuelsson, 1965). The cyclo-oxygenase enzyme is frequently termed 'prostaglandin synthetase'. PGG_2 is then converted to PGH_2, from which a number of products can result. The endoperoxides are unstable in aqueous medium and spontaneously decompose to a mixture of PGE_2 and PGD_2 (Hamberg and Fredholm, 1976). These prostaglandins, together with $PGF_{2\alpha}$, can also be formed enzymatically from the endoperoxides by an isomerase and possibly a reductase (Nugteren and Hazelhof, 1973; Hamberg *et al.*, 1974).

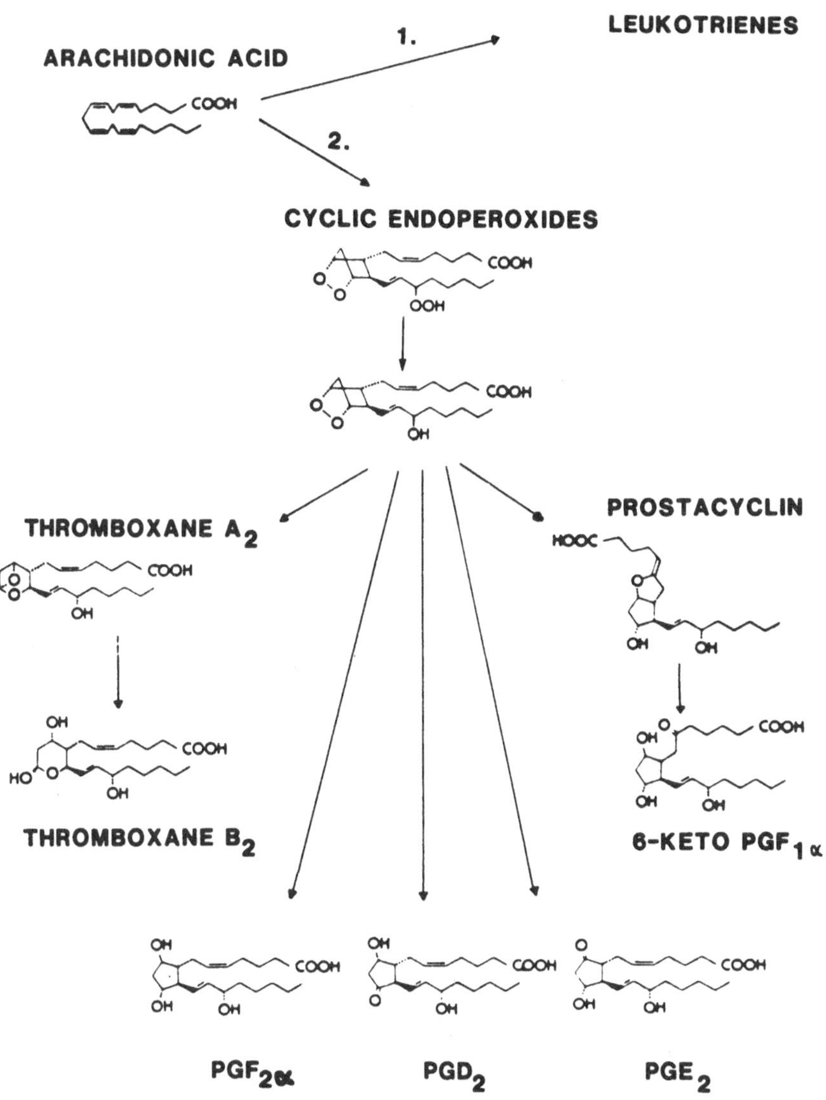

Figure 13.1 Some metabolites of arachidonic acid.

There are two other important products resulting from enzymatic conversion of the prostaglandin endoperoxides PGG_2 and PGH_2. These products, prostacyclin and thromboxane A_2 are both unstable and, unlike PGD_2, PGE_2 or $PGF_{2\alpha}$, cannot result from chemical breakdown. Each of these substances is synthesised by separate enzymes which have been termed prostacyclin synthetase (Moncada *et al.*, 1976) and thromboxane synthetase (Needleman *et al.*, 1976). The tissues in which these enzymes occur vary; for example, the major source of prostacyclin synthetase is in the vascular endothelium whereas platelets are the main location of thromboxane synthetase.

Thus a number of products with varying stability and biological activity can be derived from arachidonic acid. These are collectively termed prostanoids. First, there are the prostaglandin endoperoxides PGG_2 and PGH_2 which have a half life in aqueous media of approximately 5 min (Nugteren and Hazelhof, 1973) and are chemically degraded to the relatively stable compounds PGE_2, PGD_2 and $PGF_{2\alpha}$. Prostacyclin, which is formed enzymatically from the endoperoxides, has a half life of 2-3 min in blood at 37 °C (Dusting *et al.*, 1977) and is chemically broken down to form 6-keto prostaglandin $F_{1\alpha}$ (sometimes termed 6-oxo $PGF_1\alpha$). Similarly, thromboxane A_2, derived enzymatically from the same substrate and having a half life of 30 s (Hamberg and Samuelsson, 1974), is rapidly degraded to the stable metabolite, thromboxane B_2. Although PGE_2, PGD_2 and $PGF_{2\alpha}$ are all relatively stable in aqueous media, they are rapidly removed from the circulation *in vivo*. During passage through the lungs these prostaglandins are taken up and converted by dehydrogenases to biologically inactive metabolites (Ferreira and Vane, 1967).

Neither 6-keto $PGF_{1\alpha}$ nor thromboxane B_2 possesses significant biological activity, whereas all the other above-mentioned prostanoids have varying activities in a number of biological systems. PGE_2 and prostacyclin are both vasodilators whereas PGD_2, $PGF_{2\alpha}$ and thromboxane A_2 all possess vasoconstrictor activity. Prostaglandins also influence platelet aggregation, prostacyclin being a potent inhibitor of platelet aggregation whereas thromboxane A_2 promotes aggregation. The actions of the endoperoxides are difficult to evaluate since they vary considerably, depending on the particular tissues under investigation and their ability to produce the different prostanoids. It has been concluded, however, that the endoperoxides themselves do possess biological activity and that this is generally constrictor in nature (Moncada and Vane, 1978).

13.3 ACTIONS OF PROSTANOIDS ON EXPERIMENTAL ARRHYTHMIAS

Since PGE_1 was first reported to be antiarrhythmic by Zijlstra *et al.*, in 1972, various other prostaglandins have been shown to possess antiarrhythmic activity in a number of animal models. For example, in rats $PGF_{2\alpha}$ has been shown to be effective against calcium chloride-induced arrhythmias (Förster *et al.*, 1973) and PGA_2, PGE_1, $PGF_{2\alpha}$ and prostacyclin are effective against aconitine-induced arrhythmias (Förster, 1976; Mest and Förster, 1978). $PGE_{2\alpha}$ and $PGF_{2\alpha}$ have also been shown to be antiarrhythmic when tested against barium chloride-induced arrhythmias in rabbits (Förster *et al.*, 1973; Förster, 1976). Arachidonic acid and linoleic acid, which are prostaglandin precursors, are active in the above models whereas other fatty acids which are not prostaglandin precursors are ineffective (Mest *et al.*, 1978).

Both PGE_1 and $PGF_2\alpha$ have been reported to suppress noradrenaline-induced arrhythmias in dogs (Ito *et al.*, 1975). Other workers, however, could not demonstrate any action of these prostaglandins, or of indomethacin, on adrenaline-induced arrhythmias in halothane-anaesthetised dogs (Pace *et al.*, 1979).

PGE_1, PGE_2 and $PGF_{2\alpha}$ have been shown to protect against ouabain cardiotoxicity in the cat (Kelliher and Glenn, 1973; Somberg *et al.*, 1977; Förster *et al.*, 1973). Similarly, in rabbits, pretreatment with PGE_1 or PGE_2 reduces the arrhythmogenic potency of ouabain (Madan *et al.*, 1974).

Results from experiments such as those detailed above have led to the suggestion that prostaglandins may be endogenous antiarrhythmic agents (Förster, 1976). If prostaglandins have such a functional role then they should be effective against those arrhythmias that result from coronary artery ligation since this model probably bears a closer resemblance to the clinical situation (for example, of acute ischaemia leading to infarction) than the other models mentioned above.

There is some controversy regarding the effects of prostaglandins on arrhythmias resulting from coronary artery occlusion. In rats subject to acute coronary artery ligation Martinez and Crampton (1978) and Au *et al.* (1979) have demonstrated an antiarrhythmic effect of PGE_2. Similarly, we have shown that PGE_2 reduces both the number and the severity of the arrhythmias resulting from coronary artery ligation in anaesthetised rats; an equal infusion rate of $PGF_2\alpha$ reduces the incidence of ventricular fibrillation without altering the number of ectopic beats (Coker and Parratt, 1981).

The intravenous administration of PGE_1 is antiarrhythmic in anaesthetised cats subject to acute myocardial ischaemia, although the administration of both PGE_1 and PGA_1 via the left atrium may enhance ventricular fibrillation after occlusion of the left anterior descending coronary artery (Kelliher *et al.*, 1979). In dogs, PGE_2 and $PGF_{1\alpha}$ both reduce the incidence of premature ventricular contractions during the 25 min immediately following acute ligation of the left anterior descending coronary artery (Harvie *et al.*, 1978).

Thus it appears that in the above-mentioned experiments the intravenous administration of prostaglandins E_1, E_2 and $F_{2\alpha}$ results in antiarrhythmic actions in animals subject to acute coronary artery ligation. The conflicting results arise from left atrial administration of PGE_1 and PGA_1.

The picture with prostacyclin is less clear. It has been reported to be both antiarrhythmic (Coker and Parratt, 1981) and arrhythmogenic (Au *et al.*, 1979) in rats, to have a biphasic arrhythmogenic action in cats, depending on dosage (Dix *et al.*, 1979), and to be antiarrhythmic in dogs (Au *et al.*, 1979; DeBauche *et al.*, 1981; Ribeiro *et al.*, 1981; Starnes *et al.*, 1981).

Prostacyclin is a potent vasodilator and it is possible that exacerbation of coronary occlusion-induced arrhythmias may be caused by under-perfusion of the ischaemic myocardium as a result of systemic hypotension. Certainly this explanation may be valid for our own results in anaesthetised rats since the lower dose of prostacyclin (0.1 $\mu g\ kg^{-1}\ min^{-1}$) had a greater antiarrhythmic effect than the higher dose (1 $\mu g\ kg^{-1}\ min^{-1}$). Walker's group, however, discount systemic hypotension as a possible mechanism for their observed dose-related (0.5 and 2.0 $\mu g\ kg^{-1}\ min^{-1}$) arrhythmogenic effect of prostacyclin in rats. In our own experiments infusion rates above 1 μg kg^{-1} min^{-1} could not be examined since in some animals they precipitated excessive decreases in arterial blood pressure (to a mean < 40 mmHg) which itself resulted in rhythm disturbances.

Other workers (Dix *et al.*, 1979), who observed an arrhythmogenic effect of prostacyclin in cats subject to coronary artery ligation, also reported a marked dose-dependent hypotensive action of prostacyclin but stated that there was no apparent relationship between changes in blood pressure and the severity of the arrhythmias. It is interesting that these authors infused prostacyclin via the left atrium. In previous studies in the same model they reported that left atrial infusion of PGE_1 increased the incidence of ventricular fibrillation whereas intravenous administration decreased the incidence of ventricular fibrillation (Kelliher *et al.*, 1979). This increased occurrence of ventricular fibrillation resulting from coronary artery ligation in animals pretreated with PGE_1 was found to be dependent on an intact cardiac sympathetic innervation (Kelliher *et al.*, 1978).

Although Au *et al.* (1979) found that prostacyclin increased the severity of early arrhythmias resulting from coronary artery ligation in the rat they also found that prostacyclin (0.5 μg kg^{-1} min^{-1}) had the opposite effect in dogs. No reason was suggested for the difference in the action of prostacyclin in these two species.

There are other reports of prostacyclin reducing the severity of early arrhythmias resulting from coronary artery occlusion. In anaesthetised dogs Ribeiro *et al.* (1981) found that prostacyclin, infused intravenously at a rate of 0.32 μg kg^{-1} min^{-1}, starting 17 min after coronary occlusion, reduced mortality caused by ventricular fibrillation. This group also reported that pretreatment with prostacyclin (0.5-2.0 μg kg^{-1} min^{-1} commencing 15 min prior to ligation) decreased ventricular ectopic activity and markedly reduced the incidence of ventricular fibrillation during the first 30 min after coronary artery ligation (DeBauche *et al.*, 1981). This work suggests that in this model prostacyclin is particularly effective against early life-threatening arrhythmias, whether it is administered prophylactically or therapeutically.

Starnes *et al.* (1981) have shown that in conscious instrumented dogs a low dose of prostacyclin (100 ng kg^{-1} min^{-1}), which did not significantly decrease total peripheral resistance, totally abolished ventricular fibrillation following coronary artery occlusion.

Hirche's group (see chapter 7) have recently demonstrated a protective effect of infused prostacyclin following LAD occlusion in anaesthetised pigs. This was related to a reduced increase in extracellular K^+ in the ischaemic myocardium, to a reduced noradrenaline release into coronary sinus blood and to fluorescent-histochemical evidence for the maintenance of myocardial noradrenaline stores.

Thus, in dogs, either conscious or anaesthetised, and in anaesthetised pigs, prostacyclin reduces the severity of early arrhythmias. However, evidence from other species indicates that prostacyclin may exacerbate this type of experimental arrhythmia. If catecholamines are involved in the actions of prostacyclin then these differences may be related to the level of sympathetic tone. Comparison of the results obtained in different studies is complicated not only by variations in sympathetic tone (due to differences in species and anaesthetic) but also by differences in the vehicle for prostacyclin and the dose and route of administration. These factors are detailed in table 13.1 along with the observed actions of prostacyclin on ectopic activity and on the incidence of ventricular fibrillation. This table emphasises the difficulty encountered in trying to draw general conclusions from this experimental work.

13.4 EFFECTS OF THE INHIBITION OF PROSTANOID SYNTHESIS ON ARRHYTHMIAS

Another approach that can be used to elucidate the possible role of endogenous prostanoids in arrhythmias is to study the effects of various drugs which prevent the synthesis of prostaglandins and thromboxanes.

Ibuprofen and indomethacin are cyclo-oxygenase inhibitors and thus prevent the formation of all prostanoids, that is, the endoperoxides, PGE_2, $PGF_{2\alpha}$, prostacyclin and thromboxane. These two drugs have been shown to decrease the doses of ouabain required to produce premature ventricular beats, ventricular tachycardia and ventricular fibrillation in dogs (Wilkerson and Glenn, 1977). In our own studies on anaesthetised rats subject to acute coronary artery ligation we examined the effects of pretreatment with flurbiprofen, a potent cyclo-oxygenase inhibitor. This drug had no arrhythmogenic actions itself but exacerbated ectopic activity resulting from coronary artery ligation to the extent that at the highest dose studied (1 mg kg^{-1}) all the animals died in ventricular fibrillation; mortality in the control group was 25 per cent (Coker and Parratt, 1981).

Indomethacin has been reported to abolish the protective effect of a linoleic acid-rich diet in conscious rats subject to acute coronary artery ligation whereas aspirin did not (Leprán *et al.*, 1981). These authors suggest that this effect of indomethacin indicates the involvement of increased prostaglandin synthesis in the protection offered by the diet.

Aspirin is also a cyclo-oxygenase inhibitor and there are a number of reports of its actions on experimentally induced arrhythmias including ventricular fibrillation. In anaesthetised dogs subject to experimentally induced coronary thrombosis it was observed that in all dogs receiving aspirin (by either the intravenous or the oral route) there was a significant decrease in the incidence of arrhythmias and of mortality due to ventricular fibrillation (Moschos *et al.*, 1972). Later studies from this group showed that aspirin was similarly effective in reducing arrhythmias and mortality in dogs subject to non-thrombotic coronary occlusion (Moschos *et al.*, 1978). Similar studies were performed with indomethacin but this drug was found to be ineffective; mortality was 40 per cent in indomethacin-treated animals compared with 39 per cent in controls and 5 per cent in animals pretreated with aspirin (Moschos *et al.*, 1980). Reiser *et al.* (1980) have also reported that aspirin has a protective effect during acute coronary artery occlusion and that the ventricular fibrillation threshold was higher in aspirin-treated dogs. In our own studies

Table 13.1 Prostacyclin - arrhythmogenic or antiarrhythmic?

Author	Species	Anaesthetic	Vehicle	Dose of PGI_2	Effect on no. of VEBs	Effect on incidence of VF/mortality
Au *et al.* (1979)	Rat	Pentobarbitone	Tris–saline; pH 9.5	0.5 μg kg^{-1} min^{-1} i.v.	↑	↑
				2.0 μg kg^{-1} min^{-1} i.v.	↑↑	↑↑
Coker and Parratt (1981)	Rat	Pentobarbitone	10% ethanol	0.1 μg kg^{-1} min^{-1} i.v.	↓↓	↓↓
				1 μg kg^{-1} min^{-1} i.v.	↓	↓↓
Dix *et al.* (1979)	Cat	α-Chloralose	$NaCO_3$–Na_2HCO_3, pH 8.9	2.7 pmol kg^{-1} min^{-1}*	–	–
				27 pmol kg^{-1} min^{-1}	↑	–
				270 pmol kg^{-1} min^{-1}	–	–
				2700 pmol kg^{-1} min^{-1}	↑ (n.s.)	↑
Ribeiro *et al.* (1981)	Dog	Sodium thiamylal	Tris, pH 9.4	0.32 μg kg^{-1} min^{-1}		↓↓
Starnes *et al.* (1981)	Dog	None		0.01 μg kg^{-1} min^{-1} i.v.		↓↓
Au *et al.* (1979)	Dog	Halothane–nitrous oxide	Tris–saline, pH 9.5	0.5 μg kg^{-1} min^{-1} i.v.	↓	↓

*Administered via the left atrium.

in anaesthetised greyhounds we have reported that aspirin (3 mg kg^{-1}) delayed the onset of arrhythmias and prevented the occurrence of ventricular fibrillation following coronary artery ligation (Coker *et al.*, 1981a). The number and the severity of the arrhythmias resulting from coronary artery ligation in anaesthetised rats is also reduced by aspirin (Coker and Parratt, 1981). This is in contrast to results obtained with flurbiprofen.

Thus, the results of studies with drugs which inhibit the cyclo-oxygenase enzyme are conflicting. Indomethacin, ibuprofen and flurbiprofen have all been reported to exacerbate arrhythmias whereas aspirin seems to have antiarrhythmic activity. It has been shown that aspirin can preferentially inhibit platelet cyclo-oxygenase (Smith and Willis, 1971; Roth *et al.*, 1975; Korbut and Moncada, 1978; Masotti *et al.*, 1979). Since thromboxane A_2 is the major metabolite of arachidonic acid synthesised by platelets it is possible that aspirin may prevent thromboxane formation without altering the production of other prostanoids such as prostacyclin, PGE_2 and $PGF_{2\alpha}$, which have been shown to be antiarrhythmic. There is indeed evidence for this possibility (Coker *et al.*, 1981a). Unfortunately thromboxane A_2 is very unstable and it is therefore technically difficult to perform studies which involve its direct administration. However, it has been reported that thromboxane A_2 (generated from platelets aggregated with PGH_2) causes acute myocardial ischaemia in rabbits (Morooka *et al.*, 1977, 1979). Also, a synthetic analogue of thromboxane A_2 (carbocyclic thromboxane A_2), which has similar vasoconstrictor properties, has been demonstrated to cause sudden cardiac death in rabbits (Lefer *et al.*, 1980). Similarly, trapidil, a new drug which antagonises thromboxane A_2 and also prevents its synthesis, has been shown to reduce the extent of ischaemic heart injury caused by the intra-coronary injection of thromboxane A_2 (Ohnishi *et al.*, 1981). In summary then it would appear that, in contrast to other prostanoids, thromboxane A_2 may have arrhythmogenic properties. This difference in action can provide an explanation for the antiarrhythmic effects seen with aspirin if it is assumed that treatment with aspirin (low dose) results in inhibition of thromboxane synthesis without reducing the production of other potentially antiarrhythmic prostanoids.

13.5 PROSTANOID RELEASE DURING ACUTE MYOCARDIAL ISCHAEMIA

Prostaglandins appear in increasing amounts in coronary venous (sinus) blood when a major coronary artery is occluded and when the occlusion is subsequently released (Alexander *et al.*, 1975; Kraemer *et al.*, 1976). For example, increases in $PGF_{2\alpha}$ concentrations in blood draining from the ischaemic myocardium have been found 15 min (Berger *et al.*, 1976) and 1 h (Ogletree *et al.*, 1977) after coronary artery ligation in anaesthetised dogs. Berger's group also found PGE_2 in blood draining from the normal myocardium whereas Ogletree *et al.* did not detect any significant release of PGE_2 in response to myocardial ischaemia. There is also a more recent report of increased concentration of PGE_1 and $PGF_{2\alpha}$ in blood draining from the ischaemic area after experimental myocardial infarction in dogs (Ogawa *et al.*, 1980).

In the above studies no attempt was made to relate prostaglandin release to the consequences of acute myocardial ischaemia such as arrhythmias. We have recently shown that PGE_2, $PGF_{2\alpha}$, prostacyclin and thromboxane are all released into blood draining from the acutely ischaemic myocardium following coronary artery ligation in anaesthetised greyhounds. The time course of the release, however, varies for the different prostanoids. The pattern for PGE_2 and $PGF_{2\alpha}$ is similar; their release cannot be detected until 30 min after coronary artery ligation, at which time the concentrations in blood draining from the acutely ischaemic region of the myocardium were increased (Coker *et al.*, 1981b). The release of thromboxane B_2 (the stable metabolite of thromboxane A_2) occurs rapidly following coronary artery ligation and is confined to the ischaemic area only. There is a significant increase in local coronary venous thromboxane B_2 concentrations as soon as 2 min after ligation of the left anterior descending coronary artery. Values reached a peak at 10 min and were declining by 30 min post-ligation; times after 30 min were not examined. Prostacyclin (measured as 6-keto $PGF_{1\alpha}$) was released more gradually and the concentrations were still rising 30 min post-ligation. However, this release of prostacyclin was not confined solely to local coronary venous blood draining from the acutely ischaemic area. Prostacyclin concentrations in the coronary sinus draining the essentially normal myocardium also increased following coronary ligation (Coker *et al.*, 1981c). These patterns of prostanoid release induced by acute myocardial ischaemia are illustrated in figure 13.2.

The release of thromboxane B_2 can be related to the occurrence of cardiac arrhythmias. At 2 min after coronary artery ligation, the percentage change in local coronary venous thromboxane concentrations correlates positively with the number of ventricular ectopic beats that have occurred by that time. Similarly, there is a negative correlation between prostacyclin release from the ischaemic myocardium and the number of arrhythmias (Coker *et al.*, 1981c; figure 13.3). Thus it appears that the occurrence of early arrhythmias is related to the balance between thromboxane and prostacyclin release. A balance in favour of thromboxane release is associated with the occurrence of a greater number of arrhythmias whereas fewer arrhythmias occur when the balance is in favour of prostacyclin release.

By the time that these early arrhythmias have ceased to occur (30 min post-ligation), coronary venous thromboxane concentrations are decreasing, whereas prostacyclin, PGE_2 and $PGF_{2\alpha}$ concentrations are still increasing. It is possible that the cessation of ectopic activity may be related to this shift in the balance in favour of potentially antiarrhythmic prostaglandins, such as prostacyclin, PGE_2 and $PGF_{2\alpha}$.

The administration of aspirin (3 mg kg^{-1}) prior to coronary artery ligation delayed the onset of arrhythmias and prevented the occurrence of ventricular fibrillation (Coker *et al.*, 1981a). This action may result from the ability of aspirin to inhibit the synthesis of thromboxane A_2. In these animals there was no evidence of thromboxane release at any time during the first 30 min following coronary

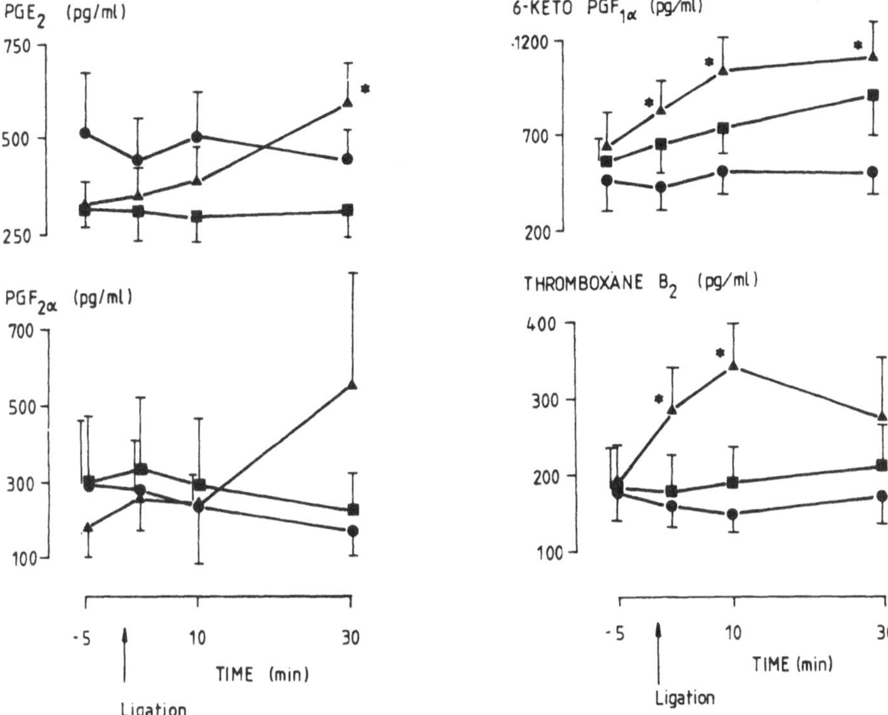

Figure 13.2 The effect of ligation of the left anterior descending coronary artery on prostanoid concentrations in the aorta (●), coronary sinus (■) and a local coronary vein draining the ischaemic region (▲) in anaesthetised greyhounds. Each point represents the mean ± S.E.M.; $n = 9$ for PGE_2, TXB_2 and 6-keto $PGF_{1\alpha}$; $n = 5$ for $PGF_{2\alpha}$. (Modified from Coker *et al.* (1981b, c).)

artery ligation whereas the release of prostacyclin followed a pattern similar to that observed in the corresponding control group (Coker *et al.*, 1981a).

Thus it seems probable that thromboxane A_2 is a contributory factor in the genesis of early arrhythmias that result from acute myocardial ischaemia. This substance is released solely from the ischaemic area of the myocardium; the magnitude of its release can be correlated with the number of arrhythmias which occur (at least during the first 2 min of ischaemia) and aspirin prevents both thromboxane release and early arrhythmias.

13.6 POSSIBLE MECHANISMS OF ACTION OF PROSTANOIDS IN RELATION TO ARRHYTHMIAS

The evidence presently available indicates that PGE_2 and $PGF_{2\alpha}$ both possess some antiarrhythmic activity. Unfortunately there are few direct *in vitro* studies of the

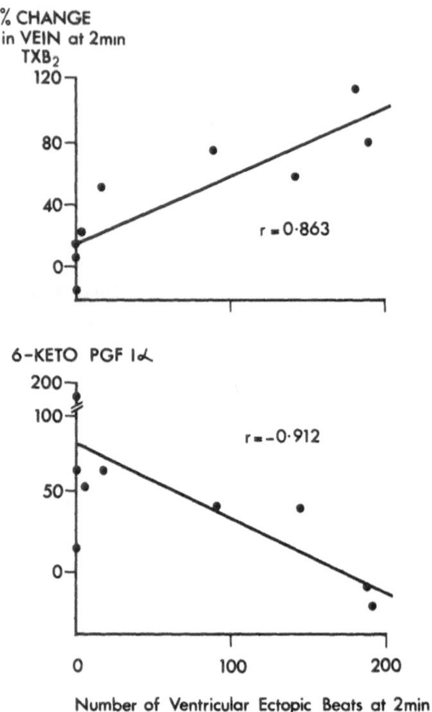

Figure 13.3 Correlations between early arrhythmias and the local release of thromboxane B_2 and 6-keto $PGF_{1\alpha}$ from the acutely ischaemic region of the myocardium in anaesthetised greyhounds. (Adapted from Coker *et al.* (1981c).)

electrophysiological effects of these compounds, although PGE_1 has been shown to reduce the rate of rise of the cardiac transmembrane action potential in atrial and ventricular tissue from a variety of species (Kecskemeti *et al.*, 1973). PGE_2 and $PGF_{2\alpha}$ have both been shown to prolong intra-atrial and atrioventricular conduction times and the functional refractory periods of the atrium and the atrioventricular conducting system (Bayer and Förster, 1978). These effects are markedly diminished by both vagotomy and reserpinisation, suggesting the involvement of the parasympathetic and the sympathetic nervous systems.

In a study in which prostacyclin was found to reduce mortality in dogs subject to coronary artery ligation this result was attributed to the fact that, while prostacyclin did not prevent the occurrence of ventricular tachycardia, the cycle length of the tachycardia was significantly increased, thus attenuating progression to ventricular fibrillation (DeBauche *et al.*, 1981).

PGE_2 and PGE_1 have similar actions regarding their effects on the release of noradrenaline from sympathetic nerve terminals. Both substances reduce the release of noradrenaline from sympathetically stimulated isolated perfused rabbit hearts. In contrast, $PGF_{2\alpha}$ has no effect on the turnover of noradrenaline (Hedqvist and Wennmalm, 1971). Prostacyclin has also been reported to inhibit the release of noradrenaline from sympathetic nerves (Weitzell *et al.*, 1978; Wennmalm, 1978), although it is not as potent as PGE_2. These effects on noradrenaline release may partially account for the antiarrhythmic actions of these prostanoids.

If prostacyclin is indeed antiarrhythmic there are several other possible actions which may contribute to this effect. Prostacyclin is a potent vasodilator and it inhibits platelet aggregation (Dusting *et al.*, 1978; Moncada *et al.*, 1976). It can also reduce the release of lysosomal enzymes (Lefer *et al.*, 1978). Further evidence that prostacyclin may be capable of preserving cellular integrity has been provided by Ogletree *et al.* (1979), who have shown that prostacyclin reduces the changes in myocardial and plasma creatine phosphokinase activity that occur as a result of myocardial ischaemia. Recently it has been reported that prostacyclin prevents ischaemia-induced increases in lactate and cyclic AMP in the myocardium (Rösen *et al.*, 1981). This is of particular relevance to possible mechanisms of antiarrhythmic action since marked elevations in cyclic AMP have been reported to occur immediately before the onset of ventricular fibrillation (Podzuweit *et al.*, 1978, and reviewed by Podzuweit in chapter 11).

In contrast to the primary prostaglandins and prostacyclin, thromboxane A_2 may have direct actions on the cardiac action potential, whilst its ability to cause platelet aggregation and coronary vasoconstriction could certainly contribute indirectly to the genesis of arrhythmias. Both these factors would reduce blood flow to localised areas of the vulnerable ischaemic myocardium. This could precipitate arrhythmias as a result of a decreased supply of oxygen and other nutrients or a decreased washout of potentially harmful products, for example, cyclic AMP or potassium ions.

The studies which have been reviewed in this chapter suggest that several conclusions may be reached regarding the influence of prostanoids on early arrhythmias. First, it is likely that thromboxane A_2 and prostacyclin are the two most important prostanoids in this respect since they are both released from the acutely ischaemic myocardium at times when early ventricular arrhythmias are evident. Secondly, all the evidence obtained so far indicates that thromboxane A_2 is arrhythmogenic and so may be an important contributory factor in early arrhythmias. Thirdly, it appears that endogenously released prostacyclin is associated with antiarrhythmic activity, although it must be borne in mind that there is some evidence that exogenously administered prostacyclin can exacerbate arrhythmias. However, the bulk of the evidence seems to favour an antiarrhythmic action of prostacyclin. This obviously requires further investigation in order to clarify the possible role of prostacyclin in early arrhythmias. There are a number of factors which would have to be carefully controlled in future studies, such as anaesthesia, vehicle and perhaps most importantly the dosage and route of administration of prostacyclin. If this information becomes available it should be possible to proceed to determine the extent of the role that prostanoids may play in the control of early arrhythmias. It seems likely that the local release of thromboxane A_2 is a contributory factor in early arrhythmias. However, the relative importance of this release in comparison with the other substances also involved in local myocardial ischaemia (and reviewed in the previous six chapters) remains to be elucidated.

ACKNOWLEDGEMENT

The author wishes to acknowledge the support given by the Scottish Hospitals Endowment Research Trust (HERT to Parratt, Ledingham and Zeitlin).

REFERENCES

Alexander, R. W., Kent, K. M., Pisano, J. J., Keiser, H. R. and Cooper, T. (1975). Regulation of postocclusive hyperemia by endogenously synthetised prostaglandins in the dog heart. *J. clin. Invest.*, **55**, 1174-81

Au, T. L. S., Collins, G. A., Harvie, C. J. and Walker, M. J. A. (1979). The actions of prostaglandin I_2 and prostaglandin E_2 on arrhythmias produced by coronary occlusion in the rat and dog. *Prostaglandins*, **18**, 707-20

Bayer, B. L. and Förster, W. (1978). Effects of prostaglandins on conduction time and refractory period before and after vagotomy and reserpine pretreatment in the cat heart *in situ*. *Acta biol. med. germ.*, **37**, 831-2

Berger, H. J., Zaret, B. L., Speroff, L., Cohen, L. S. and Wolfson, S. (1976). Regional cardiac prostaglandin release during myocardial ischemia in anaesthetised dogs. *Circulation*, **38**, 566-71

Bergström, S. and Sjövall, J. (1960). The isolation of prostaglandin F from sheep prostate glands. *Acta chem. scand.*, **14**, 1693-701

Bergström, S., Danielson, H. and Samuelsson, B. (1964). The enzymatic formation of prostaglandin E_2 from arachidonic acid. Prostaglandins and related factors. *Biochim. biophys. Acta*, **90**, 207-10

Coker, S. J. and Parratt, J. R. (1981). The effects of PGE_2, $PGF_{2\alpha}$, prostacyclin, flurbiprofen and aspirin on arrhythmias resulting from coronary artery ligation in anaesthetised rats. *Br. J. Pharmac.*, **74**, 155-9

Coker, S. J., Ledingham, I. McA., Parratt, J. R. and Zeitlin, I. J. (1981a). Aspirin inhibits the early myocardial release of thromboxane B_2 and ventricular ectopic activity following acute coronary artery occlusion in dogs. *Br. J. Pharmac.*, **72**, 593-5

Coker, S. J., Marshall, R. J., Parratt, J. R. and Zeitlin, I. J. (1981b). Does the local myocardial release of prostaglandin E_2 or $F_{2\alpha}$ contribute to the early consequences of acute myocardial ischaemia? *J. molec. cell. Cardiol.*, **13**, 425-34

Coker, S. J., Parratt, J. R., Ledingham, I. McA. and Zeitlin, I. J. (1981c). Thromboxane and prostacyclin release from ischaemic myocardium in relation to arrhythmias. *Nature, Lond.*, **291**, 323-4

DeBauche, T. L., Brandon, T. A., Ribeiro, L. G. T., Holyfield, K. and Miller, R. R. (1981). Effect of prostacyclin on ventricular arrhythmias and intracardiac conduction in myocardial ischemia. *Am. J. Cardiol.*, **47**, 437

Dix, R. K., Kelliher, G. J., Jurkiewicz, N. and Lawrence, T. (1979). The influence of prostacyclin on coronary occlusion induced arrhythmia in cats. *Prostaglandins Med.*, **3**, 173-84

Dusting, G. J., Moncada, S. and Vane, J. R. (1977). Prostacyclin (PGX) is the endogenous metabolite responsible for relaxation of coronary arteries induced by arachidonic acid. *Prostaglandins*, **13**, 3-15

Dusting, G. J., Chapple, D. J., Hughes, R., Moncada, S. and Vane, J. R. (1978). Prostacyclin (PGI_2) induces coronary vasodilatation in anaesthetised dogs. *Cardiovasc. Res.*, **12**, 720-30

Euler, U. S. von (1934). Zur Kenntnis der pharmakologischen Wirkungen von Nativsekreten und Extrackten männlicher accesscrischer Geschlechtsdrusen. *Naunyn-Schmeidebergs Arch. exp. Path. Pharmak.*, **175**, 78-84

Euler, U. S. von (1935). Über die spezifische blutdrucksenkende Substanz des Menschlichen prostata und Samenblasensekretes. *Klin. Wschr.*, **14**, 1182-3

Euler, von U.S. (1936). On the specific vasodilating and plain muscle stimulating substances from accessory genital glands in man and certain animals (prostaglandin and vesiglandin). *J. Physiol., Lond.*, **88**, 213-34

Ferreira, S. H. and Vane, J. R. (1967). Prostaglandins: their disappearance from and release into the circulation. *Nature, Lond.*, **216**, 868-73

Förster, W. (1976). Prostaglandins and prostaglandin precursors as endogenous antiarrhythmic principles of the heart. *Acta biol. med germ.*, **35**, 1101-12

Förster, W., Mest, H.-J. and Mentz, P. (1973). The influence of $PGF_{2\alpha}$ on experimental arrhythmias. *Prostaglandins*, **3**, 895-904

Goldblatt, M. W. (1933). A depressor substance in seminal fluid. *J. Soc. chem. Ind., Lond.*, **52**, 1056-7

Hamberg, M. and Fredholm, B. B. (1976). Isomerization of prostaglandin H_2 into prostaglandin D_2 in the presence of serum albumin. *Biochim. biophys. Acta*, **431**, 189-193

Hamberg, M. and Samuelsson, B. (1974). Novel transformations of arachidonic acid in human platelets. *Proc. natn. Acad. Sci. U.S.A.*, **71**, 3400-4

Hamberg, M., Svensson, J., Wakabayashi, T. and Samuelsson, B. (1974). Isolation and structure of two prostaglandin endoperoxides that cause platelet aggregation. *Proc. natn. Acad. Sci. U.S.A.*, **71**, 345-9

Harvie, C. J., Collins, G. A., Miyagishima, R. T. and Walker, M. J. A. (1978). Action of prostaglandin E_2 and $F_{1\alpha}$ on myocardial ischaemia-infarction arrhythmias in the dog. *Prostaglandins*, **16**, 885-900

Hedqvist, P. and Wennmalm, A. (1971). Comparison of the effects of PGE_1, E_2 and $F_{2\alpha}$ on the sympathetically stimulated rabbit heart. *Acta physiol. scand.*, **83**, 156-62

Ito, T., Nakamura, T., Wakamatsu, Y., Yamamoto, M., Yoshida, M., Okubo, M., Kakizawa, N., Mizutani, K., Miyagishima, Y., Suzuki, Y., Ogawa, K. and Yamazaki, N. (1975). Antiarrhythmic and antilipolytic effect of prostaglandin E_1 (PGE_1) and $F_{2\alpha}$ ($PGF_{2\alpha}$). *Jap. Circulation J.*, **39**, 1052

Kecskemeti, V., Kelemen, K. and Knoll, J. (1973). Effect of prostaglandin E_1 on the cardiac transmembrane potentials. *Eur. J. Pharmac.*, **24**, 289-95

Kelliher, G. J. and Glenn, T. M. (1973). Effect of PGE_1 on ouabain induced arrhythmias. *Eur. J. Pharmac.*, **24**, 410-4

Kelliher, G. J., Lawrence, T., Jurkiewicz, N. and Dix, R. K. (1978). Role of sympathetic nervous system in prostaglandin-induced ventricular arrhythmias. *Pharmacologist*, **20**, 233

Kelliher, G. J., Lawrence, T., Jurkiewicz, N. and Dix, R. K. (1979). Comparison of the effects of prostaglandin E_1 and A_1 on coronary occlusion induced arrhythmia. *Prostaglandins*, **17**, 163-77

Korbut, R. and Moncada, S. (1978). Prostacyclin (PGI_2) and thromboxane interaction *in vivo*. Regulation by aspirin and relationship with antithrombotic therapy. *Thrombosis Res.*, **13**, 489-500

Kraemer, R. S., Phernetton, T. M. and Folts, J. D. (1976). Prostaglandin-like substances in coronary venous blood following myocardial ischaemia. *J. Pharmac. exp. Ther.*, **199**, 611-9

Lands, W. E. M. (1979). The biosynthesis and metabolism of prostaglandins. *A. Rev. Physiol.*, **41**, 633-52

Lefer, A. M., Ogletree, M. L., Smith, J. B., Silver, M. J., Nicolaou, K. C., Barnette, W. E. and Gasic, G. P. (1978). Prostacyclin: a potentially valuable agent for preserving myocardial tissue in acute myocardial ischaemia. *Science, N.Y.*, **200**, 52-4

Lefer, A. M., Smith, E. F., III, Araki, H., Smith, J. B., Aharony, D., Claremon, D. A., Magolda, R. L. and Nicolaou, K. C. (1980). Dissociation of vasoconstrictor and platelet aggregatory activities of thromboxane by carbocyclic thromboxane A_2, a stable analog of thromboxane A_2. *Proc. natn. Acad. Sci. U.S.A.*, **77**, 1706-10

Leprán, I., Nemecz, Gy., Koltai, M. and Szekeres, L. (1981). Effect of a linoleic acid-rich diet on the acute phase of coronary occlusion in conscious rats: influence of indomethacin and aspirin. *J. cardiovasc. Pharmac.*, **3**, 847-53

Madan, B. R., Gupta, R. S. and Madan, V. (1974). Actions of prostaglandins E_1, E_2, $F_{1\alpha}$ and $F_{2\alpha}$ in ouabain-induced arrhythmia and maximal electroshock seizures. *Ind. J. med. Res.*, **62**, 1647-51

Mann, D. (1976). Action of prostaglandins on heart arrhythmias. *Acta biol. med. germ.*, **35**, 1113-7

Mann, D., Meyer, H.-G. and Förster, W. (1973). Preliminary clinical experience with the antiarrhythmic effect of $PGF_{2\alpha}$. *Prostaglandins*, **3**, 905-12

Martinez, T. T. and Crampton, J. M. (1978). The effect of post-ligation infusion of prostaglandin E_2 on arrhythmias produced by coronary artery ligation in rat. *Pharmacologist*, **20**, 148

Masotti, G., Galanti, G., Poggesi, L., Abbate, R. and Neri Serneri, G. G. (1979). Differential inhibition of prostacyclin production and platelet aggregation by aspirin. *Lancet*, *ii*, 1213

Mest, H.-J. and Förster, W. (1978). The antiarrhythmic action of prostacyclin (PGI_2) on aconitine induced arrhythmia in rats. *Acta biol. med. germ.*, **37**, 827-8

Mest, H.-J., Blass, K. E. and Förster, W. (1978). Effects of arachidonic, linoleic, linolenic and oleic acid on experimental arrhythmias in cats, rabbits and guinea-pigs. *Prostaglandins*, **14**, 163-72

Mohr, D. N., Davis, S. and Markis, J. E. (1981). Clinical evidence of prostaglandin E_2 antiarrhythmic properties. *Am. Heart J.*, **102**, 123-4

Moncada, S. and Vane, J. R. (1978). Pharmacology and endogenous roles of prostaglandin endoperoxides, thromboxane A_2 and prostacyclin. *Pharmac. Rev.*, **30**, 293-331

Moncada, S., Gryglewski, R. J., Bunting, S. and Vane, J. R. (1976). An enzyme isolated from arteries transforms prostaglandin endoperoxides to an unstable substance that inhibits platelet aggregation. *Nature, Lond.*, **263**, 663-5

Morooka, S., Kobayashi, M. and Shimamoto, T. (1977). Experimental ischaemic heart disease induced by thromboxane A_2 in rabbits. *Jap. Circulation J.*, **41**, 1373-9

Morooka, S., Kobayashi, M., Takahashi, T., Takashima, Y., Sakamoto, M. and Shimamoto, T. (1979). Experimental ischaemic heart disease - effects of synthetic thromboxane A_2. *Exp. molec. Path.*, **30**, 449-57

Moschos, C. B., Haider, B., De La Cruz, C., Lyons, M. M. and Regan, T. J. (1978). Antiarrhythmic effects of aspirin during non-thrombotic coronary occlusion. *Circulation*, **57**, 681-4

Moschos, C. B., Haider, B., Escobinas, A. J., Gandhi, A. and Regan, T. J. (1980). Chronic use of aspirin versus indomethacin during non-thrombotic myocardial ischemia: effects on survival. *Am. Heart J.*, **100**, 647-52

Moschos, C. B., Lahiri, K., Peter, A., Jesrani, M. U. and Regan, T. J. (1972). Effect of aspirin upon experimental coronary and non-coronary thrombosis and arrhythmia. *Am. Heart J.*, **84**, 525-30

Needleman, P., Moncada, S., Bunting, S., Vane, J. R., Hamberg, M. and Samuelsson, B. (1976). Identification of an enzyme in platelet microsomes which generates thromboxane A_2 from prostaglandin endoperoxides. *Nature, Lond.*, **261**, 558-60

Nugteren, D. H. and Hazelhof, E. (1973). Isolation and properties of intermediates in prostaglandin biosynthesis. *Biochim. biophys. Acta*, **326**, 448-61

Ogawa, K., Ito, T., Enomoto, I., Hashimoto, H., Kai, I. and Satake, T. (1980). Increase of coronary flow and levels of PGE_1 and $PGF_{2\alpha}$ from ischaemic area of myocardial infarction. *Adv. Prostaglandin Thromboxane Res.*, 7, 665-70

Ogletree, M. L., Flynn, J. T., Feola, M. and Lefer, A. M. (1977). Early prostaglandin release from the ischemic myocardium in the dog. *Surgery Gynec. Obstet.*, **144**, 734-40

Ogletree, M. L., Lefer, A. M., Smith, J. B. and Nicolaou, K. C. (1979). Studies on the protective effect of prostacyclin in acute myocardial ischaemia. *Eur. J. Pharmac.*, **56**, 95-103

Ohnishi, H., Kosuzume, H., Hayashi, Y., Yamaguchi, K., Suzuki, Y. and Itoh, R. (1981). Effects of trapidil on thromboxane A_2-induced aggregation of platelets, ischaemic changes in heart and biosynthesis of thromboxane A_2. *Prostaglandins Med.*, **6**, 269–81

Pace, N. L., Ohmura, A. and Wong, K. C. (1979). Epinephrine induced arrhythmias: effects of exogenous PGs and PG synthesis inhibition during halothane O_2 anaesthesia in the dog. *Anaesthesia Analgesia*, **58**, 401

Piper, P. J. and Vane, J. R. (1971). The release of prostaglandins from lung and other tissues. *Ann. N.Y. Acad. Sci.*, **180**, 363–85

Podzuweit, T., Dalby, A. J., Cherry, G. W. and Opie, L. H. (1978). Tissue levels of cyclic AMP in ischaemic and non-ischaemic myocardium following coronary artery ligation. *J. molec. cell. Cardiol.*, **10**, 81–94

Ramwell, P. W., Shaw, J. E. and Douglas, W. W. (1966). Efflux of prostaglandins from adrenal glands stimulated with acetylcholine. *Nature, Lond.*, **210**, 273–4

Ramwell, P. W., Leovey, P. M. K. and Sintetos, A. L. (1977). Regulation of the arachidonic acid cascade. *Biol. Reprod.*, **16**, 70–87

Reiser, J., Gough, W. B. and Anderson, G. J. (1980). Protective effect of aspirin following acute coronary artery occlusion. *Am. J. Cardiol.*, **45**, 424

Ribeiro, L. G. T., Brandon, T. A., Hopkins, D. G., Reduto, L. A., Taylor, A. A. and Miller, R. R. (1981). Prostacyclin in experimental myocardial ischemia: effects on hemodynamics, regional myocardial blood flow, infarct size and mortality. *Am. J. Cardiol.*, **47**, 835–40

Rösen, R., Rösen, P., Ohlendorf, R. and Schrör, K. (1981). Prostacyclin prevents ischaemia-induced increase of lactate and cyclic AMP in ischaemic myocardium. *Eur. J. Pharmac.*, **69**, 489–91

Roth, G. J., Stanford, N. and Majerus, P. W. (1975). Acetylation of prostaglandin synthetase by aspirin. *Proc. natn. Acad. Sci. U.S.A.*, **72**, 3073

Samuelsson, B. (1965). On the incorporation of oxygen in the conversion of 8,11,14-eicosatrienoic acid to prostaglandin E_1. *J. Am. chem. Soc.*, **87**, 3011–3

Smith, J. B. and Willis, A. L. (1971). Aspirin selectively inhibits prostaglandin production in human platelets. *Nature new Biol.*, **231**, 235–7

Somberg, J. C., Bounous, H., Cagin, N., Anagnostopoulos, L. and Levitt, B. (1977). The influence of prostaglandins E_1 and E_2 on ouabain cardiotoxicity in the cat. *J. Pharmac. exp. Ther.*, **203**, 480–4

Starnes, V. A., Primm, K. R., Woosley, R. L., Oates, J. A. and Hammon, J. W. (1981). Effects of low dose prostacyclin on ventricular arrhythmias following experimental coronary occlusion. *Circulation*, **62**, Suppl. III, 309

Van Dorp, D. A., Beerthuis, R. K., Nugteren, D. H. and Vonheman, H. (1964). The biosynthesis of prostaglandins. *Biochim. biophys. Acta*, **90**, 204–7

Wennmalm, A. (1978). Prostaglandin mediated inhibition of noradrenaline release: V. A comparison of the neuroinhibitory effects of three prostaglandins E_1, I_2 and 6-keto $PGF_{1\alpha}$. *Prostaglandins Med.*, **1**, 49–54

Weitzell, R., Steppler, A. and Starke, K. (1978). Effects of prostaglandin E_2, prostaglandin I_2 and 6-keto-prostaglandin $F_{1\alpha}$ on adrenergic neurotransmission in the pulmonary artery of the rabbit. *Eur. J. Pharmac.*, **52**, 137–41

Wilkerson, R. D. and Glenn, T. M. (1977). Influence of non-steroidal anti-inflammatory drugs on ouabain toxicity. *Am. Heart. J.*, **94**, 454-9

Zijlstra, W. G., Brunsting, J. R., Ten Hoor, P. and Vergrosen, A. J. (1972). Prostaglandin E_1 and cardiac arrhythmia. *Eur. J. Pharmac.*, **18**, 392-5

14

The Effect of Non-steroidal Anti-inflammatory Drugs and of a Linoleic Acid-rich Diet on Early Arrhythmias Resulting from Myocardial Ischaemia

L. Szekeres, I. Leprán, E. Boros, I. Takáts and M. Koltai

14.1 INTRODUCTION

The fact that 50 per cent of deaths due to ischaemic heart disease (IHD) occur before the patients reach hospital emphasises the importance of preventive hospital therapy. Recently, increasing attention has been paid to the non-steroid anti-inflammatory drugs (NSAIDs) as potential cardioprotective agents, although the results of clinical studies have been conflicting. Thus, the Aspirin Myocardial Infarction Study Research Group (1980) found no conclusive evidence for a beneficial effect of long term aspirin against sudden coronary death. Elwood and Sweetnam (1979) observed a 22 per cent decrease in mortality from IHD of patients treated with aspirin, although this difference in mortality between aspirin and control groups was not statistically significant. According to the Anturane Reinfarction Trial (1980), sulphinpyrazone exerts some preventive effect when given early after an acute myocardial infarction. Fatal complications of coronary disease have been reported to decrease by about 25 per cent in the latest report of the Persantine-Aspirin Reinfarction Study Research Group (1980). The significance of this and other similar trials has recently been discussed by Sherry (1980).

Another possible way to prevent sudden death due to post-infarction arrhythmias is through a long term change in dietary lipids. This possibility is based on the laboratory observations that such a change in diet is capable of altering the lipid content of cell membranes, thus influencing their physical and functional properties (Brivio-Haugland *et al.*, 1976; Awad and Zepp, 1979). The use of a diet rich in mackerel derives from the observation that Greenland Eskimos have a low incidence of cardiovascular disease, favourable plasma lipid and lipoprotein levels and an increased tendency to bleeding, perhaps due to decreased platelet aggregability

(Dyerberg and Bang, 1978). This protection is linked to an excessive intake of eicosapentaenoic acid and Miettinen *et al.* (1972) have proposed that a diet rich in soybean oil, which contains linoleic acid, should also be protective.

In view of the beneficial effect of sulphinpyrazone (as a representative of NSAIDs) and the favourable clinical experiences with linoleic acid (LA)-rich diets, we decided to study the effect of such pretreatment in a well established experimental model of coronary artery occlusion in conscious rats. The effect of sulphinpyrazone treatment and LA-rich diet on some *in vitro* electrophysiological parameters was also investigated.

14.2 MATERIALS AND METHODS

Animals and diet

Randomly bred male Sprague-Dawley CFY rats weighing 180-250 g were used throughout. They were fed commercially available food pellets containing 5 per cent mixed fat and were allowed to drink tap water *ad libitum*. LA-rich diet was started on weaning; this diet contained 12 per cent sunflower seed oil supplementing mixed fat in the standard chow.

Coronary occlusion

Our technique (Leprán *et al.*, 1979; Kane *et al.*, 1980) was a modification of that used by Selye *et al.* (1960). In a preliminary surgical operation, under ether anaesthesia, the chest wall was opened, the heart exposed and a loose ligature of atraumatic silk placed around the left anterior descending coronary artery. The ends of the silk loop were pulled through a short polyethylene tube which was left inside the thorax. Negative intrathoracic pressure was restored by compression on the chest wall, the wound was closed and the ends of the silk slipped into the tissue beneath the skin. Seven to eight days after recovery, the animals were re-anaesthetised with ether, the ends of the silk were freed through a small incision and subcutaneous safety-pin electrodes were applied to both sides of the chest wall for recording the electrocardiogram. Three to four hours later acute coronary occlusion was produced, without anaesthetic, by tightening the loose ligature. The survival rate and the occurrence of arrhythmias were established during the first 20 min after occlusion.

Electrophysiological studies

Intracellular action potentials were recorded using isolated left atrial preparations electrically driven (100 min^{-1}, 1 ms duration and twice threshold intensity; Szekeres and Vaughan Williams, 1962). The incubation medium (Locke's solution at 32 °C) was gassed with 5 per cent CO_2 in 95 per cent O_2. Hypoxia was induced by substituting nitrogen for oxygen.

Drug treatment

A single dose of 2, 10 or 50 mg kg^{-1} sulphinpyrazone (Ciba-Geigy), suspended in 0.5 ml of 1 per cent methylcellulose, was administered through a stomach tube 1 h before starting the experiments.

Statistical evaluation

The χ^2 method was used for the statistical analysis of the survival rate and the occurrence of arrhythmias. For comparison of the other parameters, the unpaired Student's *t* test was applied.

14.3 RESULTS

Coronary occlusion

Within 5-10 min of coronary artery occlusion severe arrhythmias occurred and resulted in death in 67 per cent of the control group (table 14.1). Oral pretreatment with a single dose of sulphinpyrazone markedly increased the survival rate (table 14.1). This effect was significant after 10 or 50 mg kg^{-1}. The protection was characterised by the decreased occurrence of life-threatening ventricular fibrillation and by an increasing number of animals without arrhythmias.

Table 14.1 The protective effect of sulphinpyrazone in the acute phase of coronary artery occlusion in conscious rats

Dose		Survived		Occurrence of ventricular dysrhythmias (per cent)		
(mg kg^{-1})	*n*	No.	Percentage	None	Fibrillation	Tachycardia
Vehicle	18	6	33	0	78	94
2	10	5	50	0	50	80
10	10	8	80*	10	20**	80
50	20	13	65*	20*	15***	80

Asterisks denote significant difference from control group, calculated by χ^2 method: *$P < 0.05$, **$P < 0.01$, ***$P < 0.001$.

Table 14.2 The development of the protective effect of LA-rich diet in conscious rats subjected to coronary artery occlusion

Treatment time	*n*	Survived		Occurrence of ventricular dysrhythmias (per cent)		
		No.	Percentage	None	Fibrillation	Tachycardia
Control	26	5	19	0	88	96
1 week	15	9	60**	20*	47**	53***
2 weeks	11	7	64**	18	36**	64**
4 weeks	11	7	64**	27**	36**	64**
12 weeks	21	17	81***	43***	28***	48***

Signs and symbols as in table 14.1.

The development of the effect of LA-rich diet is shown in table 14.2. A significant protection against severe arrhythmias and death due to coronary occlusion appeared as early as 1 week after commencing the diet. This protective effect was even more marked following 12 weeks on the diet. Long term LA-rich diet resulted in an exchange of *n*-6 fatty acids (mainly arachidonic and docosahexaenoic acids) for *n*-3 fatty acids in the membrane phospholipids (table 14.3).

Table 14.3 Alteration of the *n*-6/*n*-3 fatty acid ratio during LA-rich diet

Diet	Duration weeks	*n*-6/*n*-3 ratio[1]	Reference
Control	–	6.3[2]	Kramer (1980)
Corn oil	1	18.0[2]	Kramer (1980)
Corn oil	16	27.3[2]	Kramer (1980)
Control	–	4.8[3]	Leprán *et al.* (1981b)
Sunflower seed oil	4	24.5[3]	Present authors' unpublished data
Sunflower seed oil	12	31.9[3]	Leprán *et al.* (1981b)

[1] *n*-6 fatty acids include 18 : 2, 20 : 4, 22 : 4, 22 : 5; *n*-3 fatty acids are 18 : 3, 22 : 5, 22 : 6.
[2] Fatty acid ratio in phosphatidylcholine fraction comprising 34.5 per cent of total heart lipids.
[3] Fatty acid ratio in total heart phospholipids.

Electrophysiological studies

There were no differences in intracellularly recorded atrial action potentials from control rats and rats pretreated with sulphinpyrazone. Sulphinpyrazone pretreatment also did not modify the hypoxia-induced shortening of action potential duration (APD) and reduction in the maximum rate of depolarisation (dV/dt). In contrast, pretreatment with a LA-rich diet for 4 weeks did shorten APD and decreased dV/dt (table 14.4). This quinidine-like effect was also present under hypoxic conditions (table 14.4).

Table 14.4 Effect of LA-rich diet on basal and hypoxic intracellular electrophysiological parameters *in vitro* obtained for atrial muscle

	Control, $n = 9$			LA-rich diet, $n = 10$		
	Basal value	Hypoxia (min)		Basal value	Hypoxia (min)	
		5	10		5	10
50 per cent APD	22.3 ± 0.51	19.5 ± 0.41	14.3 ± 0.47	13.9 ± 0.17***	12.3 ± 0.23***	10.8 ± 0.19***
90 per cent APD	52.3 ± 1.13	44.3 ± 1.00	35.9 ± 1.00	34.4 ± 0.63***	29.2 ± 0.63***	24.0 ± 0.52***
dV/dt	62.0 ± 2.16	55.5 ± 1.65	55.0 ± 1.92	53.6 ± 1.45*	39.1 ± 1.07***	44.8 ± 1.16**

APD = action potential duration (in milliseconds); dV/dt = maximum rate of depolarisation of the action potential (in volts per second).

Asterisks denote significant difference from the corresponding control value, calculated by unpaired Student's *t* test. $^*P < 0.05$, $^{**}P < 0.01$, $^{***}P < 0.001$. Results are mean ± S.E.M.

14.4 DISCUSSION

The present results demonstrate that pretreatment with a single dose of sulphinpyrazone and prolonged treatment with a LA-rich diet both offer marked protection against life-threatening arrhythmias resulting from coronary artery occlusion and significantly increased survival. These data are in general agreement with the findings obtained with various NSAIDs in experimental animals. For example, in anaesthetised cats, ibuprofen (Lefer and Polansky, 1979; Lefer and Crossley, 1980), flurbiprofen (Smith *et al.*, 1980) and sulphinpyrazone (Kelliher *et al.*, 1980) produce beneficial effects in acute myocardial infarction. Similarly in dogs, aspirin (Moschos *et al.*, 1973, 1978), salicylic acid (Vik-Mo and Mjos, 1977) and sulphinpyrazone (Povalski *et al.*, 1980; Moschos *et al.*, 1980) protect the myocardium against ischaemic cell damage. Brunner *et al.* (1980) have demonstrated that prolonged treatment with sulphinpyrazone reduces mortality in the late phase of myocardial ischaemia in the rat and our recent studies, performed in conscious rats, have clearly demonstrated the protective effects of single doses of such NSAIDs as sulphinpyrazone, aspirin, salicylic acid and indomethacin (Leprán *et al.*, 1981a).

Our present and recent observations with LA-rich diet (Szekeres *et al.*, 1980; Leprán *et al.*, 1981b) generally support findings in man (Keys, 1970; Miettinen *et al.*, 1972; Morris *et al.*, 1977; Turpeinen *et al.*, 1979; Lewis, 1980; Shekelle *et al.*, 1981) that diet can profoundly modify the progress and consequences of coronary heart disease. The mechanism of this protective action exerted both by sulphinpyrazone and by the LA-rich diet seems to be different from that produced by standard antiarrhythmic drugs, such as the β-adrenoceptor blocking agents and local anaesthetics. These drugs produce prominent electrophysiological and biochemical changes which can adequately account for their protective effects (Szekeres, 1978a, b).

Although the cardioprotective effects of NSAIDs and of the LA-rich diet are certainly complex, a common pathway might be involved. Thus, it has been shown that local ischaemia, induced by partial obstruction of blood vessels, results in platelet aggregation (Folts *et al.*, 1976), and it is likely that this is also involved in myocardial infarction (Moschos *et al.*, 1973; Moore, 1976; Vik-Mo, 1978; Leinberger, *et al.*, 1979); NSAIDs of course prevent platelet aggregation (O'Brien, 1968). It may be relevant that there is a close correlation between the fatty acid composition of platelets and their ability to aggregate (Renaud *et al.*, 1970). Diets rich in LA reduce platelet aggregability (Hornstra, 1975; Jakubowski and Ardlie, 1978). Platelet aggregation in and around the ischaemic region can be induced by catecholamines (Haft *et al.*, 1972) and ADP (Jorgensen *et al.*, 1967) and this aggregatory effect is, at least in part, brought about by thromboxane (TxA_2) production. A stable metabolite of TxA_2 (TxB_2) can be detected in the effluent blood of the acutely ischaemic myocardium of anaesthetised greyhounds (Coker *et al.*, 1981) and TxA_2 itself is a highly active vasoconstrictor (Ellis *et al.*, 1976). Coker *et al.* (1981) have shown that aspirin inhibits the early myocardial release of TxA_2 and the ventricular ectopic activity which results from acute coronary occlusion in dogs. This mechanism (that is, inhibition of platelet aggregation and TxA_2 production) may be the common pathway by which NSAIDs and LA-rich diet exert their cardioprotective effects.

There are, however, other explanations for the protection offered by LA-rich diet. In rats this diet induces an exchange of long chain saturated fatty acids to polyunsaturated fatty acids in the membrane phospholipids and increases the ratio of *n*-6/*n*-3 fatty acids (Kramer, 1980; Leprán *et al.*, 1981b). It is pertinent to consider that this change in fatty acid composition leads to an increased availability of substrate for PG production. This is supported by the finding that indomethacin (but not aspirin) inhibits the protection offered by LA-rich diet (Leprán *et al.*, 1981a); this could be due to inhibition of PGI_2 production. This difference between indomethacin and aspirin is because aspirin acts on platelet cyclo-oxygenase rather than that of the endothelial cells (Schrör *et al.*, 1980; Shaikh *et al.*, 1980). These results suggest the superiority of aspirin over indomethacin in the prevention of myocardial infarction. Other NSAIDs should certainly be thoroughly investigated.

On the basis of these results one may speculate that during the administration of a LA-rich diet more PGI_2 than TxA_2 is produced. This shift is in accordance with the decreased aggregability of platelets. It should be kept in mind that archidonic acid is metabolised in divergent pathways in the platelets and endothelial cells (Bunting *et al.*, 1976; Moncada *et al.*, 1976) and the resultant overproduction may lead to an entirely different outcome as far as myocardial infarction is concerned. The control mechanisms regulating the balance of TxA_2 and PGI_2 production are not yet known; however, some recent findings have shown that the dietary intake of 20 : 5 fatty acid protects against platelet aggregation, either by competitively inhibiting TxA_2 synthesis or by generating PGs which prevent thrombocyte aggregation (Dyerberg and Bang, 1978). In fact, diet rich in this fatty acid reduces the production of platelet TxA_2 (Hornstra and Hemker, 1979) and decreases the severity of experimental myocardial infarction in dogs (Culp *et al.*, 1980).

In respect of a favourable human diet, it would seem reasonable to avoid such *n*-3 polyunsaturated fatty acids. By using a LA-rich diet (Szekeres *et al.*, 1980; Leprán *et al.*, 1981b) the *n*-6/*n*-3 fatty acid ratio is increased. This is in contrast to marine fish oil diet (Gudbjarnason and Hallgrimsson, 1975; Gudbjarnason *et al.*, 1978; Siess *et al.*, 1980; Culp *et al.*, 1980).

REFERENCES

Anturane Reinfarction Trial Group (1980). Sulphinpyrazone in the prevention of sudden death after myocardial infarction. *New Engl. J. Med.*, **302**, 250-6

Aspirin Myocardial Infarction Study Research Group (1980). A randomised, controlled trial of aspirin in persons recovered from myocardial infarction. *J. Am. med. Assoc.*, **243**, 661-9

Awad, A. B. and Zepp, E. A. (1979). Alteration of rat adipose tissue lipolytic response to norepinephrine by dietary fatty acid manipulation. *Biochem. Biophys. Res. Commun.*, **86**, 138-44

Brivio-Haugland, R. P., Louis, S. L., Musch, K., Waldeck, N. and Williams, M. A. (1976). Liver plasma membranes from essential fatty acid deficient rats. *Biochem. biophys. Acta*, **433**, 150–63

Brunner, L., Stepanek, J. and Brunner, H. (1980). Reduction of mortality by sulphinpyrazone after experimental myocardial infarction in the rat. *J. Pharm. Pharmac.*, **32**, 714-5

Bunting, S., Gryglewski, R., Moncada, S. and Vane, J. R. (1976). Arterial walls generate from prostaglandin endoperoxides a substance (prostaglandin X) which relaxes strips of mesenteric and coeliac arteries and inhibits platelet aggregation. *Prostaglandins*, **12**, 897-913

Coker, S. J., Ledingham, I. McA., Parratt, J. R. and Zeitlin, I. J. (1981). Aspirin inhibits the early myocardial release of thromboxane B_2 and ventricular ectopic activity following acute coronary artery occlusion in dogs. *Br. J. Pharmac.*, **72**, 593–5

Culp, B. R., Lands, W. E. M., Lucchesi, B. R., Pitt, B. and Romson, J. (1980). The effect of dietary supplementation of fish oil on experimental myocardial infarction. *Prostaglandins*, **20**, 1021–31

Dyerberg, J. and Bang, H. O. (1978). Dietary fat and thrombosis. *Lancet*, *i*, 152

Ellis, E. F., Oelz, O., Roberts, L. J., Payne, N. A., Sweetman, B. J., Nies, A. S. and Oates, J. A. (1976). Coronary arterial smooth muscle contraction by a substance released from platelets: evidence that it is thromboxane A_2. *Science, N. Y.*, **193**, 1135-7

Elwood, P. C. and Sweetman, P. M. (1979). Aspirin and secondary mortality after myocardial infarction. *Lancet*, *ii*, 1313–5

Folts, J. D., Crowell, E. D. and Rowe, G. G. (1976). Platelet aggregation in partially obstructed vessels and its elimination with aspirin. *Circulation*, **54**, 365–70

Gudbjarnason, S., Doell, B. and Oskarsdottir, G. (1978). Docosahexaenoic acid in cardiac metabolism and function. *Acta biol. med. germ.*, **37**, 777–84

Gudbjarnason, S. and Hallgrimsson, J. (1975). The role of myocardial membrane lipids in the development of cardiac necrosis. *Acta med. scand.*, Suppl. 587, 17–26

Haft, J. I., Kranz, P. D., Albert, F. J. and Fani, K. (1972). Intravascular platelet aggregation in the heart induced by norepinephrine. *Circulation*, **46**, 698–708.

Hornstra, G. (1975). Specific effects of types of dietary fat on arterial thrombosis. In *The Role of Fat in Human Nutrition* (ed. R. Vergroeson), Academic Press, London, pp. 303–6

Hornstra, G. and Hemker, H. C. (1979). Clot promoting effect of platelet-vessel wall interaction: influence of dietary fats and relation to arterial thrombus formation in rats. *Haemostasis*, **8**, 211–26

Jakubowski, J. A. and Ardlie, N. G. (1978). Modification of human platelet function by a diet enriched in saturated or polyunsaturated fat. *Atherosclerosis*, **31**, 335–44

Jorgensen, L., Rowsell, H. C., Hovig, T., Glynn, M. F. and Mustard, J. F. (1967). Adenosine diphosphate induced platelet aggregation and myocardial infarction in swine. *Lab. Invest.*, **17**, 616–44

Kane, K. A., Leprán, I., McDonald, F. M., Parratt, J. R. and Szekeres, L. (1980). The effects of prolonged oral administration of a new antidysrhythmic drug (Org 6001) on coronary artery ligation dysrhythmias in conscious and anaesthetised rats. *J. cardiovasc. Pharmac.*, **2**, 411-23

Kelliher, G. J., Dix, R. K., Jurkiewicz, N. and Lawrence, T. L. (1980). Effect of sulphinpyrazone on arrhythmias and death following coronary occlusion in cats. In *Cardiovascular Actions of Sulphinpyrazone: Basic and Clinical Research* (ed. M. McGregor, J. R. Mustard, M. F. Oliver and S. Sherry), Symposia Specialists Inc., Miami, pp. 193-207

Keys, A. (1970). Coronary heart disease in seven countries. *Circulation*, **41**, Suppl. I, 174

Kramer, J. K. G. (1980). Comparative studies on composition of cardiac phospholipids in rats fed different vegetable oils. *Lipids*, **15**, 651-60

Lefer, A. M. and Crossley, K. (1980). Mechanisms of the optimal protective effects of ibuprofen in acute myocardial ischaemia. *Adv. Shock Res.*, **3**, 133-41

Lefer, A. M. and Polansky, E. W. (1979). Beneficial effects of ibuprofen in acute myocardial ischaemia. *Cardiology*, **64**, 265-79

Leinberger, H., Suehiro, G. T. and McNamara, J. J. (1979). Myocardial platelet trapping after coronary ligation in primates (*Papio anubis*). *J. surg. Res.*, **27**, 36-40

Leprán, I., Siegmund, W. and Szekeres, L. (1979). A method of acute coronary occlusion in anaesthetised closed chest rats. *Acta physiol. hung.*, **53**, 190

Leprán, I., Koltai, M. and Szekeres, L. (1981a). Effect of non-steroid anti-inflammatory drugs in experimental myocardial infarction in rats. *Eur. J. Pharmac.*, **69**, 235-8

Leprán, I., Nemecz, Gy., Koltai, M. and Szekeres, L. (1981b). Effect of linoleic acid rich diet on the acute phase of coronary occlusion in conscious rats. Influence of indomethacin and aspirin. *J. cardiovasc. Res.*, **3**, 847-53

Lewis, B. (1980). Dietary prevention of ischaemic heart disase - a policy for the '80s. *Br. med. J.*, *ii*, 177-80

Miettinen, M., Turpeinen, O., Karvonen, M. J., Elosuo, R. and Paavilainen, E. (1972). Effect of cholesterol-lowering diet on mortality from coronary heart disease and other causes. *Lancet*, *ii*, 835-8

Moncada, S., Gryglewski, R. J., Bunting, S. and Vane, J. R. (1976). An enzyme isolated from arteries transforms prostglandin endoperoxides to an unstable substance that inhibits platelet aggregation. *Nature, Lond.*, **263**, 663-5

Moore, S. (1976). Platelet aggregation secondary to coronary obstruction. *Circulation*, **53**, Suppl. I, 66-9

Morris, J. N., Marr, J. W. and Clayton, D. G. (1977). Diet and heart: a postscript. *Br. med. J.*, *ii*, 1307-14

Moschos, C. B., Lahiri, K., Lyons, M., Weisse, A. B., Oldewurtel, H. A. and Regan, T. J. (1973). Relation of microcirculatory thrombosis to thrombus in the proximal coronary artery: effect of aspirin, dipyridamole and thrombolysis. *Am. Heart J.*, **86**, 61-86

Moschos, C. B., Haider, B., De La Cruz, C., Lyons, M. M. and Regan, T. J. (1978). Antiarrhythmic effects of aspirin during non-thrombotic coronary occlusion. *Circulation*, **57**, 681-4

Moschos, C. B., Escobinas, A. J. and Jorgensen, O. B. (1980). Effects of sulphinpyrazone on ischaemic myocardium. In *Cardiovascular Actions of Sulphinpyrazone: Basic and Clinical Research* (ed. M. McGregor, J. F. Mustard, M. F. Oliver and S. Sherry), Symposia Specialists Inc., Miami, pp. 175-87

O'Brien, J. R. (1968). Effects of salicylates on human platelets. *Lancet*, *i*, 779-83

Persantine-Aspirin Reinfarction Study Research Group (1980). Persantine and aspirin in coronary heart disease. *Circulation*, **62**, 449-61

Povalski, H. J., Olson, R., Kopia, S. and Furness, P. (1980). Comparative effects of sulphinpyrazone and aspirin in the coronary occlusion-reperfusion dog model. In *Cardiovascular Actions of Sulphinpyrazone: Basic and Clinical Research* (ed. M. McGregor, J. F. Mustard, M. F. Oliver, and S. Sherry), Symposia Specialists Inc., Miami, pp. 153-70

Renaud, S., Kuba, K., Goulet, G., Lemire, Y. and Allard, C. (1970). Relationship between fatty-acid composition of platelets and platelet aggregation in rat and man. Relation to thrombosis. *Circulation Res.*, **26**, 553-64

Schrör, K., Sauerland, S., Kuhn, A. and Rösen, R. (1980). Different sensitivities of prostaglandin-cyclooxygenases in blood platelets and coronary arteries against non-steroidal anti-inflammatory drugs. *Naunyn-Schmiedebergs Arch. Pharmac.*, **313**, 69-76

Selye, H., Bajusz, E., Grasso, S. and Mendell, P. (1960). Simple techniques for the surgical occlusion of coronary vessels in the rat. *Angiology*, **11**, 398-407

Shaikh, B. S., Bott, S. J. and Demers, L. M. (1980). The differential inhibition of prostaglandin synthesis in platelets and vascular tissue in response to aspirin. *Prostaglandins Med.*, **4**, 439-47

Shekelle, R. B., Shryock, A. M., Paul, O., Lepper, M., Stamler, J., Liu, S. and Raynor, W. J. (1981). Diet, serum cholesterol, and death from coronary heart disease. The Western Electric study. *New Engl. J. Med.*, **304**, 65-70

Sherry, S. (1980). Drug trials in myocardial infarction. Lessons to be learned from the anturane reinfarction trial. *Eur. J. clin. Pharmac.*, **17**, 401-7

Siess, W., Scherer, B., Böhlig, B., Roth, P., Kurzmann, I. and Weber, P. C. (1980). Platelet-membrane fatty acids, platelet aggregation, and thromboxane formation during a mackerel diet. *Lancet*, *i*, 441-4

Smith, E. F., Carrow, B. A. and Lefer, A. M. (1980). Effects of flurbiprofen on myocardial cell damage in acute myocardial ischaemia. *Res. Commun. chem. Path. Pharmac.*, **28**, 413-33

Szekeres, L. (1978a). Principles of the pharmacotherapy of early arrhythmias occurring in myocardial infarction. *Proc. VIIIth Wld Congr. Cardiol.*, 933-8

Szekeres, L. (1978b). Theoretical considerations concerning drug treatment of dysrhythmias due to coronary insufficiency. *Adv. Pharmac. Ther.*, **6**, 257-75

Szekeres, L. and Vaughan Williams, E. M. (1962). Antifibrillatory action. *J. Physiol., Lond.*, **160**, 470-82

Szekeres, L., Lépran, I. and Koltai, M. (1980). Influence of linoleic acid rich diet on the incidence of arrhythmias and death in the acute phase of myocardial infarction in conscious rats. In *Prostaglandins and Thromboxanes* (ed. W. Förster), Gustav Fischer Verlag, Jena, pp. 33-6

Turpeinen, O., Karvonen, M. J., Pekkarinen, M., Miettinen, M., Elosuo, R. and Paavilainen, E. (1979). Dietary prevention of coronary heart disease: the Finnish mental hospital study. *Int. J. Epidemiol.*, **8**, 99-118

Vik-Mo, H. (1978). Platelet accumulation in the myocardium during acute non-thrombotic coronary artery occlusion in dogs. *Scand. J. Haematol.*, **21**, 225-32

Vik-Mo, J. and Mjøs, O. D. (1977). Effect of sodium salicylate and acetyl-salicyclic acid on epicardial ST-segment elevation during coronary occlusion in dogs. *Scand. J. clin. Lab. Invest.*, **37**, 287-94

15

The Effects of Sodium Channel Inhibitors on Early Arrhythmias Associated with Acute Myocardial Ischaemia

R. J. Marshall and Eileen Winslow

15.1 INTRODUCTION

The initial discovery that a compound possesses antiarrhythmic activity is usually made in simple screening models involving the use of arrhythmogenic chemicals like aconitine, chloroform or ouabain. If promising results are obtained in these tests then the potential antiarrhythmic drug may be tested (usually in conscious dogs) for its ability to suppress ventricular ectopic activity ensuing 1-2 days after the production of myocardial ischaemia. Historically this sequence of events holds especially for the group of drugs variously described as 'membrane stabilisers', 'sodium channel blockers' or 'class 1 agents' (Vaughan Williams, 1970). Consequently, there is comparatively little literature describing the effects of sodium channel blocking agents on the early experimental ventricular arrhythmias and fibrillation which occur within minutes of the onset of myocardial ischaemia. The reasons for this are many but surely include the difficulties involved in producing a consistent quantitative model in which to assess the protective actions of putative antiarrhythmic drugs. For instance, our own experiences have shown that one-stage coronary artery ligation does not produce ventricular ectopic activity in every species - rabbits and guinea-pigs being particularly resistant. In addition even in those species which demonstrate early ventricular arrhythmias (for example, the dog), ligation of the same coronary artery can be associated with a range of incidence of ventricular fibrillation (VF) of between zero and 100 per cent depending on the laboratory (see Stephenson *et al.*, 1960, for review of early literature, and chapter 6 of this book). Although some of the factors involved in this variability, such as the proportion of pre-existing collateral coronary vessels (Meesmann *et al.*, 1976) and the anaesthetics used (Au *et al.*, 1979a; Marshall and Parratt, 1980a) have already been identified, there still remains some controversy as to which is the best experimental animal model for testing the activity of drugs against early ventricular arrhythmias produced by myocardial ischaemia (for example, the need for a 'pog' or a 'dig'; Janse, 1978).

15.2 INHIBITORS OF THE CARDIAC FAST SODIUM CHANNEL

The romantic discovery of the protective effects of quinine against atrial fibrillation (Wenckeback, 1914) resulted 4 years later in the prototype of antiarrhythmic drugs, quinidine. However, it was not until the late 1950s, with the development of intracellular recording, that it was shown that quinidine's major action was to reduce the maximum rate of depolarisation (MRD) in cardiac cells (Vaughan Williams, 1958) without affecting the resting membrane potential. Indeed this is the one common property shared by the group of drugs (table 15.1) under discussion here and which

Table 15.1 Na^+ channel blocking agents possessing antiarrhythmic activity in animals and man. For explanation of groups A, B and C, see text

Group A	Group B	Group C
	Quinidine	Prenylamine
Lignocaine	Procainamide	Perhexilene
Mexiletine	Disopyramide	Bepridil
Tocainide	Encainide	Amiodarone
Org 6001	Flecainide	D,L-Propranolol
Diphenylhydantoin	Lorcainide	
	Aprindine	

are collectively described as 'inhibitors of the fast Na^+ channel', 'quinidine-like' or 'membrane stabilisers'. For recent reviews of the electrophysiology of antiarrhythmic drugs see Hauswirth and Singh (1978) and Vaughan Williams (1980). The structures of some of the drugs under review are shown in figure 15.1.

As workers in the antiarrhythmic field will be aware, there has been considerable discussion surrounding the classification of this group of drugs. The original classification of Vaughan Williams (1970) pools these drugs together on the basis that they all share the common property of reducing MRD. Other workers (Hoffman and Bigger, 1971; Rosen and Hoffman, 1973) have modified this classification in recognition of the fact that some of these agents (for example disopyramide and quinidine) markedly slow conduction velocity and increase action potential duration whereas others (lignocaine, mexiletine) have little, or opposite, effects on these parameters. A separation of these two groups of drugs has also been put forward by Arnsdorf (1976) on the basis that the primary action of quinidine and procainamide in normal fibres is to reduce sodium conductance, whereas lignocaine and diphenylhydantoin mainly act by increasing potassium conductance. Whichever of these classifications is the most useful, it is clear that some of these drugs (group B, table 15.1) are clinically effective against both atrial and ventricular arrhythmias whereas those in group A (table 15.1) are mainly effective against arrhythmias of ventricular origin (see Opie, 1980).

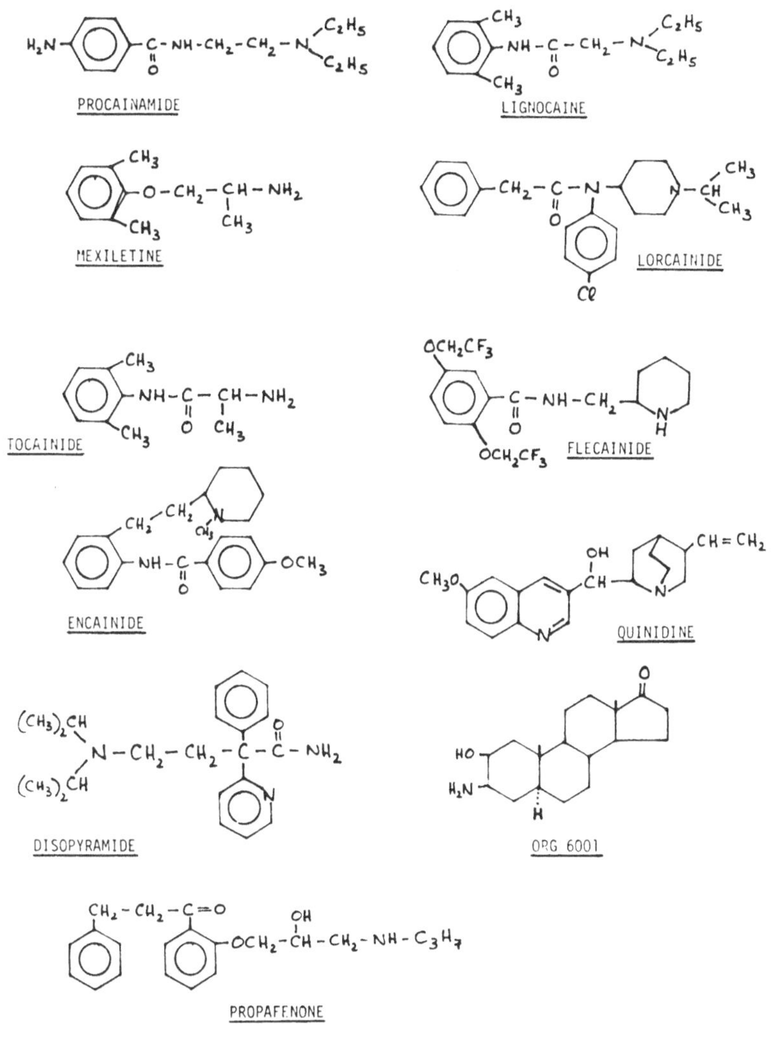

PROCAINAMIDE LIGNOCAINE

MEXILETINE LORCAINIDE

TOCAINIDE FLECAINIDE

ENCAINIDE QUINIDINE

DISOPYRAMIDE ORG 6001

PROPAFENONE

Figure 15.1 The chemical structures of some Na^+ channel blocking drugs.

The third group of drugs (C) shown in table 15.1 is of inhibitors of the fast sodium channel which possess other important pharmacological actions. For instance, in cardiac muscle, perhexilene, prenylamine and bepridil inhibit the slow inward current (carried by Ca^{2+} and or Na^+) at concentrations showing a class 1 action (Vogel *et al.*, 1979; Kane and Winslow, 1980; Vaughan Williams, 1980). D, L - Propranolol is also, of course, a potent competitive antagonist at cardiac β-adrenoceptors (class II of Vaughan Williams' classification) and the major cardiac effect of amiodarone is to markedly increase the duration of the cardiac action potential (class III effect; Singh and Vaughan Williams, 1970). Although the effectiveness of these drugs in suppressing early post-ischaemia arrhythmias has been reported (Marshall and Parratt, 1977a; Collett *et al.*, 1980; Kane and Winslow, 1980; Marshall and Muir, 1981), it is obviously difficult to decide what contribution to their protective actions is made by effects on the fast sodium channel.

15.3 THEORETICAL CONSIDERATIONS AS TO WHY SODIUM CHANNEL INHIBITORS SHOULD PREVENT EARLY VENTRICULAR ARRHYTHMIAS

The theoretical properties desirable for effective suppression of ventricular arrhythmias following myocardial ischaemia have been delineated previously (Vaughan Williams, 1979), and are summarised in table 15.2. All drugs with a main action in blocking fast sodium channels would fulfill the first two criteria (table 15.2). Their

Table 15.2 Theoretical desirable profile of drugs expected to suppress 'early' ventricular arrhythmias associated with myocardial ischaemia and relevant properties of Na^+ channel blockers (after Vaughan Williams, 1979)

Desirable properties for effective suppression of post-infarct arrhythmias

(1) Render central infarcted region electrically silent
(2) Render normal myocardium more refractory
(3) Reduce residual ectopic activity in border zone, associated with 'short' APs

Relevant properties of Na^+ channel blockers

(1) Retardation of fast inward current (MRD) – already affected by changes in K^+, H^+ and p_{O_2}
(2) Raise the electrical threshold of normal myocardium
(3) Lengthening of APD (but not lignocaine or mexiletine).

effectiveness in modifying the action potentials of short duration found in the ischaemic myocardium might theoretically depend on their individual effects on action potential duration. Such an analysis would predict that drugs which shorten duration (like lignocaine, mexiletine and the aminosteroid Org 6001) would be arrhythmogenic in this area whereas drugs which increase action potential duration (quinidine, procainamide and disopyramide) would be expected to be effective in suppressing ectopic activity in this border zone. An alternative argument claims that although lignocaine (Wittig *et al.*, 1973) and Org 6001 (Salako *et al.*, 1976) do shorten action potential duration (APD), this effect is especially marked in preterminal Purkinje fibres, in which APD is normally longest. The net effect of these two agents therefore is to make APD more homogeneous along the conducting system and perhaps also result in an increased conduction velocity. That this latter effect may be antiarrhythmic has been rigorously challenged (Vaughan Williams, 1980) and indeed has not been confirmed in experimental studies with lignocaine in whole animal models (see below).

There is now good evidence that early disturbances of ventricular rhythm following myocardial ischaemia are associated with a progressively delayed activation of ischaemic muscle (for references see Elharrar and Zipes, 1977; Kaplinsky *et al.*, 1979). It would thus seem that the early ventricular arrhythmias following myocardial ischaemia (which frequently terminate in ventricular fibrillation) involve re-entry mechanisms. This is in contrast to the ventricular arrhythmias seen 1-2 days later, which are due to increased automaticity in surviving Purkinje fibres (Scherlag *et al.*, 1970; Lazzara *et al.*, 1974).

Immediately following ischaemia it is conceivable that such delays in impulse propagation coupled to inhomogenous refractoriness may establish an area of unidirectional block (Arnsdorf, 1976). Theoretically this can be converted into a bidirectional block (electrically silent area) by drugs which further depress conduction velocity (for example, group B) or alternatively normal conduction can be restored by drugs, like lignocaine, which enhance conduction (figure 15.2). Whether these theoretical considerations are borne out by present experimental evidence will be discussed later.

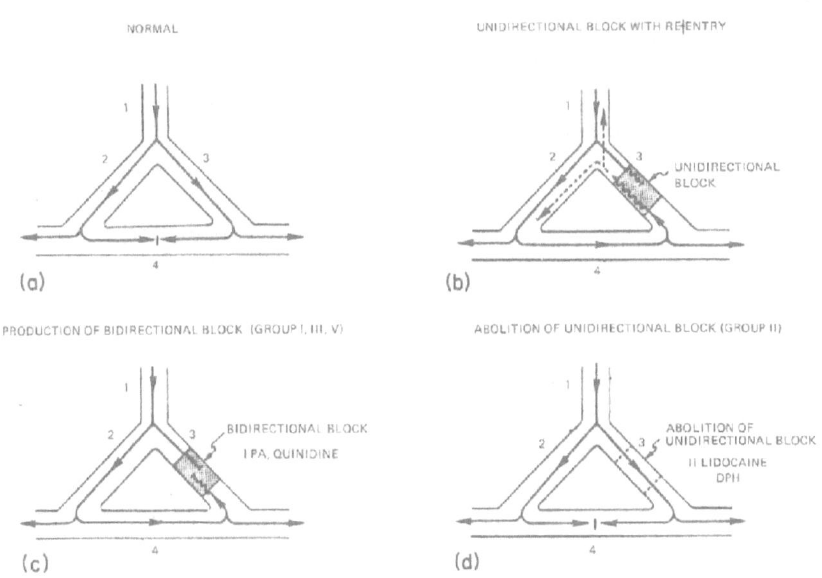

Figure 15.2 Effect of Na^+ channel blockers on re-entry. (a) Normal Purkinje fibre showing impulse spreading into branches (2 and 3) and activating ventricular tissue (4). (b) Segment 3 with unidirectional antegrade block and slow retrograde conduction (produced by ischaemia). Impulse can only propagate down branch 2 into ventricular muscle (4). If limb 2 has recovered excitability this impulse may re-enter limb 2 by passing retrogradely through area of block thus setting up a re-entry beat. (c) Na^+ channel blockers which markedly slow conduction further (group B, table 15.1) may convert the unidirectional to bidirectional block. (d) Alternatively lignocaine-type agents (group A, table 15.1) may overcome unidirectional block by improving conduction preferentially in this area. (From Arnsdorf (1976).)

15.4 THE EFFECTS OF SODIUM CHANNEL BLOCKING AGENTS ON EARLY POST-MYOCARDIAL ISCHAEMIA VENTRICULAR ARRHYTHMIAS

Lignocaine

The local anaesthetic lignocaine was first administered as an antiarrhythmic agent in 1950 (Southworth *et al.*, 1950). Thirty years on, this drug remains the agent of choice for the treatment of post-infarction arrhythmias in man (see chapter 20). Although there are instances where severe post-infarction arrhythmias are not adequately controlled by lignocaine (Benett *et al.*, 1970; Bleifeld *et al.*, 1972; Geddes *et al.*, 1972), many clinical studies have demonstrated a good response to this agent following myocardial infarction (MI) in patients who survive to reach hospital (Jewitt *et al.*, 1968; Harrison and Alderman, 1972; Büssman *et al.*, 1980). However, the effectiveness of lignocaine in preventing sudden death has not been demonstrated clinically and indeed a recent article by Pentecost *et al.* (1981), reviewing their own use of lignocaine over a 12 year period, states, 'Experience suggests that the use of lignocaine to suppress ventricular ectopic activity observed in the first few hours of admission to hospital with acute MI has no therapeutic value'. The effectiveness of lignocaine during the pre-hospital phase of MI remains to be clarified. Ribner *et al.* (1979) reported that intramuscular administration of lignocaine appeared to reduce the risk of ventricular tachyarrhythmias and sudden death over the 1-1.5 h period following administration, whereas Adgey *et al.* (1971) reported that intravenous therapeutic doses of lignocaine were ineffective in suppressing arrhythmias in 67 per cent of patients requiring therapy within 1 h of the onset of symptoms. Thus, although lignocaine has proven efficacy against arrhythmias which are seen from the time of hospital admission and during the subsequent few days, its effectiveness against very early arrhythmias remains to be demonstrated (see chapter 20).

Experimentally the effectiveness of lignocaine against very early post-infarction arrhythmias is also controversial. Borer *et al.* (1976) reported that pretreatment of dogs with a 2 mg kg^{-1} bolus injection followed by a slow infusion (70-100 $\mu g\ kg^{-1}\ min^{-1}$) to give plasma levels of 1.2-5.5 $\mu g\ ml^{-1}$ significantly reduced the incidence of spontaneous ventricular fibrillation (VF) during the first 30 min after one-stage simultaneous occlusion of the left anterior descending (LAD) and septal coronary arteries. Interestingly four dogs with high plasma levels ($>6.3\ \mu g\ ml^{-1}$) all fibrillated. In these experiments post-ligation administration of lignocaine reversed the reduction in ventricular fibrillation threshold (VFT) consequent upon coronary occlusion in six out of eight animals. A similar effect on the fall in VFT, recorded during 45 min of ligation of one to two branches of the LAD in the dog, has also been reported by Allen *et al.* (1977) in association with mean plasma levels of 1.7 $\mu g\ ml^{-1}$. In this study lignocaine was also reported to induce an increase in VFT of non-ischaemic myocardium. Lignocaine (10 mg kg^{-1} + 5 mg $kg^{-1}\ h^{-1}$) has also been shown to protect against coronary artery ligation-induced VF in the anaesthetised rat (Clark *et al.*, 1980) during the 30 min post-ligation period. In these experiments ligation of the main left coronary artery was performed 15 min after commencement of the infusion.

In contrast to these apparent beneficial effects of lignocaine, Marshall and Parratt (1980b) were unable to show a reduction in the incidence of VF in the anaesthetised greyhound during the first 30 min following ligation of the LAD in animals infused intravenously with lignocaine (1 mg kg^{-1} min^{-1} commenced 10 min prior to ligation) to a total dose of 30 mg kg^{-1} (figure 15.3). They did, however, report a significant reduction in the number of premature ventricular ectopic beats (VEBs), but only during the 11-30 min post-ligation period. Stephenson *et al.* (1960), using an infusion rate of 77 μg kg^{-1} min^{-1}, were also unable to demonstrate a protective effect of lignocaine against very early post-infarction VF in the dog.

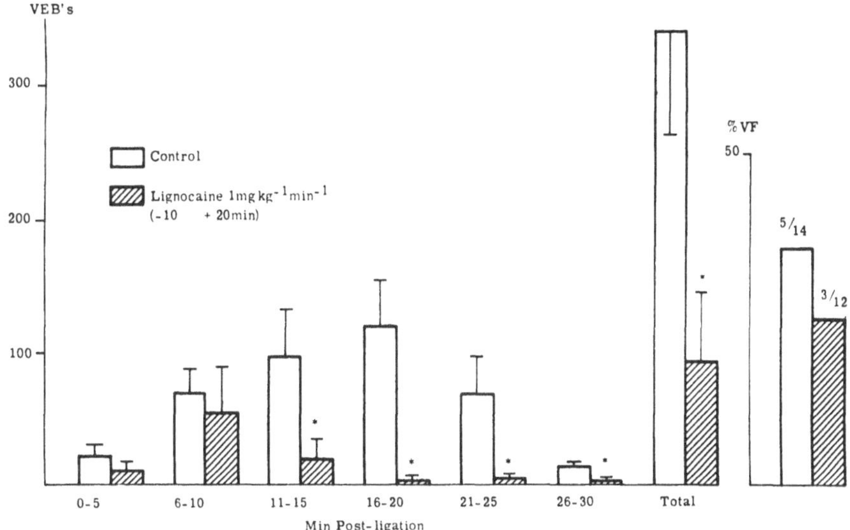

Figure 15.3 The effects of pretreatment with lignocaine on the number of premature ventricular ectopic beats (VEBs) and on the incidence of ventricular fibrillation (VF) in the first 30 min following acute coronary artery ligation in chloralose-anaesthetised greyhounds. (From Marshall and Parratt (1980b).)

Very recently one of the most detailed experimental studies on the effects of lignocaine on primary VF and ventricular fibrillation thresholds (VFTs) in anaesthetised dogs has been reported (Kramer *et al.*, 1981). These workers have shown that at plasma levels up to 0.5 μg ml^{-1}, lignocaine neither increased VFT in normal myocardium nor prevented the fall in VFT occurring within 15 min of acute ligation of the LAD. In addition, this dosage regime of lignocaine (2 mg kg^{-1} bolus + 50 μg kg^{-1} min^{-1}) did not modify the incidence of VF (100 per cent) produced by ligation of the LAD in animals which had few observable collaterals at autopsy. The conclusion reached by these workers was that clinically recommended doses of lignocaine do not protect anaesthetised dogs from primary VF during the early phase of arrhythmias following acute coronary occlusion, although some evidence of protection (increase in VFT) was observed with higher doses.

Exacerbation of early arrhythmias by lignocaine has also been reported. Zipes and Troup (1978) found that $1\,mg\,kg^{-1}\,min^{-1}$ increased the incidence of VF in dogs subjected to coronary artery ligation whilst Dughman and Cohn (1973) reported a lignocaine-induced reduction in post-infarction VFT. A similar accentuation of ligation-induced arrhythmias by lignocaine during the 45 min to 3 h period following coronary artery ligation has also been seen in the cat; Gamble and Cohn (1972) evaluated ischaemia-induced increases in automaticity by analysing the frequency of escape beats following intravenous acetylcholine. Susceptibility to re-entry was assessed by counting the number of repetitive beats induced by a premature electrical stimulus delivered to the ventricle. Lignocaine in a dose of 2–4 mg kg^{-1} consistently suppressed automaticity whereas re-entry was only abolished in six out of 17 animals. Indeed, lignocaine increased re-entry in the remaining 11 animals and induced VF in one. These deleterious effects were seen when the plasma levels were in the lower therapeutic range. McDonald (1980) has also recorded an increased mortality in rats subjected to coronary artery ligation following administration of subthreshold antiarrhythmic doses of lignocaine. Further evidence for facilitation of re-entrant arrhythmias by lignocaine comes from the work of Scherlag *et al.* (1980). Using dogs, with both LAD and circumflex coronary arteries occluded for 12-75 days, these workers showed that re-entrant arrhythmias were much more easily induced by ventricular pacing following lignocaine administration. This was associated with continuous electrical activity in the epicardium and in the endocardium. They concluded that lignocaine unmasks the potential for lethal arrhythmias to develop during chronic MI by selectively slowing conduction in tissue with latent abnormalities and thus enhances the induction of re-entrant VT.

More direct evidence for facilitation of re-entrant arrhythmias by lignocaine during the very early phase of MI has come from studies in which bipolar electrograms are used to record the electrical activity in ischaemic and non-ischaemic myocardium. A number of studies have suggested the development of a marked delay in activation time recorded in the subepicardium of the ischaemic zone and/ or the persistence of electrical activity beyond the T-wave of the electrocardiogram (reviewed by Elharrar and Zipes, 1977). These electrical changes are seen within 5 min of coronary artery occlusion. Such delayed conduction has been associated with the development of arrhythmias. Williams *et al.* (1974) found that the conduction delay followed an exponential curve from the time of ligation of the LAD to the time of occurrence of ventricular arrhythmias and that maximum conduction delay invariably preceded the onset of VT. Thus drugs which further delay conduction would be expected to facilitate re-entrant arrhythmias. In a study conducted by Nakaya *et al.* (1980), acute myocardial ischaemia was produced in the dog by complete occlusion of the LAD for 5 or 10 min. The resulting conduction delay in the ischaemic zone was enhanced by lignocaine ($2\,mg\,kg^{-1} + 4.3\,mg\,kg^{-1}\,h^{-1}$) given prior to occlusion. However, Kupersmith *et al.* (1975) found that although lignocaine increased ischaemia-induced conduction delay in the dog, the incidence of arrhythmias was reduced.

In contrast, Hope *et al.* (1974) found that lignocaine hastened the time course of conduction delay in the ischaemic zone but reduced, although not significantly, the time to the onset of ventricular arrhythmias. In this context, the work of Ogawa *et al.* (1979) is of interest. In this study acute coronary artery ligation in the dog was performed and electrical activity recorded in the normal and in the ischaemic myocardium. The results of this study suggested that the early arrhythmias were of two types: (1) acute immediate ventricular arrhythmias associated with epicardial re-entry and seen 2-10 min post ligation and (2) acute delayed ventricular arrhythmias which appear to originate from deeper muscle layers and are clearly independent of epicardial re-entry. These later arrhythmias develop 15-25 min after ligation. The two phases are separated by a 3-12 min period of quiescence (see also chapter 6 of this book). If lignocaine, as the current literature tends to suggest, does not oppose re-entrant arrhythmias, then the results obtained by Ogawa *et al.* may explain the findings (Marshall and Parratt, 1980b) that lignocaine does not reduce the number of arrhythmias during the 0-11 min post-infarction period in the dog.

Using the pig, whose coronary tree more closely resembles that of man, Cardinal *et al.* (1980) recorded the effect of 1 and 5 μg ml^{-1} lignocaine on transmembrane and DC-extracellular potentials and on patterns of activation at 60 sites in the ischaemic zone (IZ) and in nearly normal areas during arrhythmias induced by LAD occlusion in isolated perfused hearts. They found that the magnitude of the depression of action potential upstroke characteristics in the IZ seen during control occlusions was exaggerated, and its time course accelerated, during occlusion in the presence of lignocaine. Patterns of activation characteristic of a 'focal' mechanism, possibly due to injury current across the ischaemic border and present at the onset of ventricular tachycardia, were not affected by lignocaine. Lignocaine did not prevent large circus movements (diameter 10-20 mm) in the IZ which were responsible for continuation of VT. However, the high concentration of the drug prevented fractionation into multiple micro re-entrant circuits (diameter 5 mm) which is characteristic of fibrillation. This effect was due to conversion of areas of unidirectional block and slow conduction into areas of total block. VF occurred in only one of 13 hearts in the presence of 5 μg ml^{-1} lignocaine whereas the incidence of VF during control occlusions was eight out of 13; VT occurred in 11 and 12 hearts respectively. It was concluded from this study that lignocaine suppresses only the mechanism responsible for VF during ischaemia (see chapter 4).

The conflicting results concerning the efficacy of lignocaine against very early post-infarction arrhythmias may possibly reflect the relative tissue concentrations achieved in the ischaemic and non-ischaemic areas. It may be that local concentrations sufficient to convert unidirectional to bidirectional block in the ischaemic portion are necessary to eliminate re-entrant arrhythmias whereas lower concentrations, which only further delay conduction but do not prevent it, may enhance re-entry. It is also conceivable that re-entry may be enhanced whilst VF is reduced, the latter depending on the suppression of micro re-entry within the ischaemic zone.

The electrophysiological actions of lignocaine have been summarised in detail by various authors (Rosen *et al.*, 1975; Hauswirth and Singh, 1978; Vaughan Williams,

1978). The main electrophysiological effects of lignocaine which are considered to be responsible for its antiarrhythmic activity are its ability to reduce the maximum rate of rise of phase 0 of the transmembrane action potentials, to depress membrane responsiveness and to slow conduction velocity. Theoretically, selectively depressed conduction in the ischaemic area could transform areas of unidirectional block to bidirectional block, thereby abolishing re-entry. Sasynuik and Kus (1974) have, in fact, reported that lignocaine exerts more marked electrophysiological effects on surviving fibres taken from severely ischaemic myocardium than on normal myocardium. Maximum diastolic potential is also reduced by lignocaine in these ischaemic fibres.

Lignocaine exerts effects on the action potential duration (APD) and the effective refractory period which are not shared by disopyramide, procainamide or quinidine and which has led to some controversy regarding the mechanism by which lignocaine exerts its antiarrhythmic effects. Vaughan Williams (1978) demonstrated that lignocaine shortened the action potential duration throughout the cardiac conducting system, including ventricular muscle, but preferentially shortened APD in those areas where it is normally longest (false tendon) so that APD became more uniform. A dramatic shortening of the effective refractory period of Purkinje fibres (Bigger and Mandel, 1970) is also seen. Again the magnitude of this is dependent on the location (Wittig *et al.*, 1973). APD is, however, shortened more than the effective refractory period so that the relative refractory period is prolonged. It has been claimed that accelerated repolarisation associated with a relatively faster conduction of premature impulses may contribute to the antiarrhythmic action of lignocaine (Wittig *et al.*, 1973). Such an action could eliminate the unidirectional conduction block of early premature impulses which initiate re-entry rendering premature action potentials less likely to initiate sustained re-entrant tachycardias. This hypothesis has not yet been verified experimentally and Vaughan Williams (1978) puts forward convincing arguments to suggest that lignocaine is antiarrhythmic despite these actions and not because of them. Indeed such actions could equally well be arrhythmogenic and may contribute to the exacerbation of re-entrant arrhythmias seen in several studies following MI. A recent study by Wald *et al.* (1980) may shed further light on the mechanism by which lignocaine exerts its antiarrhythmic effects. In this study, asymmetric conduction properties were produced in sheep Purkinje fibres either by asymmetric segmental cooling or crushing. Lignocaine (1-5 μg ml^{-1}) (as well as procainamide, propranolol, quinidine and diphenylhydantoin) all induced reversible deterioration of conduction and converted unidirectional block to bidirectional block irrespective of the external potassium concentration (5.4 or 3.0 mM). Conversion of unidirectional block to bidirectional conduction was never seen. Thus, as Vaughan Williams (1978) has suggested, rendering of ischaemic areas to complete electrical silence may be an important action for the antiarrhythmic effectiveness of lignocaine.

Mexiletine

Mexiletine is an orally active analogue of lignocaine which has been shown to be effective in suppressing arrhythmias of varying aetiology in animals (Allen *et al.*,

1970, 1972; Okuma *et al.*, 1976) and in man (Talbot *et al.*, 1973; Campbell *et al.*, 1973; Pozenel, 1977; Esser and Kikis, 1978). To date few controlled studies of the effects of mexiletine on post-infarction arrhythmias in man have been reported. A study by Merx *et al.* (1978) on 57 patients admitted to hospital within 24 h of the onset of MI indicated that intravenously administered mexiletine (given to half the patients) reduced ectopic activity. Campbell *et al.* (1978) reported a reduction in ventricular tachycardia and in R on T phenomena in 44 patients given oral mexiletine within 12 h of MI as compared to 53 patients given placebo. In these studies effective therapeutic concentrations were between 0.5 and 2.0 $\mu g\ ml^{-1}$. More recently, it has been shown that mexiletine (200 mg + 0.5-1.0 mg min^{-1}) is superior to lignocaine (100 mg + 2-3 mg min^{-1}) in the prevention of ventricular extrasystoles occurring within 48 h of onset of MI (Horowitz *et al.*, 1981). Some relevant data is also available from animal experiments. Like lignocaine, mexiletine has been found to reverse the fall in VFT observed within 45 min of ligation of one to two side branches of the LAD in the anaesthetised dog (Allen *et al.*, 1977) and to increase VFT in the non-ischaemic myocardium. In this study the mean plasma level of mexiletine was 2.3 $\mu g\ ml^{-1}$. Some effects against early post-infarction arrhythmias have also been seen by Marshall *et al.* (1981) in the anaesthetised rat. In this study, 1 mg kg^{-1} mexiletine given intravenously 15 min prior to ligation, or 50 mg kg^{-1} given orally 1 h before ligation, prevented the development of VF and significantly reduced the number of VEBs which normally result from main left coronary artery occlusion. As in the dog, VFT of the non-ischaemic rat myocardium is increased by intravenous mexiletine (Marshall *et al.*, 1981).

In contrast to these reported beneficial effects of mexiletine, Gerin and Kulbertus (1978) found that 15 mg kg^{-1} mexiletine (given in divided doses over an 11 min period prior to occlusion) *increased* the incidence of VT and VF in the anaesthetised dog. In these experiments 6 min occlusions of the LAD were performed together with an increase in the basal pacing rate of 120 to 150 and 200 per min, the increased pacing rates being maintained for periods of 30 s. The deleterious effects of mexiletine were more marked when pacing was increased 9 min after occlusion as compared to 48 min after occlusion. Gerin and Kulbertus also demonstrated a prolongation of the QRS interval and a significantly increased conduction delay in the subepicardium of the ischaemic zone in the mexiletine-treated animals. Similar effects were observed in response to quinidine, aprindine and lorcainide. These workers concluded that any drug which significantly increases the ischaemia-induced conduction delay may increase the incidence of ligation-induced arrhythmias. This is presumably associated with a high myocardial content of antiarrhythmic agent, a high heart rate and an occlusion performed in the presence of an otherwise normal circulation. Gerin and Kulbertus stated that clinically these conditions are probably rare. However, at least in the very early stages of MI and in the presence of a high degree of sympathetic activity, these conditions could be encountered and may be relevant to the prophylactic use of antiarrhythmic drugs.

Whereas Gerin and Kulbertus have associated exacerbation of ligation-induced arrhythmias with high levels of mexiletine, Marshall *et al.* (1981) have provided indirect evidence to suggest that the reverse may be true, at least in the anaesthetised rat. Twelve hours after a single oral dose of 100 mg kg^{-1}, at a time when plasma levels were assumed to be low, mortality from ligation-induced VF increased from 7 per cent in the controls to 67 per cent in the mexiletine group. This high mortality was associated with a significantly lower VFT of the non-ischaemic myocardium compared to controls. A further fall in VFT was seen in both groups of animals 3-4 min after coronary artery ligation. Thus, like lignocaine, aggravation of arrhythmias by mexiletine, as well as amelioration in the very early phase of MI, has been encountered experimentally. The reasons for the conflicting experimental results may reside in the cardiac drug levels and their associated electrophysiological actions.

The effects of mexiletine on cardiac transmembrane action potentials have been described by Singh and Vaughan Williams (1972), by Yamaguchi *et al.* (1978), by Yamada *et al.* (1978) and by Arita *et al.* (1979). Essentially, the electrophysiological actions of mexiletine are similar to those of lignocaine, although conflicting results have been reported for the effects of mexiletine on APD. Vaughan Williams (1977) found that mexiletine, like lignocaine, preferentially shortened APD in that part of the conducting system where it is normally longest, whereas Yamaguchi *et al.* (1978) found that the degree of shortening of APD was similar throughout the conducting tissue. Low concentrations of mexiletine (2 μg ml^{-1}) have been reported to shorten the ERP of Purkinje tissue, whereas higher concentrations prolong ERP (Yamada *et al.*, 1978; Arita *et al.*, 1979). In ventricular muscle, Yamada *et al.* (1978) reported that unlike lignocaine, ERP was slightly prolonged in the absence of a significant change in APD. Arita *et al.* (1979) also found a prolongation of ERP but reported inconsistent changes in APD. The latter group also found that mexiletine increased V_{max} of propagated premature action potentials by shifting the takeoff potential to more negative levels in both Purkinje and ventricular tissue. Weld *et al.* (1979) further reported that mexiletine shortened APD of sheep Purkinje fibres at concentrations lower than those required to reduce V_{max}. Whether these actions are antiarrhythmic or arrhythmogenic remains to be demonstrated.

The ability of lignocaine and of mexiletine to suppress diastolic depolarisation and automatic impulse formation in Purkinje fibres (Singer *et al.*, 1967; Wit *et al.*, 1974; Rosen *et al.*, 1975; Yamada *et al.*, 1978; Arita *et al.*, 1979; Weld *et al.*, 1979) in concentrations which do not suppress sinus automaticity (Rosen *et al.*, 1975; Yamaguchi *et al.*, 1978) may contribute to the reported antiarrhythmic effects against early post-infarction arrhythmias seen in some studies and may also account for the selective action of lignocaine on the second phase (1b) of early arrhythmias reported by Marshall and Parratt (1980a) in which re-entry may not be the mechanism responsible (Ogawa *et al.*, 1979).

Lorcainide (R 15889; Ro 13-1042; NO(4-chlorophenyl)-*N*-(1-methylethyl)-4-piperidenylbenzene acetamide HCl)

Lorcainide is a new and potent antiarrhythmic agent with a novel structure (figure 15.1). The drug is effective against premature ventricular systoles (PVS), complex PVS and VT in man following both intravenous and oral administration (Kesteloot and Stroobandt, 1977; Cocco and Strozzi, 1978; Meinertz *et al.*, 1979; Morganroth *et al.*, 1980; Somani, 1980a). Somani (1980a) reported that in six patients, in whom arrhythmias were suppressed by 98 per cent for 20-24 h following intravenous lorcainide, peak plasma concentrations were 0.31-1.14 $\mu g\ ml^{-1}$ (mean 0.52 $\mu g\ ml^{-1}$) whilst Meinertz *et al.* (1980a) reported a 90 per cent suppression in 11 of 12 patients receiving 200-600 mg kg^{-1} p.o. per day (plasma concentrations of only 0.13-0.27 $\mu g\ ml^{-1}$). However, little is known of the effect of lorcainide against early post-infarction arrhythmias either in animals or in man. The previously mentioned study of Gerin and Kulbertus (1978) indicating that lorcainide (like quinidine, aprinidine and mexiletine) may increase the incidence of very early post-infarction arrhythmias is, to our knowledge, the only published experimental study of this kind.

Electrophysiologically, lorcainide shows a similar profile to quinidine. It exerts class I actions and prolongs the transmembrane action potential duration and the refractory period of Purkinje tissue (unpublished data quoted by Cocco and Strozzi, 1978). Automaticity is also suppressed. Similar effects are seen on ventricular and atrial muscle (Carmeliet *et al.*, 1978). Carmeliet and Zaman (1979) reported that in the perfused guinea-pig heart, lorcainide preferentially slowed conduction through the ventricular conducting system and in this respect was more selective than lignocaine. Lorcainide was the more potent by a factor of approximately 10. This agent also markedly decreased conduction of premature stimuli. In cat papillary muscle, the refractory period increased progressively over a 3 h contact period with lorcainide (Carmeliet *et al.*, 1978), an effect similar to that seen with aprindine (Carmeliet and Verdonck, 1974) but different to that of lignocaine (maximum effects reached within 15-30 min). From a qualitative point of view, lorcainide appears also selectively to depress conduction in the ventricular conducting system in man (Bar *et al.*, 1978; Manz *et al.*, 1978). The antiarrhythmic effects in man are associated with prolongation of the PR, QRS and QT intervals (Myburgh *et al.*, 1980; Somani, 1980a).

Tocainide (W36095; 2-amino-2′, 6′-propionoxylidide hydrochloride)

Tocainide (figure 15.1) is an analogue of lignocaine with a high oral bioavailability, a plasma half life of 8-12 h and an elimination half life of 12-22 h (Coltart *et al.*, 1974; Lalka *et al.*, 1976; McDevitt *et al.*, 1976). In rats, tocainide is completely absorbed up to a dose of 15 mg kg^{-1} p.o. or i.p. (Venkataramanan and Axelson, 1980). Clinically, oral tocainide has been shown to suppress ventricular ectopic activity for up to 8-12 h after administration (McDevitt *et al.*, 1976; Woosley *et al.*, 1977). It is about half as potent as lignocaine, with antiarrhythmic activity associated with plasma levels of 3-11 $\mu g\ ml^{-1}$ (Anderson *et al.*, 1978; Roden *et al.*, 1980a). Le Winter *et al.* (1980) reported that seven of 10 patients, eight of whom had coronary atherosclerosis and a previous history of MI, responded to oral tocainide (400-800 mg kg^{-1} t.i.d.) whereas they were unresponsive to other antiarrhythmic agents.

Again, little is known of the antiarrhythmic effects of this agent against the early arrhythmias resulting from ischaemia. A study by Coltart *et al.* (1974), using a conscious dog model in which arrhythmias were induced by slow constriction of the proximal LAD and circumflex coronary arteries, showed that oral tocainide completely suppressed ectopic activity for 0.25–5 h. Effective plasma levels were 15–30 $\mu g\ ml^{-1}$. However, the earliest time that the drug was given in this study was 6 h after commencement of the experiment.

The effects of tocainide on transmembrane action potentials (d'Alnoncourt *et al.*, 1980) and its clinical electrophysiology (Anderson *et al.*, 1978) are similar to those of lignocaine.

Experimentally, moderate cardiac depression as evidenced by long lasting bradycardia and reductions in $(dP/dt)_{max}$ and aortic flow has been observed in the dog following oral administration (Coltart *et al.*, 1974) whereas cardiac depression at plasma levels of 5.3 $\mu g\ ml^{-1}$ was not seen in the clinical setting in patients with valvular heart disease (Ryan and Karliner, 1979). Roden *et al.* (1980a) reported a high incidence of drug allergy in a 19 patient study and a narrow toxic therapeutic ratio, effects which may limit its use in chronic treatment. A similar conclusion was reached by Sonnhag (1980). Wasenmiller and Aronow (1980), who conducted an 8 week oral clinical study (300 mg given four times daily) concluded that quinidine was more effective, benefited a larger number of patients, and induced fewer adverse effects than 600 mg t.i.d. tocainide.

Identified metabolites to tocainide are a glucuronide of *N*-carboxytocainamide and lactoxylidide. The latter probably does not contribute to the observed antiarrhythmic or adverse effects of tocainide (Ronfelt *et al.*, 1980).

Encainide (MJ 9067; 4-methoxy-2′-(2-(1-methyl-2-piperidyl)ethyl)benzanilide)

Encainide (figure 15.1) is a new antiarrhythmic agent which is effective against ventricular ectopic activity in animals (Byrne *et al.*, 1977) and in man (Kesteloot and Stroobandt, 1979). Clinically, the drug is orally active, appears to be well tolerated during long term treatment (6–30 months) and is often effective against VT refractory to other therapy (Mason and Peters, 1980; Roden *et al.*, 1980a,b).

Again, there are few studies relating to the effects of encainide during early myocardial infarction although it has been shown to be effective against late arrhythmias occurring 48 h post infarction (Byrne *et al.*, 1977). One study (Ro *et al.*, 1979) using open-chest anaesthetised dogs, has shown that encainide prolongs conduction to a greater extent in infarcted than in non-infarcted tissue and that this effect is seen in the subendocardium and in the epicardium. The effective refractory period is prolonged only in the infarcted area. Thus encainide, by suppressing conduction in ischaemic tissue, may convert a unidirectional to a bidirectinal block and eliminate re-entrant arrhythmias. On the other hand, the results of Carmeliet (1980), using perfused guinea-pig hearts, suggest that conduction velocity in the ventricular conducting system was depressed more than the effective refractory period. This may indicate a potential to facilitate re-entry by shortening the impulse wavelength.

Electrophysiologically, encainide shares some but not all of the actions of lignocaine. Depression of V_{max} of atrial and Purkinje tissue is more frequency dependent and less potential dependent in the presence of encainide (Carmeliet, 1980). Encainide does not slow the rate of diastolic depolarisation at high levels of membrane potential of Purkinje fibres suggesting that, unlike lignocaine or lorcainide, it is without effect on the i_{K_2} current (Arnsdorf and Bigger, 1972; Weld and Bigger, 1976). In papillary muscle, encainide prolongs the effective refractory period while the APD is unchanged or lengthened. Thus the electrophysiological effects of encainide bear a closer resemblance to those of quinidine than to lignocaine (Carmeliet, 1980).

Clinically, the antiarrhythmic effects of encainide appear to correlate with QRS lengthening (Mason and Peters, 1980). Jackman *et al.* (1980) found that oral encainide (100-300 mg day^{-1}) given for at least 3 days slowed conduction in the AV nodal and His-Purkinje systems and increased atrial, ventricular and accessory pathway refractoriness, effects which were not seen following single intravenous doses. It was concluded that these effects on conduction were due to a metabolite, probably the *O*-demethylated form (Wang and Woosley, 1980).

Oral encainide does not appear to be cardiodepressant (DiBianco *et al.*, 1980; Roden *et al.*, 1980a). The latter group concluded that although drug elimination is rapid ($t_{1/2}$ = 1.9-3.8 h), the drug shows a sufficiently high therapeutic ratio to allow a 6-12 h dosing schedule.

Flecainide (R 818; (2,5-bis-2,2,2-trifluoroethoxyl-*N*-(2-piperidylmethyl)benzamide acetate))

Structurally, flecainide does not resemble other antiarrhythmic agents (see figure 15.1).

Schmid *et al.* (1975) reported that flecainide was effective orally and also intraperitoneally in antagonising experimental arrhythmias of varying aetiology. Orally, this drug was seven to 12 times more potent than quinidine, procainamide or lignocaine in mice and two or three times more potent following intravenous administration to dogs. Canine ventricular arrhythmias were completely suppressed by 3.7 mg kg^{-1} i.v. Clinically, intravenous flecainide (2 mg kg^{-1}) has been reported to suppress PVS for 6-24 h (average 13 h) at plasma levels of 0.16-0.39 μg ml^{-1} (Somani, 1980b). An excellent response to oral treatment (200-600 mg day^{-1} for 3 days) was also found by Duff *et al.* (1980) in which PVS and tachycardia were reduced by 98 and 100 per cent respectively.

Verdouw *et al.* (1979) have studied the effects of flecainide against early post-infarction arrhythmias in the pig. In this model, reduction of flow in the LAD coronary artery to 25 per cent of control values for 30 min results in a 33 per cent incidence of VF and a 42 per cent incidence of VT. Flecainide (2 mg kg^{-1} i.v. given 25 min prior to occlusion) reduced these to 12.5 and 0 per cent respectively. The total number of PVS was also significantly lower in the drug-treated group. However, when the LAD was completely occluded VF occurred in all animals (control and drug-treated). Verdouw *et al.* (1979) concluded that the effectiveness of flecainide in this model was comparable to that of aprindine, lignocaine and Org 6001.

Micro-electrode studies suggest that flecainide exerts effects similar to those of lignocaine in that myocardial cellular membrane responsiveness is reduced, APD is shortened and adrenaline-induced increases in phase 4 depolarisation are eliminated (L. D. Davis cited by Hodess *et al.*, 1979). In the intact canine heart, a dose-dependent prolongation of AV conduction and refractoriness is seen (Hodess *et al.*, 1979), effects which are quantitatively similar to those of quinidine and procainamide. However, clinically no changes in PR, QRS or QT intervals were observed by Somani (1980b) in response to intravenous flecainide in man, whereas in the oral study of Duff *et al.* (1980) effective antiarrhythmic therapy was accompanied by lengthening of the PR, QRS and QT_c intervals by 29, 27 and 11 per cent respectively. Seipel *et al.* (1980) reported a slowing of intracardiac conduction in man especially in the ventricular conducting system, together with a slight prolongation of atrial, AV nodal and ventricular refractoriness.

In the anaesthetised pig, Verdouw *et al.* (1979) found that 2 mg kg^{-1} i.v., given over 2 min, resulted in a sharp fall in LV $(dP/dt)_{max}$ and mean blood pressure. Transient coronary vasodilatation and more prolonged QRS widening was seen; heart rate remained unchanged. Some 25 min after flecainide administration, the QRS width was still slightly prolonged (by about 10 per cent) and cardiac output, left ventricular pressure and LV $(dP/dt)_{max}$ were reduced by 10, 9 and 18 per cent respectively. Despite these negative inotropic effects, the haemodynamic consequences of coronary artery ligation were no more marked in the drug-treated animals than in controls. Clinically, Duff *et al.* (1980) found no deterioration in exercise tolerance or ejection fraction at effective antiarrhythmic doses. In this study side effects were limited to blurring of vision in three out of 10 patients and these disappeared on reducing the dosage. Somani (1980b) also reported negligible side effects (tingling sensation and feeling of skin warmth for 15 min in one of 10 patients).

Duff *et al.* (1980) also reported adequate control of PVS during out-patient therapy using a 12 hourly dosage schedule.

Flecainide appears to be a long-acting, potent, orally effective and safe antiarrhythmic agent which is also effective against early experimental post-infarction arrhythmias.

Org 6001 (3α-amino-5α-androstan-2β-ol-17-one HCl) - amafalone

Org 6001 is a new antiarrhythmic agent currently undergoing clinical trial. Experimentally, this aminosteroid has been shown to be effective in antagonising the development of early post-infarction arrhythmias in the dog (Marshall and Parratt, 1975), pig (Verdouw *et al.*, 1978) and rat (Au *et al.*, 1979b; Clark *et al.*, 1980). The results of these studies have been previously reviewed by Parratt (1979). In the dog, intravenous administration of Org 6001 (1 mg kg^{-1}, 15 min prior to ligation of the anterior descending branch of the left coronary artery) reduced the number of VEBs from 904 ± 260 in control animals to 210 ± 132; deaths from VF were reduced from 33 to 20 per cent. A dose of 10 mg kg^{-1} i.v., given either 15 min or

1.5 h prior to ligation, again significantly reduced the number of VEBs to 43 ± 13 and 116 ± 43 respectively; corresponding mortalities from VF were 17 and 0 per cent. Oral Org 6001 (50 mg kg^{-1} given 4 h before ligation) also markedly protected against the development of post-infarction arrhythmias. The mean number of VEBs in orally treated animals was 78 ± 29 and VF was absent.

Complete occlusion of the LAD in the pig results in death from VF within 2 h. Verdouw *et al.* (1978) reported that 5 or 10 mg kg^{-1} Org 6001 infused at a rate of 1 mg kg^{-1} min^{-1}, 30 min prior to occlusion, increased survival to 22 and 40 per cent respectively. When coronary flow is reduced to 25 per cent in this model, VEBs, tachycardia and VF develop in 100, 47 and 30 per cent of the animals respectively. Of 19 pigs pretreated with 5 or 10 mg kg^{-1} intravenous Org 6001, only one developed VT, none fibrillated and eight were free from arrhythmias. Similar protection against arrhythmias evoked by coronary artery ligation in the rat following 5-10 mg kg^{-1} i.v. or 10 mg kg^{-1} + 2.5 mg kg^{-1} h^{-1} has also been reported (Au *et al.*, 1979b; Clark *et al.*, 1980).

Org 6001 is also orally active in the rat (Kane *et al.*, 1980; Marshall *et al.*, 1981). In these latter studies, conducted in our own laboratories, ligation of the main left coronary artery resulted during the 0-30 min post-ligation period, in a mean number of VEBs of 1458 ± 206 and an incidence of ventricular fibrilloflutter ('VF') of 44 per cent in control animals. One hour after 20 mg kg^{-1} p.o. Org 6001, the ectopic count was reduced to 547 ± 161 and 'VF' did not develop following ligation. Oral mexiletine is ineffective at this dose while doses in excess of 50 mg kg^{-1} of disopyramide or propafenone are necessary to completely prevent the development of 'VF'. In this model, 100 mg kg^{-1} p.o. mexiletine is active for less than 3 h whereas 18 h after a similar oral dose of Org 6001 the expected number of VEBs is reduced by 85 per cent and 'VF' is absent. This protective effect of Org 6001 is associated with prevention of the fall in VFT seen 3-4 min after coronary artery ligation.

Protection against post-infarction arrhythmias in rats is seen at mean plasma levels of 0.335 ± 0.068 μg ml^{-1} (Kane *et al.*, 1980, 1982). The corresponding myocardial content of Org 6001 was 2.94 ± 0.408 μg g^{-1}.

Org 6001 reduced V_{max} of cardiac transmembrane action potentials (Salako *et al.*, 1976; E. Carmeliet, unpublished; Kane, 1980), an effect which is more pronounced at high stimulation frequencies (E. Carmeliet, unpublished). Salako *et al.* (1976) reported that this effect, like that of lignocaine, was reduced by lowering the external potassium concentration; Carmeliet was unable to demonstrate such a potassium-dependent effect.

Org 6001 shortens APD of Purkinje fibres whereas its effects on APD of ventricular muscle has been variably reported as a slight prolongation (Salako *et al.*, 1976), or a slight shortening (Kane, 1980). In atrial muscle, Salako *et al.* (1976) found a slight prolongation whereas E. Carmeliet (unpublished) found no effect. Like lignocaine, Org 6001 has been reported preferentially to shorten APD of the ventricular conducting system in those areas where it is normally longest (Salako *et al.*, 1976).

Kane *et al.* (1980) have provided evidence to suggest that the antiarrhythmic effects of Org 6001 *in vivo* are related to depression of V_{max} of atrial and of papillary muscle taken from chronically treated rats. These effects were associated with a reduction in the incidence of VF following coronary artery ligation 1 h after the last dose. Twenty-four hours after the last dose was given, and at a time when myocardial drug levels were low, there was no demonstrable protection against ligation-induced arrhythmias. V_{max} was similar to that seen in control tissue whereas APD was still shortened in the papillary muscle. This would suggest that shortening of APD does not play a part in the antiarrhythmic actions of Org 6001.

Org 6001 slows intracardiac conduction velocity especially in the His-Purkinje system (Salako *et al.*, 1976; McDonald, 1980; E. Carmeliet, unpublished). McDonald (1980) concluded that this effect was more similar to that of quinidine than to lignocaine. Carmeliet further showed that conduction of premature action potentials is slowed to a greater extent than conduction of the normal impulse.

Org 6001 slightly prolongs the effective and functional refractory periods of the AV node but does not prolong the relative or absolute refractory periods of Purkinje or cardiac muscle cells (E. Carmeliet, unpublished; Kane, 1980). Its effects on pacemaker activity appear to be minimal (E. Carmeliet, unpublished).

Experimentally Org 6001 exerts only minimal haemodynamic effects at antiarrhythmic doses (Marshall and Parratt, 1975; Vargaftig *et al.*, 1975; Verdouw *et al.*, 1978). In the dog, Marshall and Parratt (1975) reported that rapid intravenous administration of 1 or 10 mg kg^{-1} resulted in immediate, transient and apparently dose-dependent decreases in diastolic blood pressure and in left ventricular $(dP/dt)_{max}$ and increases in heart rate and coronary blood flow. However 10 min after administration there were no significant changes in blood pressure, heart rate, cardiac output, left ventricular $(dP/dt)_{max}$, LVEDP, coronary blood flow, myocardial oxygen consumption or external cardiac work. Coronary and peripheral vascular resistance and whole body oxygen consumption were unaffected. Org 6001 did not modify the haemodynamic consequences of coronary artery ligation.

In the pig, Verdouw *et al.* (1978) also reported small transient changes in coronary flow and mean aortic pressure but a more sustained reduction in LV $(dP/dt)_{max}$ (for at least 30 min) in response to 5 or 10 mg kg^{-1} i.v. Lignocaine (2.75-3.5 mg kg^{-1}) did not have significant haemodynamic effects. During ischaemia there was only an additional minor depression of contractility in the Org 6001-treated animals, whereas in the animals receiving lignocaine a large fall in LV $(dP/dt)_{max}$ was seen, rendering similar values for contractility in the two drug-treated groups. Transient haemodynamic changes in response to Org 6001 have also been seen in the rat (Marshall *et al.*, 1981).

The drug appears to have a wide safety margin. The only obvious sign of toxicity in mice given Org 6001 in an oral dose equivalent to 10 times its oral ED_{50} value (for antagonising aconitine-induced arrhythmias) was ptosis (Winslow, 1980). In this study quinidine was the drug next best tolerated whilst lignocaine, mexiletine, aprindine, propafenone and disopyramide induced motor inco-ordination or convulsions in oral doses equivalent to 3.5 to five times their oral ED_{50} values. Vargaftig *et al.* (1975) found the therapeutic ratio of intravenously administered Org 6001 in rats to be much higher than that of lignocaine. The antiarrhythmic ED_{50} value for Org 6001 was approximately seven times lower than that for lignocaine (14 mg kg^{-1}) whilst the LD_{50} values were 147 and 28.5 mg kg^{-1} respectively.

Org 6001 has a reasonably long duration of action. Antiarrhythmic activity is seen for at least 6 h after oral administration to mice (Winslow, 1980), 16-18 h in rats (Vargaftig *et al.*, 1975; Marshall *et al.*, 1981), and for at least 4 h in dogs (Marshall and Parratt, 1975).

Procainamide

In 1951, it was reported that procainamide provided protection against cyclopropane-adrenaline-induced arrhythmias in the dog and successfully terminated ventricular tachycardia in 13 of 15 patients (Mark *et al.*, 1951). Since this time numerous studies have confirmed the usefulness of procainamide in the treatment of ventricular and supraventricular arrhythmias in man (reviewed by Caracta and Damato, 1975).

Although in 1952 it was demonstrated independently by two groups that procainamide is effective in reducing the frequency of rapid ventricular ectopic beats occurring 1-2 days after coronary ligation in dogs (Harris *et al.*, 1952; Stern *et al.*, 1952), the effects of the drug on early ventricular arrhythmias were not reported until the studies of Stephenson *et al.* (1960). These workers demonstrated that procainamide (4.6 mg kg^{-1} i.v.) reduced the incidence of VF produced by ligation of the LAD from 26 to 11 per cent and, in addition, reduced the proportion of animals succumbing to VF on release of the occlusion (from 71 to 58 per cent).

In these respects procainamide was superior to lignocaine, which did not protect against ligation-induced VF. A similar superiority of procainamide over lignocaine was reported by Weisse *et al.* (1971) who produced ventricular arrhythmias and VF in conscious dogs by creating a thrombus, 4 h previously, in either the anterior descending or circumflex branch of the left coronary artery. This technique was associated with an incidence of VF of 90 per cent which was reduced to 20 per cent by the administration of procainamide (15-25 mg kg^{-1} in divided doses) immediately the arrhythmias commenced. In contrast 55 per cent of animals treated with lignocaine (10-11 mg kg^{-1}, as divided doses) fibrillated during the experimental period. Gamble and Cohn (1972) demonstrated that procainamide (5-15 mg kg^{-1}) abolished the early ventricular arrhythmias associated with coronary occlusion in the cat, whether these were due to increased automaticity (induced by vagal stimulation) or to re-entry mechanisms (induced by premature stimuli). In contrast, results obtained in pentobarbitone-anaesthetised dogs suggest that procainamide (10 mg kg^{-1}) is only effective against automaticity-induced arrhythmias and is ineffective in abolishing the re-entrant beats induced by premature stimuli shortly after coronary occlusion (Han *et al.*, 1974). The reason for this disparity is not clear but may be related to the findings in chloralose-anaesthetised cats that doses of procainamide (>0.25 mg kg^{-1}) which possess atropine-like properties, may exacerbate the number of early ventricular beats and also the incidence of VF induced by LAD occlusion (Corr *et al.*, 1978). Studies in conscious dogs, in which temporary myocardial ischaemia was induced by balloon occlusion of the LAD, have shown that a 'high therapeutic dose' of procainamide is capable of markedly reducing the incidence of VF (from 53 to 6 per cent; Lown and Wolf, 1971). Interestingly, treatment with procainamide also protected animals from VF following deflation of the balloon.

Other studies of the effects of various antiarrhythmic drugs on the extent of conduction delay and incidence of ventricular arrhythmias in anaesthetised dogs have indicated that procainamide, when administered in therapeutic doses before coronary ligation, modified neither the time to onset of early ventricular arrhythmias nor the extent and time course of conduction delay in the epicardial ischaemic zone (Hope *et al.*, 1974). This is in contrast to the clinical findings of Giardina and Bigger (1973), who demonstrated that procainamide was capable of gradually prolonging conduction in the depressed portion of a re-entrant pathway until bidirectional block finally occurred and the arrhythmia was abolished (see figure 15.2). There is some experimental evidence to support this mechanism of action of procainamide against early re-entrant arrhythmias (Rosen *et al.*, 1973).

One of the major toxic manifestations of chronic procainamide therapy is the development of a syndrome resembling systemic lupus erythematosis. Since this side effect has been attributed to the aromatic primary amino group in the molecule, studies have been performed on the antiarrhythmic efficacy of the *N*-acetyl metabolite (NAPA). In anaesthetised dogs NAPA and procainamide have been shown to suppress ventricular arrhythmias produced either by ouabain or by coronary ligation 48 h previously, that is, late arrhythmias (Bagwell *et al.*, 1976). More recently NAPA, when administered at an intravenous dose of 20 mg kg^{-1} 10 min prior to simultaneous ligation of the left anterior descending and septal coronary arteries, was shown to reduce the incidence of VF from 77 per cent in the control dogs to 40 per cent (Reynolds and Kamath, 1979). This antiarrhythmic effect of NAPA was associated with a decrease in heart rate of 11 per cent.

Although the electrophysiological studies in Purkinje tissue clearly showed that procainamide is a blocker of the fast Na^+ channel, that is, it decreases $(\mathrm{d}V/\mathrm{d}t)_{max}$, decreases automaticity and slows conduction velocity (Kayden *et al.*, 1957), it remains uncertain how relevant these properties are to abolition of early re-entrant arrhythmias. Bigger and Heissenbuttel (1969) reported that procainamide increased Purkinje fibre effective refractory period more than action potential duration and suggested that these effects could modify the relationship between conduction and refractoriness existing in re-entrant circuits and thereby be an important mechanism in the termination of re-entry arrhythmias. Similar findings have been reported for NAPA by Bagwell *et al.* (1976), although Jaillon *et al.* (1979) claim that NAPA and procainamide possess different electrophysiological properties while Dangman and Hoffman (1978) have demonstrated that prolongation of the action potential is the only major electrophysiological effect of NAPA in Purkinje fibres.

Quinidine

The activity of the prototype antiarrhythmic, quinidine, in suppressing the 'late' ventricular arrhythmias induced by coronary ligation in experimental animals is well documented (Harris *et al.*, 1951; Winbury and Hemmer, 1955; Madan *et al.*, 1960; Mokler and Van Arman, 1962; Cosnier *et al.*, 1971). However, there is still some controversy as to the clinical effectiveness of quinidine in the early post-infarction period (see Jones *et al.*, 1974, for references).

Quinidine, when administered intravenously in a dose of 15 mg kg^{-1} 10 min after LAD ligation in anaesthetised dogs, has been shown to significantly reduce the incidence of VF, from 26 per cent (in the control group) to 7 per cent (Stephenson *et al.*, 1960). Similar, but less marked, antifibrillatory effects have been described for quinidine in conscious dogs in which myocardial ischaemia was produced by balloon occlusion of a coronary artery (Lown and Wolf, 1971). Studies in conscious pigs (Hurst *et al.*, 1967) have shown that continuous treatment with quinidine (5-10 mg kg^{-1} per 6 h period for 72 h) significantly reduced VF and ventricular arrhythmias ensuing after myocardial ischaemia produced by gradual Ameroid-induced constriction of the LAD. In this study only three control animals (15 per cent) survived the 72 h experimental period whereas survival in the group treated with the high dose of quinidine was 35 per cent. Such an antifibrillatory effect of quinidine had already been suggested by Levine in 1932, who demonstrated that quinidine produced an increase in the myocardial fibrillatory threshold in decerebrate cats. Quinidine (10 mg kg^{-1}) has also been shown to reduce the ventricular arrhythmias and to abolish VF produced by acute coronary ligation in the pentobarbitone-anaesthetised rat (Kane *et al.*, 1981).

Many experimental studies have demonstrated that quinidine, in concentrations likely to be encountered clinically (1-10 μg ml^{-1}), decreases $(dV/dt)_{max}$ in atrial, ventricular and Purkinje fibres (Weidmann, 1955; Johnson and McKinnon, 1957; Vaughan Williams, 1958; West and Amory, 1960). Moreover these effects of quinidine are clearly rate-dependent but are not dependent on membrane potential (see Chen *et al.*, 1975, for references). Since quinidine has also been shown to slow intraventricular conduction in closed-chest dogs (Wallace *et al.*, 1966) and in man (Josephson *et al.*, 1974), it might theoretically convert unidirectional block into bidirectional block and thus suppress re-entry pathways, especially in an environment of elevated extracellular potassium (Watanabe *et al.*, 1963) and/or decreased pH (Nattel *et al.*, 1981). However, as far as we are aware there has been only one study published on the effects of quinidine on conduction velocity in the ischaemic myocardium immediately after coronary artery ligation (Zipes *et al.*, 1977a). In this study treatment with quinidine (8 mg kg^{-1}, i.v.) had very little effect on the degree of conduction delay in the area made ischaemic by LAD ligation and, in the dogs that developed ventricular tachycardia or VF in response to electrical pacing after ligation, progressive conduction delay in the ischaemic zone was no different from the conduction delay which occurred before drug administration. In line with these observations, quinidine did not modify the incidence of ventricular tachycardia or of VF.

Disopyramide

Although the basic cardiovascular pharmacology of disopyramide was described as long ago as 1962 (Mokler and Van Arman, 1962; Sekiya and Vaughan Williams, 1963), it is only in the last few years that the drug has been extensively used clinically in the treatment of arrhythmias of various aetiologies. Disopyramide administered intravenously or orally is effective in preventing the potentially serious arrhythmias in patients with acute myocardial infarction (see Danilo and Rosen, 1976; Ankier *et al.*, 1977; Yu, 1979, for references). However, there are relatively few reports on the effects of disopyramide on early ventricular arrhythmias and VF produced by coronary ligation in experimental animals. Some studies (Cosnier *et al.*, 1971; Dean, 1975; Kus and Sasyniuk, 1976) focused on late (24–48 h) post-infarction ventricular arrhythmias and demonstrated that disopyramide was approximately equi-active with quinidine in suppressing ventricular ectopics.

In 1979, it was reported (Marshall and Parratt, 1979) that disopyramide, when administered intravenously (2.5-5.0 mg kg^{-1}) 15 min before ligation of the LAD in trichlorethylene-anaesthetised greyhound dogs, significantly reduced the number of ventricular arrhythmias that occur in the initial 30 min post-ligation period and also abolished the development of VF. However, these protective antiarrhythmic effects were accompanied by marked cardiodepression. Similar activity of disopyramide in pentobarbitone-anaesthetised dogs has been reported by Dean *et al.* (1979). They found that 5 mg kg^{-1} disopyramide reduced the number of animals exhibiting ventricular arrhythmias (from 100 to 67 per cent) and completely prevented VF produced by occlusion of the LAD for 20 min. This dose of disopyramide also significantly reduced the incidience of VF on release of the occlusion. Disopyramide (10 mg kg^{-1} i.v.) has also been shown to reduce the number of early ventricular ectopics and to abolish VF produced by coronary ligation in the pentobarbitone-anaesthetised rat (Kane and Winslow, 1980).

In contrast, using an experimental model of re-entrant ventricular tachycardia induced by premature ventricular stimuli in conscious dogs 2–4 days after coronary artery ligation, it has been shown that only high ($>7\ \mu g\ ml^{-1}$) plasma concentratins of disopyramide prevent ventricular tachycardia (Patterson *et al.*, 1980). Indeed, at lower steady state plasma concentrations ($1\ \mu g\ ml^{-1}$) disopyramide improved depressed conduction in the ischaemic zone and increased the rate and duration of ventricular tachycardia. That 'subthreshold concentrations' of antiarrhythmic agents can facilitate re-entry arrhythmias is not unique to disopyramide and has been demonstrated in animals with verapamil (El-Sherif and Lazzara, 1979) and in patients with procainamide (Reddy *et al.*, 1977). It is interesting to note that disopyramide and procainamide both possess marked antimuscarinic properties at cholinoceptors (Mirro *et al.*, 1979; Corr *et al.*, 1978) and that these are apparent at subthreshold antiarrhythmic concentrations.

Electrophysiological studies have demonstrated that disopyramide exerts typical class I effects, that is, depression of $(dV/dt)_{max}$, membrane responsiveness and automaticity without changes in membrane potential (Sekiya and Vaughan Williams,

1963; Yeh *et al.*, 1973; Danilo *et al.*, 1977a). More recently (Kojima, 1981) has shown that low concentrations (2 μM) of disopyramide prolong action potential duration (APD) in guinea-pig papillary muscles without changing $(dV/dt)_{max}$ (a class III effect). Tenfold higher concentrations were required to exert a classical quinidine-like action, that is, depression of $(dV/dt)_{max}$ associated with lengthening of APD. Kus and Sasynuik (1978) have reported that disopyramide prolongs APD in such a way that action potential duration becomes more homogeneous throughout the ventricular conducting system. This may explain the finding of Levites and Anderson (1979) that disopyramide reduced both the number of ventricular ectopic beats and the disparity of refractory periods between ischaemic and non-ischaemic areas of myocardium in pigs subjected to acute coronary ligation.

Ethmozin (EN-313)

Ethmozin is the ethyl ester hydrochloride of 10-(2-morpholinopropionyl)phenothiazine-2-carbamic acid. This drug has been used clinically in the USSR for the treatment of arrhythmias of varying aetiology (Vikhliaev *et al.*, 1981; Kaverina *et al.*, 1972). Effective plasma levels are 0.6 μg ml^{-1} (Morganroth *et al.*, 1979).

Experimentally, ethmozin has been shown to suppress late ventricular arrhythmias following two-stage ligation of the LAD in the dog and orally is more effective than quinidine in this respect (Danilo *et al.*, 1977b). It also suppresses arrhythmias induced by epinephrine 2-4 days after infarction.

Again few studies describe the effects of ethmozin against very early arrhythmias. Ruffy *et al.* (1977) reported that ethmozin (3-5 mg kg^{-1} i.v.) increased by 50 per cent the incidence of VF produced by 5 min occlusion of the LAD coronary artery in dogs. Ethmozine was given during the ischaemic episode and was found to increase conduction time between the right ventricle and ischaemic zone. The duration of the ischaemic electrocardiogram was prolonged. The refractory period of the non-ischaemic myocardium (left or right atria or left ventricle) was unaltered but the left ventricular excitability threshold was increased. However, Fox *et al.* (1980) using conscious dogs failed to demonstrate an ethmozin-induced increase in VFT and reported that the defibrillation threshold was increased by this drug. These results cast some doubt on the antifibrillatory efficacy of ethmozine.

Danilo *et al.* (1977b) reported that in blood-superfused Purkinje fibres, ethmozine at therapeutic concentrations reduced V_{max} and APD and slightly decreased maximum diastolic potential. No significant effect on phase 4 depolarisation was seen in normal fibres, whereas the slope of phase 4 was decreased in ischaemic fibres.

In the canine heart *in vivo*, Shenoy *et al.* (1977) found that ethmozine increased the effective refractory period of the AV node but did not alter refractoriness of atrial or ventricular muscle. Ruffy *et al.* (1977) found no change in AV conduction time. Taken together, these studies would suggest that the electrophysiological profile of ethmozine is more similar to that of lignocaine than to quinidine.

Aprindine (*N*-(3-diethylamino)propyl-*N*-phenyl-2-indanamine; AC1802; Amidonal)

Intravenous or oral aprindine is clinically effective in suppressing arrhythmias of varying aetiology including those following MI (Hagemeijer and Hugenholtz, 1974; Geltman *et al.*, 1978; Hai *et al.*, 1979; Malini *et al.*, 1979).

Experimentally, aprinidine has been shown to be effective against late post-infarction arrhythmias in the dog (Ueda *et al.*, 1975; Nattel *et al.*, 1979) but is ineffective against adrenaline-induced arrhythmias in cats (Ueda *et al.*, 1975). Effective plasma levels are in the region of 0.5-1.8 μg ml^{-1} (Malini *et al.*, 1979).

As with lignocaine, the results of studies relating to the effects of aprindine against early post-infarction arrhythmias are conflicting. Verdouw *et al.* (1977) demonstrated that aprindine was effective against arrhythmias in the pig occurring during the first 30 min of partial occlusion of the LAD (flow reduced to 25 per cent of control values). In these experiments aprindine was infused at a rate of 2 mg kg^{-1} h^{-1} for 1 h and then at 0.8 mg kg^{-1} h^{-1} for the remainder of the experiment to maintain therapeutic plasma levels. Aprindine reduced the incidence of VF and VEBs and completely prevented the development of VT (of 22 control occlusions, 10 resulted in VT). Georges *et al.* (1973) reported that aprindine (1.5 mg kg^{-1} i.v.) given 33 min after ligation of the LAD abolished VEBs in one dog (the only observation made). On the other hand, Kroll and Lucchesi (1975) failed to demonstrate a protective effect of aprindine against acute ligation-induced arrhythmias in the dog. Nattel *et al.* (1979) found in dogs that intravenous aprindine given prior to occlusion of the LAD *increased* the incidence of VT/VF from 10 per cent in the controls to 49 per cent, whereas post-occlusion administration did not change the incidence of VT/VF. Nattel and co-workers measured the aprindine content in the ischaemic and non-ischaemic zones at times up to 70 min following dosing. Their results indicated that pre-occlusion administration resulted in similar drug levels in both zones at the time of occlusion, but thereafter drug content in the non-ischaemic zone decreased more rapidly than in the ischaemic zone. In contrast, dogs given aprindine post-ligation attained very low drug levels in the ischaemic zone but these levels remained fairly constant. It was concluded that aprindine levels in the ischaemic zone greater than or equal to levels in the non-ischaemic zone were associated with exacerbation of arrhythmias. Elharrar *et al.* (1977) also found that in dogs subjected to 6 min occlusions of the LAD, administration of aprindine (2.85 mg kg^{-1}) led to a marked increased in the incidence of VT/VF (seen in one of 11 control occlusions compared to eight out of 11 occlusions after aprindine). This was associated with a more marked depression of conduction in the ischaemic zone compared to controls.

Aprindine exerts effects on transmembrane cardiac action potentials which are similar to those of lignocaine. It induces a potassium-dependent reduction in V_{max}, shortens APD, slows conduction in quiescent Purkinje fibres and depresses phase 4 depolarisation (Greenspan *et al.*, 1974; Neuss and Buss, 1978). Verdonk *et al.* (1974) found that these actions were long lasting and less marked in contractile tissue and that tissue concentrations became 10 times greater than the concentrations in the bathing medium.

In the anaesthetised dog, aprindine slows intracardiac conduction at all levels.

Cabedo *et al.* (1978) reported that a cumulative dose of 2 mg kg^{-1} i.v. decreased cardiac rate by 8.5 per cent and increased sinus node recovery time and the refractory period of the AV node by 8.5 and 4.9 per cent respectively. S-A, A-H and H-V conduction intervals were increased by 33, 14.9 and 31.4 per cent respectively. Aprindine also blocks accessory bypass-tract conduction between atria and ventricles (Zipes *et al.*, 1977b). Kesteloot *et al.* (1973) concluded that the influence of aprindine on sinus node discharge rate, on abnormal atrial pacemakers and on atrial conduction time distinguishes this agent from other local anaesthetics such as lignocaine.

Propafenone (Rytmonorm)

Clinically propafenone (figure 15.1) has been shown to suppress VEBs of varying aetiology including those associated with MI. This drug is effective following both intravenous administration of 1-2 mg kg^{-1} (Aldor and Heeger, 1976) or oral administration (Kalusche and Loenne, 1978; Meyer *et al.*, 1978; Beck and Hochrein, 1978). Effective plasma levels are approximately 0.4-0.5 μg ml^{-1} (Blanke *et al.*, 1979). Oral maintenance therapy is achieved with a dosing regime of 300 mg t.i.d. (Aldor and Heeger, 1976) or 200-250 mg t.i.d. (Blanke *et al.*, 1979).

Experimentally, the drug is effective against a variety of arrhythmias, including those induced by adrenaline infusion plus chloroform inhalation, by digoxin, by calcium chloride and by aconitine (Hapke and Prigge, 1976). Effective antiarrhythmic doses are 1 mg kg^{-1} i.v. or 2-10 mg kg^{-1} p.o. Little is known about its effects against early post-infarction arrhythmias. Hapke and Prigge (1976) reported that intravenous injection of 2 mg kg^{-1} immediately after the appearance of the first VEB induced in one dog by ligation of the ramus circumflexus completely prevented the development of further arrhythmias. An injection of 1 mg kg^{-1} was essentially ineffective. In this model, control dogs develop VF within 4-6 min of occlusion. This observation is the only one of its kind that we are aware of. Unpublished results obtained in our own laboratories have indicated that propafenone is effective in inhibiting the development of arrhythmias in the anaesthetised rat during the 0-30 min period following acute ligation of the main left coronary artery (figure 15.4). In these experiments the ectopic count in control animals was 1435 ± 214 beats and the incidence of ventricular fibrilloflutter ('VF') was 50 per cent. Intravenous propafenone (2 or 5 mg kg^{-1} given 15 min prior to ligation) significantly reduced the ectopic count to 457 ± 116 and 227 ± 130 beats respectively. The incidence of 'VF' was reduced to 14.3 and 0 per cent. Oral propafenone (50 or 100 mg kg^{-1} given 1 h prior to ligation) again significantly reduced the number of VEBs to 759 ± 152 and 513 ± 352 respectively and the incidence of 'VF' to 33 and 14.3 per cent.

Propafenone has been shown to reduce V_{max} of transmembrane action potentials of guinea-pig atrial and papillary muscle, an effect attributed to blockade of open sodium channels (Heistracher and Beck, 1979). Its effects on V_{max} are more pronounced than those of mexiletine or lignocaine (Neuss and Buss, 1978). The latter workers have reported that propafenone exerts electrophysiological actions similar

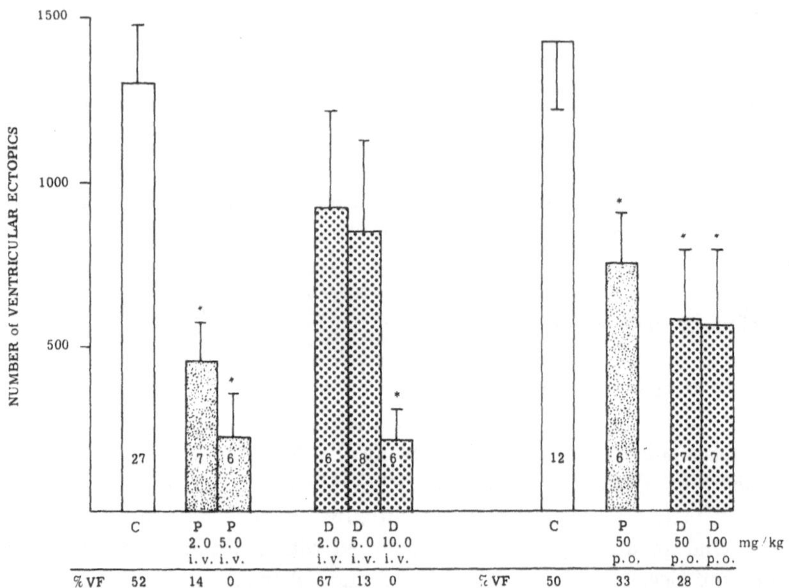

Figure 15.4 A comparison of the antiarrhythmic effects of both intravenously and orally administered propafenone (P) and disopyramide (D) in the pentobarbitone-anaesthetised rat subjected to acute coronary artery ligation. The histograms show the number of ventricular ectopic beats in the initial 30 min post-ligation period. VF = ventricular fibrillation.

to those of disopyramide in that the depression of V_{max} is potassium dependent, APD is prolonged and the drug exerts slight calcium antagonistic actions. The effects of propafenone on automaticity are unknown. Unlike disopyramide, propafenone has a β-blocking effect. In isolated tissue propafenone decreases atrial rate and prolongs the atrial functional refractory period to a greater extent than does lignocaine or mexiletine (Neuss and Buss, 1978).

Clinically, His bundle electrocardiography (Seipel *et al.*, 1975) demonstrates that propafenone (1.2-2 mg kg^{-1} i.v.) reduces cardiac rate and slows conduction at all levels of the conducting system. In this study, the effect on AV nodal conduction was dose dependent and more marked during high frequency stimulation; effects on the His-Purkinje system were independent of frequency. Atrial and AV nodal effective refractory periods were prolonged. Probst and Pachinger (1976), however, found that intra-atrial conduction time, heart rate and sinus node recovery time were not significantly changed by 2 mg kg^{-1} i.v. propafenone; the refractory period of the AV node was prolonged, PQ and QRS durations were lengthened and A-H and H-V intervals prolonged.

Beck *et al.* (1975) found that conduction delay was enhanced in patients with an impaired conducting system and sinoatrial blockade (in 14 out of 23 patients) was seen in similar patients by Seipel *et al.* (1974). Taken together, these results suggest that propafenone exerts more marked effects on atrial tissue than does lignocaine or mexiletine. Indeed, propafenone has been shown to be effective against supraventricular arrhythmias (Aldor and Heeger, 1976; Beck and Hochrein, 1978).

Diphenylhydantoin

In 1950, Harris and Kokernot showed that diphenylhydantoin (DPH) was capable of suppressing the ventricular arrhythmias which occurred 4–8 h after acute coronary artery ligation in conscious dogs. Since that time there have been sporadic and contradictory reports concerning the clinical antiarrhythmic efficacy of DPH (see Conn, 1965; Karlsson, 1975; Stone *et al.*, 1971). As regards the early ventricular arrhythmias associated with myocardial ischaemia, DPH has been shown to be moderately effective in anaesthetised dogs following thrombus occlusion (Weisse *et al.*, 1971) and in conscious dogs after balloon occlusion of the LAD (Lown and Wolf, 1971). However, in both these studies DPH was considerably less effective than procainamide, an observation confirmed in patients suffering from ventricular arrhythmias within 8 h of diagnosis of myocardial infarction (Lown and Wolf, 1971).

The mechanisms underlying the antiarrhythmic actions of DPH are controversial and probably involve a direct Na^+ channel blocking action on the heart as well as a depressant action on sympathetic centres in the central nervous system. The cardiac electrophysiological properties of DPH (reviewed by Wit *et al.*, 1975) resemble lignocaine more than quinidine, since the drug tends to improve conduction and shortens action potential duration, especially in Purkinje and ventricular fibres. Thus, theoretically, beneficial actions of DPH on early re-entry arrhythmias could be due to abolition of unidirectional block and restoration of normal conduction through the damaged conducting lines (see figure 15.2). In addition to these cardiac effects, DPH has been shown to decrease efferent sympathetic activity in cardiac nerves and this effect is thought to be partly responsible for the efficacy of DPH in suppressing ventricular arrhythmias associated with digitalis toxicity (Evans and Gillis, 1974). This central action coupled with direct electrophysiological actions on cardiac muscle probably explain why DPH was at one time proposed as the drug of choice in the treatment of digitalis-induced ventricular arrhythmias (Helfant *et al.*, 1967).

15.5 CONCLUSIONS

There seems little doubt that Na^+ channel blocking agents are extremely effective in suppressing ventricular ectopic activity which occurs several hours or days after production of myocardial ischaemic in experimental animals. At this time, Purkinje cells in the damaged area show enhanced automaticity (Lazzara *et al.*, 1974), impaired conduction and a prolongation of action potential duration. The abnormalities in the conducting system probably produce automatic and re-entrant ectopic beats which are readily suppressed by drugs (for example, Na^+ channel blockers) which reduce diastolic depolarisation (Lazzara *et al.*, 1978).

In contrast, there is considerable controversy regarding the protective actions of Na^+ channel blocking agents against the ventricular arrhythmias occurring within 30 min of myocardial ischaemia and which frequently terminate in VF. Clearly, the underlying electrophysiological changes at this time are different from those occurring several hours later and include severe impairment of conduction, especially in the epicardial layers of the ischaemic zone (Elharrar and Zipes, 1977; Kaplinsky *et al*., 1979) which facilitates re-entry circuits. Transmembrane potential recordings *in situ* have also demonstrated a marked shortening of action potential duration and a decrease in $(\mathrm{d}V/\mathrm{d}t)_{max}$ accompanied by the appearance of potentials of 'slow response' type (Cranefield *et al*., 1972; Elharrar and Zipes, 1977; Russell *et al*., 1979). These changes have been ascribed to an inactivation of rapid inward sodium current following depolarisation of the membrane caused by local release of K^+ (Prinzmetal *et al*., 1962; Kleber *et al*., 1978; Hill and Gettes, 1980). Furthermore, it has been postulated that local release of catecholamines could stimulate the slow channel (Wit and Bigger, 1975), resulting in slow responses. This hypothesis must await clear demonstration that noradrenaline is released from ischaemic myocardial cells at this time after coronary occlusion (see Marshall and Parratt, 1980a, and further discussion in chapters 8-10). If impulse propagation in ischaemic myocardium is mediated by the slow calcium current, then drugs like verapamil would be expected to further depress conduction. So far experimental studies have shown that verapamil is capable of *improving* conduction in ischaemic myocardium (Elharrar *et al*., 1977; Nakaya *et al*., 1980, and further discussed in chapter 18). Clearly it is difficult to know whether the action potentials observed immediately following myocardial ischaemia are true 'slow responses' or whether they represent depressed fast responses. Clearly Na^+ channel blockers could only be expected to modify the latter. This is especially so in ventricular muscle, which may be more susceptible to re-entrant activation under conditions that result in depression, but not complete inactivation, of the fast sodium channel (Lazzara *et al*., 1978).

The disparities in the reported effectiveness of Na^+ channel blockers in suppressing early arrhythmias and VF ensuing after experimental myocardial ischaemia deserve some comment. Some of the discrepancies can be explained by the different experimental protocols used. For instance, the method of drug administration is a critical factor since if drugs are given after ligation of the coronary artery, effective concentrations may not be attained in the poorly perfused area of myocardium at risk. The effectiveness of verapamil and aprindine has been shown to depend on the time of administration (that is, pre- or post-ligation) in anaesthetised dogs Kupersmith *et al*., 1976; Zipes *et al*., 1977b). However, for drugs like procainamide this does not seem to be an important factor since it has been shown that even in severely ischaemic zones (blood flow reduction of more than 90 per cent) procainamide concentrations of 40 per cent of those found in normally perfused myocardium are attained (Wenger *et al*., 1978). In addition, it should be remembered that the environmental conditions in the acutely ischaemic myocardium (increased K^+ and H^+) are known to potentiate the Na^+ channel blocking effects of antiarrhythmic drugs (see Nattel *et al*., 1981, for references) and therefore it is conceivable that concentrations, although subthreshold for the normal myocardium, may be able to exert an antiarrhythmic effect on ischaemic cells.

In anaesthetised dogs, pigs and rats, there is evidence that most Na^+ channel blocking agents (with the exception of lignocaine), when administered prior to acute ligation of the main coronary artery, can suppress the number of ventricular ectopic beats and reduce or abolish the incidence of VF. Whether this type of experimental model is relevant to the clinical situation is of course debatable, and the view has been expressed that acute coronary ligation models do not simulate the chronic electrical instability associated with sudden coronary death (Patterson *et al.*, 1980). This has led to the increasing use of experimental models of myocardial ischaemia in which re-entry ventricular arrhythmias and fibrillation are initiated by electrical pacing (Elharrar and Zipes, 1977) or by programmed premature stimuli (Patterson *et al.*, 1980). Results obtained in this setting with Na^+ channel blocking drugs have been confusing, ranging from exacerbation of arrhythmias with aprindine (Zipes *et al.*, 1977b) and disopyramide (Patterson *et al.*, 1980), through reported ineffectiveness of procainamide and quinidine (Zipes *et al.*, 1977a) to a protective action of lignocaine (Kupersmith *et al.*, 1975). It is probable that antiarrhythmic agents of this type exert diverse actions on the ischaemic and partially ischaemic myocardium and that some of these actions may be arrhythmogenic (further increase in conduction delay) while other effects may be antiarrhythmic (production of more homogeneous action potential and refractory period durations between ischaemic and non-ischaemic tissue). Haemodynamic effects of the drugs and effects on cardiac metabolism may also influence overall antiarrhythmic activity. In this respect it should be noted that there have been reports that lignocaine (Schaub *et al.*, 1977), disopyramide (Marshall and Parratt, 1979) and the aminosteroid Org 6001 (Marshall and Parratt, 1977b) all reduce the extent of myocardial injury produced by acute coronary ligation in anaesthetised dogs.

A recent study (Patterson *et al.*, 1980) has also suggested that it may be necessary to achieve high, steady state concentrations of antiarrhythmic drugs to prevent re-entry ventricular arrhythmias. Since most Na^+ channel blocking agents produce significant haemodynamic side effects (see Singh, 1977, for a review), more emphasis should perhaps be placed on those newer agents which have relatively little effect on cardiac contractility. In this respect mexiletine, lorcainide and Org 6001 would seem the best candidates.

We are entering an era in which the pharmacological prevention of sudden coronary death may soon become a reality. The task of identifying the proper agent or agents will not be a simple one, especially since there is still no good predictive animal model. However, the study of the effects of drugs on the early experimentally induced ventricular arrhythmias and VF ensuing shortly after coronary ligation will surely help in exploring the pathophysiological processes which render the myocardium vulnerable to sudden ventricular fibrillation and in studying how pharmacological agents of different types act to prevent this fatal electrical event.

ACKNOWLEDGEMENTS

We gratefully acknowledge the help of Mr I. McFarlane for assistance in literature searching and Mrs A. Jones for her careful preparation of the manuscript.

REFERENCES

Adgey, A. A. J., Allen, J. D., Geddes, J. S., James, R. G., Webb, G., Zaidi, S. W. and Pantridge, J. F. (1971). Acute phase of myocardial infarction. *Lancet, ii*, 510-4

Aldor, E. and Heeger, H. (1976). Propafenone ein neues Antarrhythmikum. *Dt. med. Wschr.*, **101**, 1318-22

Allen, J. D., James, R. G. G., Kelly, J. G., Shanks, R. G. and Zaidi, S. A. (1977). Comparison of the effects of lignocaine and mexiletine on experimental ventricular arrhythmias. *Postgrad. med. J.*, **53**, 35-45

Allen, J. D., Kofi Ekue, J. M., Shanks, R. G. and Zaidi, S. A. (1970). The effect on experimental cardiac arrhythmias of a new anticonvulsant agent, Kö 1173, and its comparison with phenytoin and procainamide. *Br. J. Pharmac.*, **39**, 183-4P

Allen, J. D., Kofi Ekue, J. M., Shanks, R. G. and Zaidi, S. A. (1972). The effect of Kö 1173, a new anticonvulsant agent on experimental cardiac arrhythmias. *Br. J. Pharmac.*, **45**, 561-73

Anderson, J. L., Mason, J. W., Winkle, R. A., Meffin, P. J., Fowles, R. E., Peters, F. and Harrison, D. C. (1978). Clinical electrophysiological effects of tocainide. *Am. J. Cardiol.*, **41**, 415

Ankier, S. I., Carmichael, D. J. S. and Kidner, P. H. (1977). Disopyramide - a review. *Scot. med. J.*, **22**, 314-9

Arita, M., Goto, M., Nagamoto, Y. and Saikawa, T. (1979). Electrophysiological actions of mexiletine (Kö 1173) on canine Purkinje fibres and ventricular muscle. *Br. J. Pharmac.*, **67**, 143-52

Arnsdorf, M. F. (1976). Electrophysiologic properties of antidysrhythmic drugs as a rational basis for therapy. *Med. Clin. N. Am.*, **60**, 213-32

Arnsdorf, M. F. and Bigger, J. T. (1972). Effect of lidocaine hydrochloride on membrane conductance in mammalian cardiac Purkinje fibres. *J. clin. Invest.*, **51**, 2252-63

Au, T. L. S., Collins, G. A., MacLeod, B. A. and Walker, M. J. A. (1979a). Arrhythmic responses to coronary occlusion in different species. *Proc. Can. Fedn. biol. Soc.*, **22**, 63

Au, T. L. S., Collins, G. A., Harvie, C. J. and Walker, M. J. A. (1979b). The actions of prostaglandins I_2 and E_2 on arrhythmias produced by coronary occlusion in the rat and dog. *Prostaglandins*, **18**, 707-20

Bagwell, E. E., Walle, T., Drayer, D. E., Reidenberg, M. M. and Pruett, J. K., (1976). Correlation of the electrophysiological and antiarrhythmic properties of the *N*-acetyl metabolite of procainamide with plasma and tissue drug concentrations in the dog. *J. Pharmac. exp. ther.*, **197**, 38-48

Bar, F., Forré, J., Gorgels, A. and Wellens, H. (1978). Electrophysiological effects of lorcainide, a new antiarrhythmic drug in man. *Circulation*, **58**, 966

Beck, O. A. and Hochrein, H. (1978). Wirksamkeit und Risiken von Propafenon bei der Akutbehandlung von Herzrhythmusstoerungen. *Dt. med. Wschr.*, **103**, 1261-5

Beck, O. A., Witt, E. and Hochrein, H. (1975). Antiarrhythmikmus Propafenon auf die intrakardiale Erregungsleitung. Klinische Untersuchungen mit Hilfe der His-Buendel-Elektrographie. *Z. Kardiol.*, **64**, 179-87

Benett, M. A., Wilner, J. M. and Pentecost, B. L. (1970). Controlled trial of lignocaine prophylaxis of ventricular arrhythmias complicating myocardial infarction. *Lancet, ii*, 909-11

Bigger, J. T. and Heissenbuttel, R. H. (1969). The use of procainamide and lidocaine in the treatment of cardiac arrhythmias. *Progr. cardiovasc. Dis.*, **11**, 515-34

Bigger, J. T. and Mandel, W. J. (1970). Effect of lidocaine on the electrophysiological properties of ventricular muscle and Purkinje fibres. *J. clin. Invest.*, **49**, 63-77

Blanke, H., Aschbrenner, B., Karsch, K. R. and Kreuger, H. (1979). Plasmaspiegel-Wirkungs-Beziehung und Organverteilung von Propafenon. *Dt. med. Wschr.*, **104**, 587-91

Bleifeld, W., Merx, W., Heinrich, K. W. and Effert, S. (1972). Lidocain zur Arrhythmieprophylaxe beim frischen Infarkt. *Verh. dt. Ges. inn. Med.*, **78**, 1035-9

Borer, J. S., Harrison, L. A., Kent, K. M., Levy, R., Goldstein, R. E. and Epstein, S. E. (1976). Beneficial effect of lidocaine on ventricular electrical stability and spontaneous ventricular fibrillation during experimental myocardial infarction. *Am. J. Cardiol.*, **37**, 860-3

Büssmann, W. D., Schreiber, S. and Kaltenbach, M. (1980). Comparison of antiarrhythmic effects of oral prajmalium bitartrate and intravenous lidocaine in acute myocardial infarction. *Am. Heart. J.*, **99**, 589-97

Byrne, J. E., Gomoll, A. W. and McKinney, G. R. (1977). Antiarrhythmic properties of MJ 9067 in acute animal models. *J. Pharmac. exp. Ther.*, **200**, 147-54

Cabedo, J. A. F., Insa Perez, L. D., Merino, V. L., Salana, S. B., Auban, A. B. and Requena, J. E. (1978). Electrophysiological effects of aprindine on A-V conduction in the dog. *Arch. int. Pharmacodyn. Thér.*, **236**, 154-63

Campbell, N. P. S., Chaturverdi, N. C., Kelly, J. G., Strong, J. E., Shanks, R. G. and Pantridge, J. F. (1973). Mexiletine (Kö 1173) in the management of dysrhythmias. *Lancet, ii*, 404-7

Campbell, R. W. F., Pottage, A., Murray, A., Achuff, S. C., Prescott, L. F. and Julian, D. G. (1978). Prophylactic mexiletine therapy in acute myocardial infarction. In *Management of Ventricular Tachycardia - Role of Mexiletine* (ed. E. Sandoe, D. G. Julian and J. W. Bell), Excerpta Medica, Amsterdam, pp. 479-83

Caracta, A. R. and Damato, A. N. (1975). Procainamide. In *Drugs in Cardiology*, Vol. 1 (ed. E. Donoso), Stratton Intercontinental, New York, pp. 1-16

Cardinal, R., Janse, M. J., d'Alnoncourt, C. N. and Durrer, D. (1980). Effects of lidocaine on ventricular potentials, activation and arrhythmias during coronary occlusion in the porcine heart. *Circulation*, **62**, Suppl. III, 345

Carmeleit, E. (1979). Electrophysiological evaluation of Org 6001 in isolated tissues. Report to Organon International, 9 July 1979

Carmeliet, E. (1980). Electrophysiological effects of encainide on isolated cardiac muscle and Purkinje fibres and on the Langendorff-perfused guinea-pig heart. *Eur. J. Pharmac.*, **61**, 247-62

Carmeliet, E. and Verdonk. F. (1974). Effects of aprindine and lidocaine on transmembrane potentials and radioactive K^+ efflux in different cardiac tissues. *Acta cardiol.*, Suppl. 18, 73-90

Carmeliet, E. and Zaman, M. Y. (1979). Comparative effects of lignocaine and lorcainide on conduction in the Langendorff-perfused guinea-pig heart. *Cardiovasc. Res.*, **13**, 439-49

Carmeliet, E., Janssen, P. A. J., Marsboom, R., Van Nueten, J. M. and Xhonneux, R. (1978). Antiarrhythmic, electrophysiologic and haemodynamic effects of lorcainide. *Arch. int. Pharmacodyn. Thér.*, **231**, 104-30

Chen, C. M., Gettes, L. S. and Katzung, B. G. (1975). Effects of lidocaine and quinidine on steady-state characteristics and recovery kinetics of (dV/dt max) in guinea-pig ventricular myocardium. *Circulation Res.*, **37**, 20-9

Clark, C., Foreman, M. I., Kane, K. A., McDonald, F. M. and Parratt, J. R. (1980). Coronary artery ligation of anaesthetised rats as a method for the production of experimental dysrhythmias and for the determination of infarct size. *J. pharmac. Meth.*, **3**, 357-68

Cocco, G. and Strozzi, C. (1978). Initial clinical experience of lorcainide (Ro 13-1042), a new antiarrhythmic agent. *Eur. J. clin. Pharmac.*, **14**, 105-9

Collett, J. T., Chew, C. Y. C., Campbell, C., Eng, C. and Singh, B. N. (1980). Abolition of early ischaemic ventricular arrhythmias in conscious dogs pretreated with amiodarone. *Clin. Res.*, **28**, 161A

Coltart, D. J., Berndt, T. B., Kernoff, R. and Harrison, D. C. (1974). Antiarrhythmic and circulatory effects of Astra W36095, a new lidocaine-like agent. *Am. J. Cardiol.*, **34**, 35-41

Conn, R. D. (1965). Diphenylhydantoin sodium in cardiac arrhythmias. *New Engl. J. Med.*, **272**, 277-82

Corr, P. B., Helke, C. J. and Gillis, R. A. (1978). Exacerbation of coronary occlusion-induced ventricular arrhythmias by the vagolytic effect of procainamide. *Cardiovasc. Res.*, **8**, 486-92

Cosnier, D., Grimal, J. and Duchene-Marullaz, P. (1971). Comparaison des effets du disopyramide, de la dihydroquinidine et du procainamide sur deux types d'arhythmies ventriculaires. *Thérapie*, **26**, 97-107

Cranefield, P. F., Wit, A. L. and Hoffman, B. F. (1972). Conduction of the cardiac impulse. III. Characteristics of very slow conduction. *J. gen. Physiol.*, **59**, 227-46

d'Alnoncourt, N. C., Cardinal, R., Janse, M. J., Luederitz, B. and Durrer, D. (1980). Effects of tocainide on ectopic impulse formation in isolated cardiac tissue. *Klin. Wschr.*, **58**, 227-31

Dangman, K. H. and Hoffman, B. F. (1978). Effects of *N*-acetylprocainamide on cardiac Purkinje fibres. *Pharmacologist*, **20**, 150

Danilo, P. R. and Rosen, M. R. (1976). Cardiac effects of disopyramide. *Am. Heart J.*, **92**, 532-6

Danilo, P., Hordof, A. J. and Rosen, M. R. (1977a). Effects of disopyramide on electrophysiologic properties of canine cardiac Purkinje fibres. *J. Pharmac. exp. Ther.*, **201**, 701-10

Danilo, P., Langan, W. B., Rosen, M. R. and Hoffman, B. F. (1977b). Effects of the phenothiazine analog EN-313 on ventricular arrhythmias in the dog. *Eur. J. Pharmac.*, **45**, 127-39

Dean, R. R. (1975). The pharmacology of Norpace. *Angiology*, **26**, Suppl. 1, Pt 2, 67-84

Dean, R. R., McDermott, D. J. and Smith, W. S. (1979). Disopyramide. In *Pharmacological and Biochemical Properties of Drug Substances* (ed. M. E. Goldberg), American Pharmaceutical Association, New York, pp. 165-85

DiBianco, R., Gottdiener, J. S., Fletcher, R. D., Singh, S., Katz, R. J. and Sauerbrunn, B. (1980). Effects of encainide on left ventricular function; assessment with treadmill exercise and radionuclide ventriculography. *Circulation*, **62**, Suppl. III, 282

Duff, H. J., Roden, D. M. and Woosley, R. L. (1980). Abolition of resistant ventricular arrhythmias by twice daily dosing with flecainide. *Circulation*, **62**, Suppl. III, 181

Dughman, S. and Cohn, K. (1973). Detrimental effect of non-homogeneous distribution of lidocaine to the myocardium. *Circulation*, **43**, Suppl. IV, 132

Elharrar, V. and Zipes, D. P. (1977). Cardiac electrophysiologic alterations during myocardial ischemia. *Am. J. Physiol.*, **233**, H329-45

Elharrar, V., Gaum, W. E. and Zipes, D. P. (1977). Effect of drugs on conduction delay and incidence of ventricular arrhythmias induced by acute coronary occlusion in dogs. *Am. J. Cardiol.*, **39**, 544-9

El-Sherif, N. and Lazzara, R. (1979). Re-entrant ventricular arrhythmias in the late myocardial infarction period. 7. Effect of verapamil and D600 and the role of the slow channel. *Circulation*, **60**, 605-15

Esser, H. and Kikis, D. (1978). Mexiletine in the suppression of ventricular ectopic activity: short and long term treatment. In *Management of Ventricular Tachycardia - Role of Mexiletine* (ed. E. Sandoe, D. G. Julain and J. W. Bell), Excerpta Medica, Amsterdam, pp. 585-93

Evans, D. E. and Gillis, R. A. (1974). Effect of diphenylhydantoin and lidocaine on cardiac arrhythmias induced by hypothalamic stimulation. *J. Pharmac. exp. Ther.*, **191**, 506-14

Fox, S., Hoffman, B., Rosen, M. and Hoffman, B. (1980). Effects of ethomozine and lidocaine on ventricular fibrillation and defibrillation in anaesthetised dogs. *Am. J. Cardiol.*, **45**, 474

Gamble, O. W. and Cohn, K. (1972). Effect of propranolol, procainamide and lidocaine on ventricular automaticity and re-entry in experimental myocardial infarction. *Circulation*, **46**, 498-506

Geddes, J. S., Webb, S. and Pantridge, J. F. (1972). Limitations of lignocaine in control of early ventricular dysrhythmias complicating acute myocardial infarction. *Br. Heart J.*, **34**, 964-5

Geltman, E. M., Campbell, M. K., Ambos, H. D. and Roberts, R. (1978). Treatment of refractory ventricular arrhythmias with oral aprindine. *Clin. Res.*, **26**, 233A

Georges, A., Horslet, A. and Duvernay, G. (1973). Pharmacological evaluation of aprindine (AC 1802) a new antiarrhythmic agent. *Acta cardiol.*, **28**, 166-91

Gerin, M. G. and Kulbertus, H. E. (1978). Effects of various antiarrhythmic agents on conduction delay and incidence of ventricular arrhythmias induced by acute coronary occlusion in the dog. In *Management of Ventricular Tachycardia - Role of Mexiletine* (ed. E. Sandoe, D. G. Julian and J. W. Bell), Excerpta Medica, Amsterdam, pp. 299-304

Giardina, E. G. and Bigger, J. T. (1973). Procainamide against re-entrant ventricular arrhythmias: lengthening of R-V intervals of coupled ventricular premature depolarization as an insight into the mechanisms of action of procainamide. *Circulation*, **48**, 959-70

Greenspan, K., Steinberg, M., Holland, D. and Freeman, A. R. (1974). Electrophysiological alterations in cardiac dysrhythmias. Antiarrhythmic effects of aprindine. *Am. J. Cardiol.*, **33**, 140

Hagemeijer, F. and Hugenholtz, P. G. (1974). Antiarrhythmic efficacy of aprindine in acute myocardial infarction. *Am. J. Cardiol.*, **33**, 142

Hai, H. A., Ostrowski, T. L. and Davison, R. (1979). Successful control of resistant ventricular tachycardia with aprindine hydrochloride. *Am. J. Cardiol.*, **43**, 358

Han, J., Goel, B. D., Yoon, M. S. and Rodgers, R. (1974). Effect of procainamide and lidocaine on ventricular automaticity and re-entry during acute coronary occlusion. *Am. J. Cardiol.*, **34**, 171-8

Hapke, H. J. and Prigge, E. (1976). Pharmakologie von 2'-[Hydroxy-3-(propylamino) propoxy]-3-phenylpropiophenon (Propafenon, SA79)-hydrochlorid. *Arzneimittel-Forsch.*, **26**, 1849-57

Harris, A. S. and Kokernot, R. H. (1950). Effects of diphenylhydantoin sodium and phenobarbital sodium upon ectopic ventricular tachycardia in acute myocardial infarction. *Am. J. Physiol.*, **163**, 505-16

Harris, A. S., Estandia, A., Ford, T. J. and Tillotson, R. F. (1951). Quinidine lactate and gluconate in the suppression of ectopic ventricular tachycardias associated with myocardial infarction. Control of toxicity by morphine. *Circulation*, **4**, 522-33

Harris, A. S., Estandia, A., Ford, T. J., Smith, H. T., Olsen, R. W. and Tillotson, R. F. (1952). The effects of intravenous procaine and procainamide (Pronestyl) upon ectopic ventricular tachycardia accompanying acute myocardial infarction. *Circulation*, **5**, 551-8

Harrison, D. C. and Alderman, E. L. (1972). The pharmacology and clinical use of lidocaine as an antiarrhythmic drug. *Mod. Treat.*, **9**, 139-75

Hauswirth, O. and Singh, B. N. (1978). Ionic mechanisms in heart muscle in relation to the genesis and the pharmacological control of cardiac arrhythmias. *Pharmac. Rev.*, **30**, 5-64

Heistracher, P. and Beck, A. (1979). Effects of propafenone on the maximum rate of rise of cardiac action potentials. *Arch. Pharmac.*, **308**, Suppl. R37, 039/474

Helfant, R. H., Scherlag, B. J. and Damato, A. N. (1967). The electrophysiological properties of diphenylhydantoin sodium as compared to procainamide in the normal and digitalis-intoxicated heart. *Circulation*, **36**, 108-18

Hill, J. L. and Gettes, L. S. (1980). Effect of acute coronary artery occlusion on local myocardial extracellular K^+ activity in swine. *Circulation*, **61**, 768-77

Hodess, A. B., Follansbee, W. P., Spear, J. F. and Moore, E. N. (1979). Electrophysiological effects of a new antiarrhythmic agent, flecainide on the intact canine heart. *J. cardiovasc. Pharmac.*, **1**, 427-39

Hoffman, B. F. and Bigger, J. T. (1971). Antiarrhythmic drugs. In *Drill's Pharmacology in Medicine*, 4th edn (ed. J. R. Di Palma), McGraw-Hill, New York, pp. 824-52

Hope, R. R., Williams, D. O., El-Sherif, N., Lazzara, R. and Scherlag, B. J. (1974). The efficacy of antiarrhythmic agents during acute myocardial ischemia and the role of heart rate. *Circulation*, **50**, 507-14

Horowitz, J. D., Anavekar, S. N., Morris, P. M., Goble, A. J., Doyle, A. E. and Louis, W. J. (1981). Comparative trial of mexiletine and lignocaine in the treatment of early ventricular tachyarrhythmias after acute myocardial infarction. *J. cardiovasc. Pharmac.*, **3**, 409-19

Hurst, V. W., Morris, J. T., Zeft, H. J., Hackel, D. B. and McIntosh, H. D. (1967). Increased survival with prophylactic quinidine after experimental myocardial infarction. *Circulation*, **36**, 294-303

Jackman, W. M., Prystowsky, E. N., Rinkenberger, R. L., Naccarelli, G. V., Heger, J. J. and Zipes, D. P. (1980). Oral encainide increases refractoriness of ventricle, atrium and accessory pathway. *Circulation*, **62**, Suppl. III, 11

Jaillon, P., Kernoff, R. and Winkle, R. (1979). *N*-Acetylprocainamide and procainamide have different electrophysiologic properties. *Am. J. Cardiol.*, **43**, 359

Janse, M. J. (1978). The ideal experimental animal model: the 'dig' or the 'pog'. In *Managment of Ventricular Tachycardia - Role of Mexiletine* (ed. E. Sandoe, D. G. Julian and J. W. Bell), Excerpta Medica, Amsterdam, p. 38

Jewitt, D. E., Kishon, Y. and Thomas, M. (1968). Lignocaine in the management of arrhythmias after acute myocardial infarction. *Lancet*, *i*, 266-70

Johnson, E. A. and McKinnon, M. G. (1957). Differential effect of quinidine and pyrilamine on the myocardial action potential at various rates of stimulation. *J. Pharmac. exp. Ther.*, **120**, 460-5

Jones, D. T., Kostuk, W. J. and Gunton, R. W. (1974). Prophylactic quinidine for the prevention of arrhythmias after acute myocardial infarction. *Am. J. Cardiol.*, **33**, 655-60

Josephson, M. E., Seides, S. F., Batsford, W. P., Weisfogel, G. M., Akhtar, M., Caracta, A. R., Lau, S. H. and Damato, A. N. (1974). Electrophysiological effects of intramuscular quinidine on the atrioventricular conducting system in man. *Am. Heart J.*, **87**, 55-64

Kalusche, D. and Loenne, E. (1978). Die therapie chronischer schwer beeinflussbarer Rhythmusstoerungen mit Propafenon. *Z. Kardiol.*, Suppl. 5, 44

Kane, K. A. (1980). Comparative electrophysiological effects of Org 6001, a new orally active antidysrhythmic agent, and lignocaine on human ventricular muscle. *Br. J. Pharmac.*, **68**, 25-31

Kane, K. A. and Winslow, E. (1980). Antidysrhythmic and electrophysiological effects of a new antianginal agent, bepridil. *J. cardiovasc. Pharmac*, **2**, 193-203

Kane, K. A., Lepran, I., McDonald, F. M., Parratt, J. R. and Szekeres, L. (1980). The effects of prolonged oral administration of a new antidysrhythmic drug

(Org 6001) on coronary artery ligation dysrhythmias in conscious and anaesthetised rats. *J. cardiovasc. Pharmac.*, **2**, 411-23

Kane, K. A., McDonald, F. M. and Parratt, J. R. (1981). What pharmacological properties are necessary for the prevention of early post-infarction ventricular dysrhythmias? *Br. J. Pharmac.*, **72**, 512-3P

Kane, K. A., McDonald, F. M., Timmer, C. J., Parratt, J. R. and Vink, J. (1982). Correlation of the antiarrhythmic effects of Org 6001 with plasma and tissue drug concentrations following oral administration in the rat. *Br. J. Pharmac.*, **75**, 319-23

Kaplinsky, E., Ogawa, S., Balke, C. W. and Dreifus, L. S. (1979). Two periods of early ventricular arrhythmia in the canine acute myocardial infarction model. *Circulation*, **60**, 397-403

Karlsson, E. (1975). Procainamide and phenytoin: comparative study of their antiarrhythmic effects at apparent therapeutic plasma levels. *Br. Heart J.*, **37**, 731-40

Kaverina, N. V., Senova, Z. P., Mitrofanov, V. S. and Runova, M. F. (1972). Pharmacology of ethmosin; a new antiarrhythmic drug. *Farmak. Toksikol.*, **35**, 182-5

Kayden, H. J., Brodie, B. B. and Steele, J. M. (1957). Procainamide. *Circulation*, **15**, 118-26

Kesteloot, H. and Stroobandt, R. (1977). Clinical experience with lorcainide (R15889), a new antiarrhythmic drug. *Arch. int. Pharmacodyn. Thér.*, **230**, 225-34

Kesteloot, H. and Stroobandt, R. (1979). Clinical experience of encainide (MJ 9067): a new antiarrhythmic drug. *Eur. J. clin. Pharmac.*, **16**, 323-6

Kesteloot, H., Van Mieghem, W. and De Geest, H. (1973). Aprindine (AC 1802), a new antiarrhythmic drug. *Acta cardiol.*, **28**, 145-65

Kleber, A. G., Janse, M. J., Van Capelle, F. J. L. and Durrer, D. (1978). Mechanism and time course of S-T and T-Q segment changes during acute regional myocardial ischemia in the pig heart determined by extracellular and intracellular recordings. *Circulation Res.*, **42**, 603-13

Kojima, M. (1981). Effects of disopyramide on transmembrane action potentials in guinea-pig papillary muscle. *Eur. J. Pharmac.*, **69**, 11-24

Kramer, B., Gülker, H. and Meesmann, W. (1981). The effects of lidocaine on the ventricular fibrillation threshold and primary ventricular fibrillation following acute experimental coronary occlusion. *Basic Res. Cadiol.*, **76**, 29-43

Kroll, D. A. and Lucchesi, B. R. (1975). Antiarrhythmic and antifibrillatory properties of aprindine. *J. Pharmac. exp. Ther.*, **194**, 427-34

Kupersmith, J., Antman, E. M. and Hoffman, B. F. (1975). *In vivo* electrophysiological effects of lidocaine in canine acute myocardial infarction. *Circulation Res.*, **36**, 84-91

Kupersmith, J., Shiang, H., Litwak, R. S. and Herman, M. V. (1976). Electrophysiological effects of verapamil in canine myocardial ischemia. *Am. J. Cardiol.*, **37**, 149

Kus, T. and Sasyniuk, B. I. (1976). Effects of disopyramide phosphate on ventricular arrhythmias in experimental myocardial infarction. *J. Pharmac. exp. Ther.*, **196**, 665-75

Kus, T. and Sasyniuk, B. I. (1978). The electrophysiological effects of disopyramide phosphate on canine ventricular muscle and Purkinje fibres in normal and low potassium. *Can. J. Physiol. Pharmac.*, **56**, 139-49

Lalka, D., Meyer, M. B., Duce, B. R. and Elvin, A. T. (1976). Kinetics of the oral antiarrhythmic lidocaine congener, tocainide. *Clin. Pharmac. Ther.*, **19**, 757-66

Lazzara, R., El-Sherif, N. and Scherlag, B. J. (1974). Early and late effects of coronary artery occlusion on canine Purkinje fibres. *Circulation Res.*, **35**, 391-9

Lazzara, R., El-Sherif, N., Hope, R. R. and Scherlag, B. J. (1978). Ventricular arrhythmias and electrophysiological consequences of myocardial ischemia and infarction. *Circulation Res.*, **42**, 740-9

Levine, H. D. (1932). Effect of quinidine sulphate in inhibiting ventricular fibrillation. *Archs int. Med.*, **49**, 808-15

Levites, R. and Anderson, G. J. (1979). Electrophysiological effects of disopyramide phosphate during experimental myocardial ischemia. *Am. Heart J.*, **98**, 339-44

Le Winter, M. M., Engler, R. L. and Karliner, J. S. (1980). Tocainamide therapy for treatment of ventricular arrhythmias: assessment with ambulatory electrocardiographic monitoring and treadmill exersie. *Am. J. Cardiol.*, **45**, 1045-52

Lown, B. and Wolf, M. (1971). Approaches to sudden death from coronary heart disease. *Circulation*, **44**, 130-42

McDevitt, D. G., Nies, A. S., Wilkinson, G. R., Smith, R. F., Woosley, R. L. and Oates, J. A. (1976). Antiarrhythmic effects of a lidocaine congener, tocainide, 2-amino-2′,6′-propionoxylidide, in man. *Clin. Pharmac. Ther.*, **19**, 396-404

McDonald, F. M. (1980). Experimental models for the production of cardiac dysrhythmias and for the assessment of activity of antidysrhythmic drugs. PhD thesis, University of Strathclyde, Glasgow

Madan, B. R., Arora, R. B. and Kapila, K. (1960). Anticonvulsant, antiveratrinic and antiarrhythmic actions of *Acorus calamus* Linn. An Indian indigenous drug. *Archs int. Pharmacodyn. Thér.*, **124**, 201-11

Malini, P. L., Ambrosioni, E., Bracchetti, D. and Magnani, B. (1979). Evaluation of clinical efficacy and plasma levels of aprindine. *Int. J. Clin. Pharmac. Biopharm.*, **17**, 396-403

Manz, M., Steinbeck, G. and Lüderitz, B. (1978). Wirkung von Lorcainid (R 15889) auf Sinusknotenfunktion und intrakardiale Erregunsleitung. *Herbsttagung dt. Ges. Kreislaufforsch.*, Abstract 78

Mark, L. C., Kayden, H. J., Steel, J. M., Dooper, J. R., Berlin, I., Rovenstine, E. A. and Brodie, B. B. (1951). The physiological disposition and cardiac effects of procainamide. *J. Pharmac. exp. Ther.*, **102**, 5-17

Marshall, R. J. and Muir, A. W. (1981). The antiarrhythmic, haemodynamic and metabolic effects of a new antianginal agent, bepridil, in the early stages of canine acute myocardial infarction. *Br. J. Pharmac.*, **72**, 114-5P

Marshall, R. J. and Parratt, J. R. (1975). Antiarrhythmic, haemodynamic and metabolic effects of 3α-amino-5α-androstan-2β-ol-17-one hydrochloride in greyhounds following acute coronary artery ligation. *Br. J. Pharmac.*, **55**, 359-68

Marshall, R. J. and Parratt, J. R. (1977a). The haemodynamic and metabolic effects of MG8926, a prospective antidysrhythmic and anti-anginal agent. *Br. J. Pharmac.*, **59**, 311-22

Marshall, R. J. and Parratt, J. R. (1977b). The antidysrhythmic aminosteroid, Org 6001, reduces the ST-segment elevation produced by coronary occlusion in the dog. *Br. J. Pharmac.*, **61**, 315-7

Marshall, R. J. and Parratt, J. R. (1979). The effects of disopyramide phosphate on early post-coronary artery ligation dysrhythmias and on epicardial ST-segment elevation in anaesthetised dogs. *Br. J. Pharmac.*, **66**, 241-50

Marshall, R. J. and Parratt, J. R. (1980a). The early consequences of myocardial ischaemia and their modification. *J. Physiol., Paris*, **76**, 699-715

Marshall, R. J. and Parratt, J. R. (1980b). Prophylactic lignocaine and early post-coronary artery occlusion dysrhythmias in anaesthetised greyhounds. *Br. J. Pharmac.*, **71**, 597-600

Marshall, R. J., Muir, A. W. and Winslow, E. (1981). A comparison of the intensity and duration of the antidysrhythmic effect of mexiletine and Org 6001 in anaesthetised rats. *Br. J. Pharmac.*, **74**, 381-8

Mason, J. W. and Peters, F. A. (1980). Antiarrhythmic efficacy of encainide in patients with refractory recurrent ventricular tachycardia. *Circulation*, **62**, Suppl. III, 153

Meesmann, W., Gülker, H., Kramer, B. and Stephan, K. (1976). Time course of changes in ventricular fibrillation threshold in myocardial infarction: characteristics of acute and slow occlusion with respect to the collateral vessels of the heart. *Cardiovasc. Res.*, **10**, 466-73

Meinertz, T., Kaspar, W., Kersting, F., Just, H., Bechtold, H. and Jahnchen, E. (1979). Lorcainide. II. Plasma concentration–effect relationship. *Clin. Pharmac. Ther.*, **26**, 187-95

Meinertz, T., Kasper, W., Kersting, F., Bechtold, H., Just, H. and Jahnchen, E. (1980a). Antiarrhythmic effect of lorcainide during chronic treatment. *Arzeimittel-Forsch.*, **30**, 1593-5

Meinertz, T., Kersting, F., Kasper, W., Just, H., Bechtold, H. and Jahnchen, E. (1980b). Haemodynamic effects of a single intravenous dose of lorcainide in patients with heart disease. *Eur. J. clin. Pharmac.*, **18**, 461-5

Merx, W., Henning, B., Franken, G. and Effert, S. (1978). Mexiletine in acute myocardial infarction. In *Management of Ventricular Tachycardia – Role of Mexiletine* (ed. E. Sandoe, D. G. Julian and J. W. Bell), Excerpta Medica, Amsterdam, pp. 472-8

Meyer, E. G., Keller, K., Beck, O. A. and Hochrein, H. (1978). Antiarrhythmische Wirksamkeit bon propafenon in Abhaengigkeit von Serumkonzentration unde Erregungsleitungshemmung. *Z. Kardiol.*, **67**, 352-6

Mirro, M. J., Watanabe, A. M. and Baily, J. C. (1979). Anticholinergic effects of quinidine and disopyramide on canine cardiac Purkinje fibres. *Clin. Res.*, **27**, 189A

Mokler, C. M. and Van Arman, C. G. (1962). Pharmacology of a new antiarrhythmic agent α-diisopropylamine-α-phenyl-α-(2-pyridyl)butyramide (SC-7031). *J. Pharmac. exp. Ther.*, **136**, 114-24

Morganroth, J., Pearlman, A. S., Dunkman, W. B., Horowitz, L. N., Josephson, M. E. and Michelson, E. L. (1979). Ethmosine - a new antiarrhythmic agent developed in the USSR. Efficacy and tolerance. *Am. Heart. J.*, **98**, 621-8

Morganroth, J., Dreifus, L. S., Michelson, E. L. and Sawain, H. S. (1980). Efficacy and tolerance of lorcainide. *Circulation*, **62**, 111-80

Myburgh, D. P., Goldman, A. P. and Schamroth, J. M. (1980). Lorcainide - an antiarrhythmic agent for ventricular arrhythmias. *S. Afr. med. J.*, **57**, 236-9

Nakaya, H., Hattori, Y. and Kanno, M. (1980). Effects of calcium antagonists and lidocaine on conduction delay induced by acute myocardial ischaemia in dogs. *Jap. J. Pharmac.*, **30**, 587-97

Nattel, S., Pederson, D. H. and Zipes, D. P. (1979). Regional myocardial aprindine concentration and effects on arrhythmia after coronary occlusion. *Am. J. Cardiol.*, **43**, 358

Nattel, S., Elharrar, V., Zipes, D. P. and Bailey, J. C. (1981). pH-dependent electrophysiological effects of quinidine and lidocaine on canine cardiac Purkinje fibres. *Circulation Res.*, **48**, 55-61

Neuss, H. and Buss, J. (1978). Wirkungsspektrum neuer Antiarrhythmika. *Internist*, **19**, 234-40

Ogawa, S., Kaplinsky, E., Balke, C. W. and Dreifus, L. S. (1979). Evidence of two periods of early ventricular arrhythmia following acute myocardial infarction. *Am. J. Cardiol.*, **43**, 371

Okuma, K., Sugiyama, S., Wada, M., Sugenoya, J., Niimi, N., Oguri, H., Toyama, J. and Yamada, K. (1976). Experimental studies on the antiarrhythmic action of a lidocaine analog. *Cardiology*, **61**, 289-97

Opie, L. H. (1980). Drugs and the heart: IV. Antiarrhythmic agents. *Lancet*, *i*, 861-8

Parratt, J. R. (1979). The search for prophylactic antidysrhythmic drugs - the place of aminosteroids. *Progr. Pharmac.*, **2**, 85-94

Patterson, E., Gibson, J. J. and Lucchesi, B. R. (1980). Electrophysiological effects of disopyramide phosphate on re-entrant ventricular arrhythmia in conscious dogs after myocardial infarction. *Am. J. Cardiol.*, **46**, 792-9

Pentecost, B. L., De Giovanni, J. V., Lamb, P., Cadigan, P. J., Everny, K. L. and Flint, E. J. (1981). Reappraisal of lignocaine therapy in management of myocardial infarction. *Br. Heart J.*, **45**, 42-7

Pozenel, H. (1977). Haemodynamic studies on mexiletine, a new antiarrhythmic agent. *Postgrad. med. J.*, **53**, 78-80

Prinzmetal, M., Toyashima, H., Ekmekci, A. and Nagaya, T. (1962). Angina pectoris. VI. Nature of ST-segment elevation and other ECG changes in acute severe ischaemia. *Clin. Sci.*, **23**, 489-514

Probst, P. and Pachinger, O. (1976). Einfluesse von Propafenone auf die Haemodynamik des linken Ventrikels und die atrioventrikulaere Ueberleitung unter besonderer Beruecksichtigung des WPW-Syndroms. *Z. Kardiol.*, **65**, 212-24

Reddy, C. P., Damato, A. N., Akhtar, M., Dhatt, M. S., Gomes, J. A. C. and Calon,

A. H. (1977). Effect of procainamide on re-entry within the His–Purkinje system in man. *Am. J. Cardiol.*, **40**, 957-64

Reynolds, R. D. and Kamath, B. L. (1979). *N*-Acetylprocainamide and ischaemia-induced ventricular fibrillation in the dog. *Eur. J. Pharmac.*, **59**, 115-9

Ribner, H. S., Isaacs, E. S. and Frishman, W. H. (1979). Lidocaine prophylaxis against ventricular fibrillation in acute myocardial infarction. *Progr. cardiovasc. Dis.*, **21**, 287-313

Ro, J., Gillon, J. and Kupersmith, J. (1979). Electrophysiologic effects of encainide following acute coronary occlusion in dogs. *Pharmacologist*, **21**, 200

Roden, D. M., Reele, S. B., Higgins, S. B., Carr, R. K., Smith, R. F., Oates, J. A. and Woosley, R. L. (1980a). Tocainide therapy for refractory ventricular arrhythmias. *Am. Heart J.*, **101**, 15-22

Roden, D.M., Reele, S.B., Higgins, S.B., Mayol, R.F., Gammans, R.E., Oates, J.A. and Woosley, R. L. (1980b). Total suppression of ventricular arrhythmias by encainide. Pharmacokinetic and electrocardiographic characteristics. *New Engl. J. Med.*, **302**, 877-82

Ronfeld, R. A. M., Wolshin, E. M. and Block, A. J. (1980). Tocainamide and metabolities: human pharmacokinetics and animal pharmacology. *Clin. Pharmac. Ther.*, **27**, 282

Rosen, M. R. and Hoffman, B. F. (1973). Mechanisms of action of antiarrhythmic drugs. *Circulation Res.*, **32**, 1-8

Rosen, M. R., Merker, C., Gelband, H. and Hoffman, B. F. (1973). Effects of procainamide on the electrophysiologic properties of the canine ventricular conducting system. *J. Pharmac. exp. Ther.*, **185**, 438-46

Rosen, M. R., Hoffman, B. F. and Wit, A. L. (1975). Electrophysiology and pharmacology of cardiac arrhythmias. V. Cardiac antiarrhythmic effects of lidocaine. *Am. Heart J.*, **89**, 526-36

Ruffy, R., Rozenshtraukh, L., Elharrar, V. and Zipes, D. P. (1977). Cardiac electrophysiologic properties of ethmozine. *Clin. Res.*, **25**, 557A

Russell, D. C., Smith, H. J. and Oliver, M. F. (1979). Transmembrane potential changes and ventricular fibrillation during repetitive myocardial ischaemia in the dog. *Br. Heart J.*, **42**, 88-96

Ryan, W. R. and Karliner, J. S. (1979). Effects of tocainide on left ventricular performance at rest and during acute alterations in heart rate and systemic arterial pressure. An echocardiographic study. *Br. Heart J.*, **41**, 175-81

Salako, L. A., Vaughan Williams, E. M. and Wittig, J. H. (1976). Investigations to characterise a new antiarrhythmic drug, Org 6001, including a simple test for calcium antagonism. *Br. J. Pharmac.*, **57**, 251-62

Sasyniuk, B. I. and Kus, T. (1974). Comparison of the effects of lidocaine on electrophysiological properties of normal Purkinje fibres and those surviving acute myocardial infarction. *Fedn Proc. Fedn Am. Socs exp. Biol.*, **33**, 476

Schaub, R. G., Stewart, G., Strong, M., Ruotola, R. and Lemole, G. (1977). Reduction of ischemic myocardial damage in the dog by lignocaine infusion. *Am. J. Path.*, **87**, 399-414

Scherlag, B. J., Herfant, R. H., Haft, J. J. and Damato, A. N. (1970). Electrophysiology underlying ventricular arrhythmias due to coronary ligation. *Am. J. Physiol.*, **219**, 1665-71

Scherlag, B. J., Harrison, L. A., Kabell, G., Brachmann, J., Harrison, L. H. and Lazzara, R. (1980). Lidocaine unmasks ventricular arrhythmias in chronic myocardial infarction. *Circulation*, **62**, 111-73

Schmid, J. R., Seeback, B. D., Hennie, C. L., Banitt, E. H. and Kuam, D. C. (1975). Some antiarrhythmic actions of a new compound, R-818, in dogs and mice. *Fedn Proc. Fedn Am. Socs exp. Biol.*, **34**, 775

Seipel, L., Breithardt, G., Both, A. and Loogen, F. (1974). Messung der 'sinuatrialen Leitungszeit' mittels verzeitiger Vorhofstimulation beim Menschen. *Dt. med. Wschr.*, **99**, 1895-900

Seipel, L., Breithardt, G. and Both, A. (1975). Elektrophysiologische Effekte der Antiarrhythmika Disopyramid und Propafenon auf das menschliche Reizleitungssystem. *Z. Kardiol.*, **64**, 731-40

Seipel, L., Abendroth, R. R. and Breithardt, G. (1980). Electrophysiological effects of flecainide R-818 in man. *Circulation*, **62**, 153

Sekiya, A. and Vaughan Williams, E. M. (1963). A comparison of the antifibrillatory actions and effects on intracellular cardiac potentials of pronethalol, disopyramide and quinidine. *Br. J. Pharmac.*, **21**, 473-81

Shenoy, P. N., Ogawa, S., Osmick, M. J. and Dreifus, L. S. (1977). Electrophysiologic effects of ethmozin (EN313), a new antiarrhythmic agent. *Clin. Res.*, **25**, 276A

Singer, D. H., Lazzara, R. and Hoffman, B. F. (1967). Interrelationships between automaticity and conduction in Purkinje fibres. *Circulation Res.*, **21**, 537-58

Singh, B. N. (1977). Side effects of antiarrhythmic drugs. *Pharmac. Ther. C*, **2**, 151-66

Singh, B. N. and Vaughan Williams, E. M. (1970). The effect of amiodarone, a new anti-anginal drug, on cardiac muscle. *Br. J. Pharmac.*, **39**, 657-68

Singh, B. N. and Vaughan Williams, E. M. (1972). Investigations of the mode of action of a new antidysrhythmic drug Kö 1173. *Br. J. Pharmac.*, **44**, 1-9

Somani, P. (1980a). Clinical pharmacology of lorcainide, a new antiarrhythmic drug in patients with cardiac dysrhythmias. *Clin. Res.*, **28**, 590A

Somani, P. (1980b). Antiarrhythmic effects of flecainide. *Clin. Pharmac. Ther.*, **27**, 464-70

Sonnhag, C. (1980). Efficacy and tolerance of tocainide during acute and long-term treatment of chronic ventricular arrhythmias. *Eur. J. clin. Pharmac.*, **18**, 301-10

Southworth, J. L., McKusick, V. A., Peine, E. L. and Rawson, F. L. (1950). Ventricular fibrillation precipitated by cardiac catheterization: complete recovery of patient after 45 mins. *J. Am. med. Assoc.*, **143**, 717-20

Stephenson, S. E., Cole, R. K., Parrish, T. F., Bauer, F. M., Johnson, I. T., Kochtitzky, M., Anderson, J. S., Hibbitt, L. L., McCarty, J. E., Young, E. R., Wilson, J. R., Meiers, H. N., Meador, C. K., Ball, O. T. and McNeely, G. R. (1960). Ventricular fibrillation during and after coronary artery occlusion. Incidence and protection afforded by various drugs. *Am. J. Cardiol.*, **5**, 77-87

Stern, H., Yelnosky, J. and Clark, B. B. (1952). Action of procainamide on ventricular tachycardia produced by coronary artery ligation. *Fedn Proc. Fedn. Am. Socs exp. Biol.*, **11**, 393

Stone, N., Klein, M. D. and Lown, B. (1971). Diphenylhydantoin in the prevention of recurring ventricular tachycardia. *Circulation*, **43**, 420-9

Talbot, R. G., Clark, R. A., Nimmo, J., Neilson, J. M. M., Julian, D. G. and Prescott, L. F. (1973). Treatment of ventricular arrhythmias with mexiletine (Kö-1173). *Lancet*, *ii*, 399-404

Ueda, M., Kimoto, S., Matsuda, S., Kawakami, M., Morishige, E., Matsumura, S. and Takeda, H. (1975). Antiarrhythmic effect of aprindine on several types of ventricular arrhythmias. *Jap. J. Pharmac.*, **25**, 549-61

Vargaftig, B. B., Sugrue, M. F., Buckett, W. R. and Van Riezen, H. (1975). Org 6001 (3α-amino-5α-androstan-2β-ol-17-one hydrochloride) a steroidal anti-arrhythmic agent. *J. Pharm. Pharmac.*, **27**, 697-9

Vaughan Williams, E. M. (1958). The mode of action of quinidine in isolated rabbit atria interpreted from intracellular records. *Br. J. Pharmac. Chemother.*, **13**, 276-87

Vaughan Williams, E. M. (1970). Classifiction of antiarrhythmic drugs. In *Symposium on Cardiac Arrhythmias* (ed. E. Sandoe, E. G. Flensted-Jensen and K. H. Olesen), Astra, Södertälje, pp. 449-72

Vaughan Williams, E. M. (1977). Mexiletine in isolated tissue models. *Postgrad. med. J.*, **53**, 30-4

Vaughan Williams, E. M. (1978). Some factors that influence the activity of anti-arrhythmic drugs. *Br. Heart J.*, **40**, 52-61

Vaughan Williams, E. M. (1979). Characterisation of new antiarrhythmic drugs. *Progr. Pharmac.*, **2**, 13-24

Vaughan Williams, E. M. (1980). *Antiarrhythmic Action and the Puzzle of Perhexilene*, Academic Press, London

Venkataramanan, R. and Axelson, J. E. (1980). Dose-dependent pharmacokinetics of tocainide in the rat. *J. Pharmac. exp. Ther.*, **215**, 231-4

Verdonck, F., Vereecke, J. and Vleugels, A. (1974). Electrophysiological effects of aprindine on isolated heart preparation. *Eur. J. Pharmac.*, **26**, 338-47

Verdouw, P. D., Remme, W. J. and Hugenholtz, P. G. (1977). Cardiovascular and antiarrhythmic effects of aprindine (AC 1802) during partial occlusion of a coronary artery in the pig. *Cardiovasc. Res.*, **11**, 317-23

Verdouw, P. D., Schamhardt, H. C., Remme, W. J. and De Jong, J. W. (1978). Antiarrhythmic, metabolic and haemodynamic effects of Org 6001 (3α-amino-5α-androstan-2β-ol-17-one hydrochloride) after coronary flow reduction in pigs *J. Pharmac. exp. Ther.*, **204**, 634-44

Verdouw, P. D., Deckers, J. W. and Conard, G. J. (1979). Antiarrhythmic and haemodynamic actions of flecainide acetate (R-818) in the ischaemic porcine heart. *J. cardiovasc. Pharmac.*, **1**, 473-86

Vikhliaev, Y. I., Kaverina, N. V., Senova, Z. P. and Vl 'Yanova Ov (1971). Relationship between structure and antiarrhythmic activity in the 10-acyl derivatives of 2-trifluoro-substituted phenothiazine and phenothiazine-2-carbamates. *Farmak. Toksikol.*, **34**, 163-7

Vogel, S., Crampton, R. and Sperelakis, N. (1979). Selective blockade of myocardial slow channels by bepridil (CERM-1978). *J. Pharmac. exp. Ther.*, **210**, 378-85

Wald, R. W., Waxman, M. B. and Downar, E. (1980). The effect of antiarrhythmic drugs on depressed conduction and unidirectional block in sheep Purkinje fibres. *Circulation Res.*, **46**, 612-9

Wallace, A. G., Cline, R. E., Sealy, W. G. and Troyer, W. J. (1966). Electrophysiological effects of quinidine. *Circulation Res.*, **19**, 960-9

Wang, T. and Woosley, R. L. (1980). Contribution of a metabolite to the ECG and antiarrhythmic actions of encainide. *Circulation*, **62**, Suppl. III, 141

Wasenmiller, J. E. and Aronow, W. S. (1980). Effect of tocainide and quinidine on premature ventricular contractions. *Clin. Pharmac. Ther.*, **28**, 431-5

Watanabe, Y., Dreifus, L. S. and Likoff, W. (1963). Electrophysiologic antagonism and synergism of potassium and antiarrhythmic agents. *Am. J. Cardiol.*, **12**, 702-10

Weidmann, S. (1955). Effect of calcium ions and local anaesthetics on electrical properties of Purkinje fibres. *J. Physiol., Lond.*, **129**, 568-82

Weisse, A. B., Moschos, C. B., Passannante, A. J., Khan, M. I. and Regan, T. J. (1971). Relative effectiveness of three antiarrhythmic agents in the treatment of ventricular arrhythmias in experimental acute myocardial ischemia. *Am. Heart J.*, **81**, 503-10

Weld F. M. and Bigger, J. T. (1976). The effect of lidocaine on diastolic transmembrane currents determining pacemaker depolarization in cardiac Purkinje fibres. *Circulation Res.*, **38**, 203-8

Weld, F. M., Bigger, J. R., Swistel, D., Bordiuk, J. and Lau, Y. H. (1979). Electrophysiological effects of mexiletine (Kö 1173) on ovine cardiac Purkinje fibres. *J. Pharmacol. exp. Ther.*, **210**, 222-8

Wenckebach, K. F. (1914). In *Die Unregalmassige Herstatigkeit Undre Ihre Bedeutung* (ed. W. Engellman), Leipzig, p. 124

Wenger, T. L., Masterton, C. E., Abou-Donia, M. B., Lee, K. L., Bache, R. J. and Strauss, H. C. (1978). Relationship between regional myocardial procainamide concentration and regional myocardial blood flow during ischemia in the dog. *Circulation Res.*, **42**, 846-51

West, T. C. and Amory, D. N. (1960). Single fibre recording of the effect of quinidine at atrial and pacemaker sites in the isolated right atrium of the rabbit. *J. Pharmacol. exp. Ther.*, **130**, 183-93

Williams, D. P., Scherlag, B. J., Hope, R. R., El-Sherif, N. and Lazzara, R. (1974). The pathophysiology of malignant ventricular arrhythmias during acute myocardial ischemia. *Circulation*, **50**, 1163-72

Winbury, M. M. and Hemmer, M. L. (1955). Action of quinidine, procaineamide and other compounds on experimental atrial and ventricular arrhythmias in the dog. *J. Pharmacol. exp. Ther.*, **113**, 402-13

Winslow, E. (1980). Evaluation of antagonism of aconitine-induced dysrhythmias in mice as a method of detecting and assessing antidysrhythmic activity. *Br. J. Pharmac.*, **71**, 615-22

Wit, A. L. and Bigger, J. T. (1975). Possible electrophysiological mechanisms for lethal arrhythmias accompanying myocardial ischemia and infarction. *Circulation*, **51**, Suppl. 3, 96–115

Wit, A. L., Rosen, M. R. and Hoffman, B. F. (1974). Electrophysiology and pharmacology of cardiac arrhythmias. II. Relationship of normal and abnormal electrical activity of cardiac fibres to the genesis of arrhythmias. A. Automaticity. *Am. Heart J.*, **86**, 515-24

Wit, A. L., Rosen, M. R. and Hoffman, B. F. (1975). Electrophysiology and pharmacology of cardiac arrhythmias. VIII. Cardiac effects of diphenylhydantoin. *Am. Heart J.*, **90**, 397–404

Wittig, J. H., Harrison, L. A. and Wallace, A. G. (1973). Electrophysiological effects of lidocaine on distal Purkinje fibres of canine heart. *Am. Heart J.*, **86**, 69–78

Woosley, R. L., McDevitt, D. G., Nies, A. S., Smith, R. F., Wilkinson, G. R. and Oates, J. A. (1977). Suppression of ventricular ectopic depolarisations by tocainide. *Circulation*, **56**, 980–4

Yamada, K., Ikeda, N., Goto, J., Okuma, K., Iwamura, N., Toyoshima, H., Toyama, J. and Hanimi, K. (1978). Electrophysiological action of mexiletine on dog Purkinje and papillary muscle fibres studies in both *in vitro* and *in situ* experiments. In *Management of Ventricular Tachycardia - Role of Mexiletine* (ed. E. Sandoe, D. G. Julian and J. W. Bell), Excerpta Medica, Amsterdam, pp. 210-6

Yamaguchi, I., Singh, B. N. and Mandel, W. J. (1978). Electrophysiological effects of mexiletine on isolated cardiac tissue. In *Management of Ventricular Tachycardia - Role of Mexiletine* (ed. E. Sandoe, D. G. Julian and J. W. Bell), Excerpta Medica, Amsterdam, pp. 197-209

Yeh, B. K., Sung, P. K. and Scherlag, B. J. (1973). Effects of disopyramide on electrophysiological and mechanical properties of the heart. *J. pharm. Sci.*, **62**, 1924–9

Yu, P. N. (1979). Disopyramide phosphate (Norpace). A new antiarrhythmic drug. *Circulation*, **59**, 236–7

Zipes, D. P. and Troup, P. J. (1978). New antiarrhythmic agents. *Am. J. Cardiol.*, **41**, 1005-24

Zipes, D. P., Elharrar, V., Noble, R. J., Gaum, W. E., Troup, P. J. and Fasola, A. (1977a). Effects of various drugs on ventricular conduction delay and ventricular arrhythmias during myocardial ischaemia in the dog. In *Re-entrant Arrhythmias. Mechanisms and Treatment* (ed. H. E. Kulbertus), Medical and Technical Press, Lancaster, pp. 312-26

Zipes, D. P., Gaum, W. E., Foster, P. R., Rosen, K. M., Wu, D., Amatyleo, F. and Noble, R. J. (1977b). Aprindine for treatment of supraventricular tachycardias: with particular application of Wolff-Parkinson-White syndrome. *Am. J. Cardiol.*, **40**, 586-96

16

The Effects of β-Adrenoceptor Blocking Drugs on Early Arrhythmias in Experimental and Clinical Myocardial Ischaemia

J. D. Fitzgerald

16.1 INTRODUCTION

In 1842, Erichsen (1842) observed 'tremulation of the ventricles' within 2 min of occlusion by ligation of the main coronary artery of rabbits and dogs. In the subsequent 140 years, the possible factors which determined the onset of ventricular fibrillation following regional ischaemia have been studied in detail. These studies have acquired enhanced clinical relevance within the last 20 years because a large number of deaths in patients with coronary artery disease are sudden, and have been attributed to 'tremulation of the ventricles' or ventricular fibrillation. Sudden death is commonest in patients with extensive coronary artery disease who smoke cigarettes. It is postulated that a transient episode occurs which suddenly alters the electrical stability of the heart, leading to lethal ventricular arrhythmias (Lown and Wolf, 1971). The precise nature and relative importance of the factors precipitating transient electrical instability of the heart, in often symptomless patients with coronary artery disease, is unknown. It is generally believed that catecholamines play an important part in precipitating ventricular fibrillation, and, since the cardiac effects of catecholamines are mediated mainly by activation of β-adrenoceptors, it is clear that the study of specific antagonists of the effect of catecholamines on these adrenoceptors (β-blockers) in clinical and experimental myocardial ischaemia may clarify the role of catecholamines as a cause of sudden death.

The involvement of catecholamines and the sympathetic nervous system in the genesis of ischaemic arrhythmias is based on a variety of experimental and clinical observations. Catecholamines enhance myocardial excitability (Hoffman and Singer, 1967) and elicit arrhythmias in dogs recovering from experimental myocardial infarction (Maling and Moran, 1957). Neural activity of the efferent sympathetic nervous system increases within 5 min of coronary occlusion in the cat, although this increase is not uniform (Gillis, 1971). Electrical stimulation of either the left stellate ganglion or the higher sympathetic centres within the hypothalamus of the dog causes ventricular fibrillation if the anterior descending coronary artery is occluded, but this does not occur in the absence of occlusion (Verrier *et al.*, 1975; Schwartz *et al.*, 1976). Furthermore, chronic surgical denervation of the heart reduces the incidence of ventricular fibrillation following coronary occlusion, although acute neural ablation or bilateral stellate ganglionectomy does not (Ebert *et al.*, 1970). Additionally, catecholamine levels are elevated in the plasma following experimental (Stazewska-Barczak and Ceremuzynski, 1968) and also clinical myocardial infarction (Richardson, 1963). These studies provide strong circumstantial evidence that there is increased sympathetic activity during acute myocardial ischaemia and that catecholamines may play a major role in promoting electrical instability of the ischaemic myocardium. If this hypothesis is correct, effective blockade of the cardiac actions of catecholamines by β-adrenoceptor blocking drugs should prevent serious ventricular arrhythmias and reduce mortality associated with acute myocardial ischaemia. This paper will summarise the results of experimental and clinical studies designed to test this hypothesis.

16.2 STUDIES IN ANIMALS

Experimental design

The widely different protocols used in studies designed to examine the effects of β-blockers in myocardial ischaemia makes it difficult to form a clear view as to their efficacy in preventing serious ventricular arrhythmias. Some of the experimental variables are listed in table 16.1. The factors of particular importance are the animal species, the use of anaesthesia, the site of experimental occlusion and the relationship between onset of occlusion and time of drug administration. In addition, the criteria used to assess the efficacy of the intervention include alterations in ventricular fibrillation threshold, the incidence and type of ventricular arrhythmia, the time to, and incidence of, ventricular fibrillation and survival following occlusion. Since the hypothesis is that catecholamine release associated with acute myocardial ischaemia leads to lethal arrhythmias, only studies of the effects of β-blockers administered within 6 h of coronary occlusion will be reviewed. In the majority of studies, the species used has been the dog and the β-blocker used has been propranolol.

Studies in dogs

Effects of β-blocking drugs on the ventricular fibrillation threshold

Stimulation of either the cardiac sympathetic nerves or the posterior hypothalamus in the dog reduces the ventricular fibrillation threshold (VFT). This reduction is

Table 16.1 Factors influencing the outcome of experimental studies of β-blockers in myocardial ischaemia

Variable	Example
Species	Cat Pig Dog Rat
Experimental conditions	Anaesthesia Conscious – stressed conditions
Anatomical	Site of occlusion Extent of collateral circulation Extent of infarction
Drug	Type and dose of β-blocker
Criteria	Fibrillation threshold Incidence and type of arrhythmia Time to (latency) and incidence of fibrillation Survival

prevented by prior administration of propranolol. Furthermore, aversive conditioning of dogs reduces the VFT and this reduction is also prevented by pretreatment with β-blockers such as tolamolol (Matta *et al.*, 1976; Lown *et al.*, 1977).

The current required to induce ventricular fibrillation is reduced 50-fold within 3 min of acute coronary occlusion in dogs. Pretreatment of dogs with propranolol not only elevates the fibrillation threshold prior to ischaemia but prevents the reduction in threshold during ischaemia (Corbalan *et al.*, 1976). This is illustrated in figure 16.1. These studies establish that β-blockade by practolol, tolamolol or propranolol will prevent the reduction in fibrillation threshold induced by stress, sympathetic nerve stimulation or acute myocardial ischaemia.

Effects of β-blockers on arrhythmias and survival

There are numerous reports concerning the effects of β-adrenoceptor blockers on the functional, electrophysiological and morphological changes in the heart following acute myocardial ischaemia (Fitzgerald, 1972). Propranolol reduces the area of myocardial necrosis and associated electrocardiographic abnormalities as well as partially reversing depressed regional contractility (Higginson *et al.*, 1977; Vatner *et al.*, 1977). Such studies have not been designed specifically to assess the effects of β-blockers on ventricular arrhythmias and survival. There are 23 reports (table 16.2) concerning the effects of six different β-blocking drugs on cardiac arrhythmias and survival within 6 h of ischaemia in conscious or anaesthetised dogs. The majority of reports concern propranolol or practolol, and only four studies involve assessment in conscious dogs. The conclusion from such studies is that β-adrenoceptor blockade will (1) increase the time (latency) to ventricular tachycardia (Rosenfeld *et al.*, 1978); (2) reduce the incidence of arrhythmias

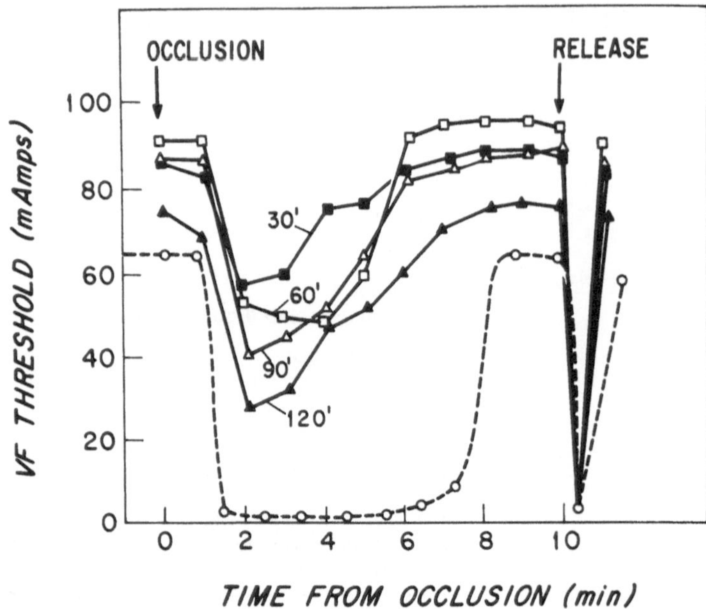

Figure 16.1 Effect of propranolol-induced β-adrenoceptor blockade on the VF threshold changes associated with coronary artery occlusions and release in 11 dogs. The number beside each curve refers to the time following drug administration. The dashed line depicts the pattern of threshold changes observed during the initial occlusion in untreated dogs. Propranolol administration increased the VF threshold by 64 per cent with the coronary circulation intact and significantly diminished the decrease in fibrillation threshold during coronary occlusion. This drug, however, was without effect on the threshold changes associated with release of occlusion.

(Khan *et al.*, 1972); (3) improve survival (Evans *et al.*, 1976). The study by Menken *et al.* (1979) provides an excellent example of the effect of β-adrenoceptor blockers in acute myocardial infarction in dogs. Dogs were pretreated for 5 days with either 2.0 or 10.5 mg kg^{-1} of atenolol given orally. The circumflex coronary artery was then ligated under urethane-chloralose anaesthesia; dogs with significant collateral circulation were excluded from the study. In this model, cardiac arrhytimias occurred either at 3-7 min (phase 1a) or 15-28 min (phase 1b) and all control dogs died from ventricular fibrillation within 30 min. Pretreatment with oral atenolol reduced the incidence of ventricular arrhythmias in phase 1a and had a dramatic effect on survival in that only two of 12 dogs died, whereas all 19 control dogs died. Plasma levels of atenolol were measured at the time of ligation and survival was associated with plasma levels of about 300 ng ml^{-1}, whereas dogs with levels of about 150 ng ml^{-1} did not survive. The effect of ischaemia on VFT was also determined and atenolol raised the control threshold level and prevented the rapid fall associated with ischaemia (see chapter 9, and especially figure 9.1).

Certain studies with propranolol have, however, failed to demonstrate a beneficial effect (table 16.3). Pentecost and Austen (1966) observed that propranolol

Table 16.2 References to studies of the effects of different β-blockers on arrhythmias and survival in dogs

Propranolol

1. Ceremuzynski *et al.* (1969)
2. Evans *et al.* (1976)
3. Fearon (1967)
4. Higginson *et al.* (1977)
5. Hope *et al.* (1974)
6. Khan *et al.* (1972)
7. Kupersmith *et al.* (1976)
8. Lown and Wolf (1971)
9. Pearle *et al.* (1978)
10. Peter *et al.* (1978)
11. Pentecost and Austen (1966)
12. Proger and Naimi (1966)
13. Reimer *et al.* (1973)
14. Reynolds *et al.* (1978)
15. Shuster *et al.* (1973)
16. Sommers (1966)

Practolol

1. Harris *et al.* (1975)
2. Khan *et al.* (1972)
3. Lown and Wolf (1971)
4. Sethi *et al.* (1973)
5. Stephan and Meesmann (1974)
6. Szekeres (1978)

Sotalol

1. Khan *et al.* (1972)
2. Kaumann and Aramendia (1968)

Nadolol

1. Evans *et al.* (1976)

Tolamolol

1. Rosenfeld *et al.* (1978)

Atenolol

1. Menken *et al.* (1979)

(0.2 mg kg^{-1}) did not significantly increase survival in anaesthetised dogs following an acute occlusion of the anterior descending coronary artery, though there was a reduced incidence of ventricular fibrillation. A lower dose of propranolol (0.08 mg kg^{-1}) did improve survival significantly in another group of dogs. Khan *et al.* (1972) observed that although a lower dose of propranolol (0.1 mg kg^{-1}) reduced

Table 16.3 Summary of studies in dogs in which propranolol was ineffective

Authors	Drug (mg kg^{-1})	Result (% survivors)
Pearle *et al.* (1978)	Practolol (1.5–2.5)	70*
	Propranolol (0.5)	15
	Control	15
Pentecost and Austen (1966)	Propranolol (0.08)	83
	Propranolol (0.2)	50*
	Control	85
Khan *et al.* (1972)	Propranolol (1.0)	20*
	Propranolol (0.1)	72
	Control	84

*Significantly different from control.

mortality from 84 to 24 per cent in conscious dogs following balloon occlusion of the circumflex coronary artery, a higher dose of propranolol (1.0 mg kg^{-1}) did not. The incidence of ventricular arrhythmias was reduced in both groups. Pearle *et al.* (1978) compared the effects of propranolol (0.25 mg kg^{-1}) with practolol (1.25–2.5 mg kg^{-1}) on survival in anaesthetised vagotomised dogs. Only one of the seven practolol-treated dogs died whereas six of seven propranolol and saline-treated dogs died. In a brief communication Proger and Nami (1966) also state that propranolol did not improve survival in anaesthetised dogs.

There is no obvious explanation for these negative findings. The lack of effect of higher doses of propranolol has not been confirmed in other studies using either anaesthetised or conscious dogs. For example, Shuster *et al.* (1973) found that propranolol (5 mg kg^{-1} by infusion over 10 min) prevented the development of ventricular fibrillation whilst 50 per cent of the animals in the control series fibrillated. The non-selective β-blockers sotalol (Kaumann and Aramendia, 1968) and nadalol (Evans *et al.*, 1976) improve survival following acute ischaemia. Further studies are required before concluding that cardioselective β-blockers are more efficacious than non-selective β-blockers in preventing ventricular fibrillation and death following acute coronary occlusion in the dog.

Studies in pigs

The effect of β-adrenoceptor blocking drugs on the incidence of arrhythmias and on survival following occlusion of the coronary artery in pigs is not clearly defined. Morris *et al.* (1967) observed that propranolol (0.2 mg kg^{-1}) prolonged survival in pigs following gradual occlusion of the anterior descending coronary artery by an ameroid constrictor. The control group survived for 28 h whereas the propranolol-treated group survived for 49 h. Skinner *et al.* (1975) have evaluated the effects of propranolol following occlusion of the LAD coronary artery in normal conscious pigs. They also examined the effects of psychological stress. Coronary occlusion in the conscious pig causes a variety of ventricular arrhythmias resembling those observed in the dog. Furthermore, they also observed two distinct periods of arrhythmia, period 1a occurring 1-4 min after occlusion followed by a quiescent period and then period 2a from 9 to 14 min after occlusion. The effect of stress and β-blockade was assessed on the basis of ventricular fibrillation latency (VFL), which is the time taken for fibrillation to develop from the onset of occlusion. The VFL in the control animals ranges from 10 to 13 min. Propranolol (2 mg kg^{-1} i.v.) caused a significant reduction in the time to fibrillation, whereas a lower dose of propranolol (0.2 mg kg^{-1}) and D-propranolol (2 mg kg^{-1}) had no effect. When pigs were adapted to the laboratory conditions the VFL increased, so that in fully adapted pigs it did not occur within the 20 min period of occlusion. When these 'laboratory-adapted pigs' were pretreated with propranolol and then underwent occlusion, the ventricular fibrillation latency was reduced from control levels. The authors conclude that β-blockade with propranolol has a deleterious effect on the VFL in normal and adapted pigs.

The situation is made more complex by the results of Muller and Opie (1980) who have compared the effects of sotalol (10 mg kg^{-1} i.v.) and metoprolol (10 mg kg^{-1}) 30 min prior to ligation of the LAD coronary artery in anaesthetised open-chest pigs. They observe that sotalol significantly reduced the duration of ventricular tachycardia (VT) from 103 s in control to 0.2 s in the treated group, whereas metoprolol did not significantly reduce it (25.9 s). However, 13 of 16 control pigs developed ventricular fibrillation, as did all six pigs in the sotalol-treated group, whereas only two of 13 pigs developed fibrillation in the metoprolol-treated group. They conclude that sotalol reduced the incidence of VT but that metoprolol significantly reduced the incidence of VF. The inference from this paper is that cardioselective antagonism by metoprolol provides greater protection against ventricular fibrillation than non-selective blockade. It should be noted that the metoprolol group received an additional dose of drug 20 min after ligation but the sotalol group did not.

Because the experimental protocols differ so greatly in the studies reported, it is not possible to draw a general conclusion as to the effect of β-adrenoceptor blockers on arrhythmias and survival during acute ischaemia in the pig.

Studies in cats

There are four reports of the effects of β-blockers on experimental ischaemia in cats. Corr and Gillis (1975) showed that propranolol reduced the incidence of ventricular arrhythmias but did not significantly alter the incidence of VF. A similar lack of effect of propranolol on ventricular fibrillation has been confirmed by others (Corr *et al.*, 1978; Sheridan *et al.*, 1980). In contrast Kelliher *et al.* (1975) showed that practolol significantly reduced the incidence of VF following coronary ligation in anaesthetised cats. The inference is that propranolol, whilst reducing the incidence of ventricular arrhythmias, does not affect VF or mortality, whereas practolol may differ from propranolol and be more effective in improving survival in cats. It has been speculated that the differing pharmacological and haemodynamic profiles of propanolol and practolol may account for these differences (Corr and Gillis, 1978). The evidence to support this speculation is insubstantial at present.

The elegant study of ischaemia-induced arrhythmias in cats by Corr *et al.* (1978) demonstrated a relationship between VF and elevation of cyclic AMP (cAMP) levels in normal and ischaemic myocardium. In this preparation, propranolol did not reduce the rise in cAMP, though it did reduce the disparity in tissue levels of cAMP between normal and ischaemic tissue in those animals which did not develop VF. Such observations suggest that either blockade of the β-receptors was incomplete (the dose of propranolol was 0.75 mg kg^{-1}) or alternative non-adrenergic factors are responsible for the rise in tissue cAMP levels in ischaemic tissue. The role of elevated tissue cAMP levels in promoting VF remains controversial since ventricular fibrillation has been observed in ischaemic hearts without a concomitant rise in cAMP concentrations. This has been discussed by Podzuweit in chapter 11. It may be concluded from these various studies that the effect of β-blockers on the incidence of arrhythmias and survival following acute ischaemia in cats is unpredictable, and that although β-blockers may reduce the incidence of arrhythmias, their effect on survival is uncertain.

Studies in rats

The effects of β-blockers on myocardial ischaemia in the rat heart have been examined both *in vitro* and *in vivo*. In the isolated perfused rat heart model, Lubbe *et al.* (1978) showed that adrenaline lowered the VFT and raised tissue cAMP levels. These effects were prevented by adding atenolol (38 μmol l^{-1}) to the perfusate. Following ligation of the left coronary artery in the same preparation, there was a sudden fall in VFT from 8.0 to 1.2 mA and this was accompanied by a significant rise in cAMP in the ischaemic tissue. Atenolol (700 μmol l^{-1}) and sotalol did not prevent the fall in VFT or the accompanying rise in tissue cAMP. In surprising contrast, racemic propranolol and both the D and L isomers (24 μmol l^{-1}) significantly prevented the reduction in VFT and the rise in tissue cAMP. The observation that atenolol and sotalol were ineffective in this model of ischaemia could be explained by their lack of membrane-stabilising properties (Fitzgerald, 1969). Lignocaine is not effective in this model either, so that the effectiveness of the isomers of propranolol must be attributed to some unusual action associated with these molecules. One possibility is that the isomers of propranolol are inhibiting the membrane transport of calcium. Elevated levels of intracellular calcium have a direct effect in increasing cAMP concentrations by an effect unrelated to activation of β-adrenoceptors. It may be that the enhanced cellular entry of calcium during ischaemia is prevented by propranolol and its isomers but not by atenolol and sotalol. In general these *in vitro* studies do not provide much evidence as to what β-blockers might do in acute myocardial ischaemia *in vivo*.

Acute ligation of the left coronary artery (LCA) in rats causes a predictable pattern of ventricular arrhythmias, ventricular fibrillation and death in about 60 per cent of animals (Kenedi and Losonci, 1973). The effects of various β-adrenoceptor blockers in this model have been assessed by Kane *et al.* (1979), Campbell and Parratt (1981) and Szekeres and coworkers (Szekeres, 1978; Siegmund *et al.*, 1979). In the study by Campbell and Parratt (1981) the effects of propranolol and practolol and its isomers were assessed in terms of their effect on the incidence and duration of ventricular ectopic beats (VEBs), ventricular tachycardia (VT) and ventricular fibrillation (VF) in the first 30 min after acute occlusion of the left coronary artery in pentobarbitone-anaesthetised animals. The assessment of efficacy depends upon which of these variables is selected. The authors conclude that membrane-stabilising activity is not important, yet show that D-oxprenolol (1 mg kg^{-1}) reduced significantly the incidence of VF from 69 to 22 per cent, and a similar effect on incidence of VF was observed with practolol (5 mg kg^{-1}). Propranolol (5 mg kg^{-1}) prevented the development of VF but had no effect on the incidence of VT. The interpretation of these experiments therefore would depend on the relative importance attached to these various arrhythmias.

The effects of prolonged pretreatment with β-blockers has also been studied. Szekeres (1978) demonstrated that pindolol (4 mg kg^{-1} daily for 14 days) reduced mortality in conscious rats, undergoing acute ligation of the coronary artery, from 74 to 40 per cent. In an analogous study Parratt *et al.* (1981) administered two differing doses of oxprenolol (2 and 50 mg b.d. for 6 weeks). The higher dose of oxprenolol markedly reduced the incidence and duration of VF and VT following ligation of the LCA in acutely anaesthetised rats.

These various studies indicate clearly that β-adrenoceptor blocking drugs given in appropriate doses will have a salutary effect on the consequences of occlusion of the left coronary artery in rats.

16.3 CLINICAL STUDIES

There are serious logistic difficulties in attempting the evaluation of the effects of β-blockers on the incidence of arrhythmias during the early phase of myocardial ischaemia in man. Two approaches have been used: first, the administration of β-blockers as soon as the patient presents with diagnostic symptoms, that is, early intervention studies; secondly, the examination of the effects of β-blockers in a population of patients who have recovered from an initial myocardial infarction but have a high risk of developing a subsequent myocardial infarction, that is, secondary prevention studies.

Early intervention studies

The effects of β-blockers on arrhythmias associated with myocardial ischaemia have been studied in all the phases of myocardial infarction including pre-hospital, coronary care, late hospital and ambulatory. Predictably there have been very few studies examining the effects of β-adrenoceptor blocking drugs on arrhythmias within the first 6 h of myocardial infarction. There have been no studies in man which replicate precisely the animal experimental studies in which the drugs have been given in the period immediately before the onset of acute regional myocardial ischaemia. In order to ensure that the onset of effect of the drugs is obtained as soon as possible within this 6 h period, it is essential to give the agent intravenously. This is particularly important in the early phase of acute myocardial infarction since it has been observed that plasma levels following oral propranolol at this time are suboptimal (Peter *et al.*, 1978). Understandably, there has been a reluctance to administer β-blockers intravenously during this acute phase because early experience with propranolol by this route showed that it could cause hypotension and bradycardia. However, with greater understanding and experience, it is now possible to select patients appropriately so that the drugs can be administered during this phase.

Rossi *et al.* (1981) have compared the effects of atenolol (5 mg i.v.) or placebo in 70 patients admitted to a coronary care unit within 12 h of the onset of chest pain. Patients were randomly allocated to either treatment or placebo group. There was a significant reduction in the total number of hours during which R on T ventricular ectopic beats were observed, and also the rate of VT was reduced from a mean of 171 to 142 beats min^{-1}. In addition, there was a reduction in the incidence of ventricular ectopic beats in the first 12 h of observation, but not over the whole 24 h period. The authors conclude that atenolol caused a reduction in the rate of VT and in the incidence of R on T ventricular ectopic beats, and also had some effect on other ectopic beats. In the study by Ahumada *et al.* (1979) the effects of acebutolol (1-20 mg i.v. 4 hourly) was examined in 22 patients; there were 22 controls. Acebutolol was given 6 h after the first rise in creatine phosphokinase (CPK), so this study does not strictly meet the requirement of intervention within 6 h of the onset of symptoms of acute myocardial infarction. The authors report a reduction in ventricular extrasystoles and complex ventricular arrhythmias due to acebutolol.

In the study by Andersen *et al.* (1979) alprenolol (10 mg intravenously) was given followed by 200 mg orally twice daily for a year. Of the 282 patients under 65 years of age, there was a significant reduction in mortality at 1 year from 28 to 15 per cent. Unfortunately, this paper makes no reference to the incidence of cardiac arrhythmias within 24 h, although, since electrocardiographic recordings were taken daily, the data is presumably available for analysis.

It is clear that despite intensive study for many years there remains a major gap in our knowledge concerning the effects of early intervention with β-blockers on the incidence of arrhythmias in acute myocardial infarction. There are two current early intervention studies examining the effects of atenolol and metoprolol in this setting, and these studies may provide an answer to this problem (see Addendum).

Secondary prevention studies

The alternative method used to assess the effects of β-blockers on the consequences of acute myocardial ischaemia is to administer the drug chronically to subjects likely to experience an acute myocardial infarction. Such studies are termed secondary prevention because the only way to select an infarction-prone population is to administer the agent to survivors of an initial myocardial infarction. There have been numerous studies in which β-blockers have been given, during either the pre-infarction or the post-infarction period, for various lengths of time under differing conditions. There have only been five double blind randomised secondary prevention trials on the effect of these drugs on mortality and on the rate of re-infarction in survivors of an initial myocardial infarction in which trial designs have met the necessary criteria. The drugs which have been studied are alprenolol (two studies), practolol, propranolol and timolol. A detailed discussion of these trials would require a separate review, so only a critical summary of the results will be given. In order to do so it is also necessary to state the criteria which should be met in the trial design. As successive trials are published, the trial design pundits forge ever more demanding criteria, this activity having reached its apogee in the recent critical appraisal of the timolol trial (Mitchell, 1981). This appraisal has been described as a mixture of classical therapeutic nihilism topped by a combination of arrogant assumption and charming naivity. Certainly a pragmatic balance ought to be struck between therapeutic nihilism and uncritical acceptance when assessing results of trials.

In appraising the design of clinical trials attention should be paid to the following points:

(1) The characterisation of the total patient population for which the trial group was selected should be considered so that the general applicability of the results can be assessed.

(2) The number of patients initially randomised to each group should be known.

(3) What is the total number of patients who continue treatment and also the total number who stopped treatment?

(4) What is the fate of all patients initially randomised, irrespective of the treatment status?

(5) Neither prospective nor retrospective sub-group stratification for analysis is permissable. Such data may only be used to define questions to be answered by a separate trial.

(6) The end-points must be easily measurable. Thus mortality is preferred as an end-point rather than sudden death or re-infarction because of the problems in accurate diagnosis with the latter. There is argument as to whether total mortality is the only acceptable criterion or whether disease-specific mortality is acceptable as an end-point.

(7) The treatment and control groups should be comparable with respect to a number of variables, including age, sex, disease state, concomitant disease and severity of coronary artery disease (including the number of incidents of heart failure and arrhythmias), as well as the number of patients with hypertension and the nature of current or previous therapy. In addition, the timing of initiation of treatment and proof that the withdrawal pattern is similar in both groups is required. Finally, data on social habits such as smoking, drinking and exercise are important.

The final interpretation of trials results can best be left to the physician as long as the results are viewed in the light of the above criteria. In the studies to be described it should be noted that β-blocking therapy was started more than 1 week after the initial infarction.

Studies with alprenolol

In the initial assessment of alprenolol on mortality and morbidity, 230 patients were selected and given either placebo or alprenolol, 400 mg daily, commencing 6 or more weeks after the initial infarction and continuing for 2 years (Wilhelmsson *et al.*, 1974). In this trial no difference in the total mortality or re-infarction rate was observed but there was a statistically significant reduction in sudden death (three of 106 patients on alprenolol versus 11 of 108 on placebo). This latter result was obtained by retrospective analysis.

In a more recent study by Andersen *et al.* (1979) the effects of alprenolol, given as early as possible, to suspected infarction cases was reported. The total number of patients studied was 480 and they received either placebo or alprenolol (5–10 mg i.v.) on admission, followed by 400 mg daily for 2 years. In this trial about 50 per cent of the patients received the first dose within 6 h of the onset of symptoms. There was no difference in total mortality but there was a significant difference in patients under 65 years of age who had been prospectively stratified by age, in that the death rates were 13 of 140 patients on alprenolol versus 29 of 142 patients on placebo. In contrast, those over 65 years of age did less well in that the death rates for the group as a whole were 61 on alprenolol and 64 on placebo, which is not significantly different. The results of these two studies are regarded by many as equivocal (Hampton, 1981), though others accept them as evidence of a beneficial effect of alprenolol (Chamberlain, 1978).

The effects of alprenolol treatment on infarct size in the under 65 age group were also determined and published in a separate study (Jurgensen *et al.*, 1981). The results show that infarct size, as determined by serial creatine phosphokinase (CPK) determinations, was reduced by alprenolol; the infarct size in the control group was 34.4 CK-equiv m^{-2} body surface compared with 20.6 CK g-equiv m^{-2} for the alprenolol group. Unfortunately no information was given on the incidence of arrhythmias during the early phase of infarction in this study.

Studies with propranolol

Following the initial claim by Snow (1965) that propranolol (30–60 mg daily) reduced in-hospital mortality in patients with acute myocardial infarction, seven further studies were carried out to assess the effects of propranolol (40–160 mg daily) given 24–48 h after onset of symptoms. There was a 1 month follow-up period and no significant reduction in mortality was detected. A further study was reported by Mitchell and his colleagues (Wilcox *et al.*, 1980) in which propranolol (120 mg daily) was given within 6–12 h of chest pain and the 88 patients followed for 1 year; no beneficial effect was observed.

Propranolol has also been investigated in two multicentre studies (Baber *et al.*,

1980), one a double-blind study involving 720 patients and the second an open study comprising 501 patients. The subjects were those who had recovered from an acute myocardial infarction and had been placed on propranolol, 40 mg three times a day commencing 2–14 days after infarction. The patients were observed for a mean period of 9 months and no reduction in total mortality or re-infarction rate was detected.

Studies with practolol

A large late entry (mean 13 days post-infarction) study of practolol was reported in 1975 (Multicentre International Study, 1977). A total of 3053 patients were given placebo or practolol (200 mg b.d.) and followed for 2 years, the end-points being mortality and non-fatal re-infarction. If the criteria of total deaths as opposed to disease specific deaths is used then there was not a significant difference between treatment and control groups. There was, however, a highly significant reduction in sudden death (48 versus 78; $P < 0.01$) and especially in patients with an anterior myocardial infarction (23 versus 50; $P < 0.01$). These latter results were obtained by retrospective analysis and have therefore been criticised by some as biased (Hampton, 1981), although accepted by others (Chamberlain, 1978). In an earlier study Barber *et al.* (1976) gave practolol (300 mg daily) or placebo to 500 patients within 12 h of the onset of chest pain and found no difference in morbidity over the 2 year follow-up period. The general point worth emphasising is that β-blockers given orally within 48 h of myocardial infarction may be inadequately absorbed (Peter *et al.*, 1978). In addition, long term studies involving small groups of post-infarction patients are less likely to show an effect, although the negative practolol results in the study by Barber *et al.* (1976) are in contrast to those with alprenolol, even though both groups contained less than 1000 patients.

Studies with timolol

The results of a large Norwegian multicentre post-infarction study (Norwegian Multicenter Study Group, 1981) have been reported in which timolol (10 mg b.d.) was given to 945 patients and compared with 939 receiving placebo. Treatment commenced 28 days after infarction and the mean follow-up time was 17 months. There were 152 deaths on placebo and 98 on timolol. The accumulative sudden death rate was 13.9 per cent on placebo versus 7.7 per cent on timolol ($P < 0.0001$). At face value these results are very impressive and one annotation contains the comments '. . . an excellent study with a splendid result' (*Lancet*, 1981).

An alternative view has been stated suggesting that the trial is lacking in performance on the following grounds:

(1) There is a lack of information on the timing of onset of infarction in relation to the timing of diagnosis.

(2) There is a lack of information on the fate of the 6970 non-infarct patients which comprise the balance from the original total of 11 125 suspected infarct subjects.

(3) There is a lack of comparability between the two groups in that the placebo group contained (a) older patients (61.4 versus 60.3 years of age); (b) more hypertensive subjects (22 versus 18); (c) more patients having had previous diuretic treatment (23 versus 18); (d) more incidence of heart failure (34 versus 32) (e) more cases of cardiomegaly (23 versus 21); (f) more arrhythmias during the index event (43 versus 36). The authors of the article claim that these differences, using the Cox model for unevenly distributed variables, do not alter the conclusion of the trial, but obviously one annotator chooses not to accept the Cox model because it cannot take account of any hidden imbalance between the groups. There is, therefore, a difference of view as to whether the groups at entry were evenly balanced or not.

(4) There is a lack of data on survival patterns between smokers and non-smokers.

It is unlikely that many of these desiderata will be forthcoming, and a view is required on the data published, bearing in mind the imperfections listed above. The issue revolves around two factors:

(1) Could the results have been arrived at by chance? A balanced, experienced pragmatic view must be that the difference between timolol treatment and placebo treatment could not be due to a 1 : 1000 chance.

(2) Could the difference be due to patient selection, such that the treatment group inherently had a better prognosis than the placebo group, irrespective of the therapeutic intervention? Again, it seems more than probable that the groups are comparable and that the differences can be attributed to timolol treatment. Until a further and more detailed report is published, the provisional and incomplete conclusion is that timolol reduces mortality in post-infarction patients.

There are now clinical trials in progress to study the effects of propranolol, oxprenolol, sotalol, pindolol, acebutolol and metoprolol on survival following acute myocardial infarction (table 16.4; Vedin and Wilhelmsson, 1979). Clearly the results of these studies are awaited with great interest, but undoubtedly they will all be lacking in one way or another in design performance. It is likely that the influence of β-blockers on survival following myocardial infarction will continue to be debated for years to come (see Addendum).

16.4 SUMMARY

The effects of β-adrenoceptor blocking drugs on early arrhythmias in experimental and clinical myocardial infarction have been reviewed. In the experimental studies, comparison is difficult because of major differences in protocol design. However, it is apparent that these drugs reduce or prevent arrhythmias secondary to acute myocardial infarction in the rat and dog, although effects in the cat and pig are less

Table 16.4 Summary of on-going studies of β-blockers in secondary prevention studies

Centre	Compound	Number of patients	Prognostic stratification	Acute i.v. injection
Multicentre, France	Acebutolol	550	–	–
Stockholm, Sweden	Metoprolol	250	+	–
Amsterdam, Netherlands	Metoprolol	500	+	–
Gothenberg, Sweden	Metoprolol	600	+	+
Multicentre, USA	Metoprolol	3 000	–	–
Multicentre, UK	Oxprenolol	1 100	–	–
Multicentre, Germany	Oxprenolol	4 000	–	–
Multicentre, Sweden–Australia	Pindolol	500	–	–
Multicentre, UK	Propranolol	500	–	–
Multicentre, USA	Propranolol	4 200	–	–
Oslo, Norway	Propranolol	500	–	–
Multicentre, northern England	Sotalol	1 600	–	–
Total		17 300		

clear. In man, it has been shown that the administration of β-blockers intravenously within the first 6 h of myocardial infarction reduces the incidence of arrhythmias and infarct size, but that the effect on long term survival is unknown. In comparison, the long term secondary prevention studies have provided conflicting results; propranolol has not been shown to be effective but practolol and alprenolol may reduce mortality, although the trial protocols have been severely criticised. The recent study with timolol shows a highly significant reduction in mortality in the treatment group but the final judgement on this trial awaits publication of further details.

REFERENCES

Ahumada, G. G., Karlsberg, R. P., Jaffe, A. S., Ambos, H. D., Sobel, B. E. and Roberts, R. (1979). Reduction in early ventricular arrhythmias by acebutolol in patients with acute myocardial infarction. *Br. Heart J.*, **41**, 654–9

Andersen, M. P., Frederikson, J., Jurgensen, H. J., Pedersen, F., Bechsgoord, P., Hansen, D. A., Neilsen, B., Pedersen-Bjergaard, O. and Rasmussen, S. L. (1979). Effect of alprenolol on mortality among patients with definite and suspected acute myocardial infarction: preliminary results. *Lancet*, *ii*, 865–7

Baber, M. S., Evans, D. W., Howitt, G., Thomas, M. and Wilson, C. (1980). Two multicentre propranolol post-infarction trials in 84 hospitals in the United Kingdom, Italy and Yugoslavia. *Br. Heart J.*, **44**, 96-100

Barber, J. M., Boyle, D. C., Chaturvedi, H. C., Singh, N. and Walsh, M. J. (1976). Practolol in acute myocardial infarction. *Acta. med. scand.*, **587**, 213-6

Ceremuzynski, L., Staszewska-Barczak, J. and Herbaczynska-Cedro, K. (1969). Cardiac rhythm disturbances and the release of catecholamines after acute coronary occlusion in dogs. *Cardiovasc. Res.*, **3**, 190-7

Campbell, C. A. and Parratt, J. R. (1981). Which properties of beta-adrenoceptor blocking drugs are important in the prevention of early post-infarction dysrhythmias? *Br. J. Pharmac.*, **74**, 195-6P

Chamberlain, D. A. (1978). Beta-adrenergic blocking agents in prevention of sudden death. *Adv. Cardiol.*, **25**, 196-205

Corbalan, R., Verrier, R. L. and Lown, B. (1976). Differing mechanisms for ventricular vulnerability during coronary artery occlusion and release. *Am. Heart J.*, **92**, 223-30

Corr, P. D. and Gillis, R. A. (1975). Effect of autonomic neural influences on the cardiovascular changes induced by coronary occlusion. *Am. Heart J.*, **89**, 766-74

Corr, P. D. and Gillis, R. A. (1978). Autonomic neural influences on the dysrhythmias resulting from myocardial infarction. *Circulation Res.*, **43**, 1-9

Corr, P. D., Witkowski, F. X. and Sobel, B. E. (1978). Mechanisms contributing to malignant dysrhythmias induced by ischemia in the cat. *J. clin. Invest.*, **61**, 109-19

Ebert, P. A., Vanderbee, R. B., Allgood, R. J. and Sabiston, D. C. (1970). Effect of chronic denervation on arrhythmias after coronary artery ligation. *Cardiovasc. Res.*, **4**, 141-7

Erichsen, J. E. (1842). On the influence of the coronary circulation on the action of the heart. *London med. Gaz.*, **30**, 561-9

Evans, D. E., Peschka, M. T., Leigh, R. J. and Laffan, R. J. (1976). Antiarrhythmic action of nadolol, a beta-adrenergic receptor blocking agent. *Eur. J. Pharmac.*, **35**, 17-27

Fearon, R. E. (1967). Propranolol in the prevention of ventricular fibrillation due to experimental coronary artery occlusion. *Am. J. Cardiol.*, **20**, 222-8

Fitzgerald, J. D. (1969). Perspectives in adrenergic beta-receptor blockade. *Clin. Pharmac. Ther.*, **10**, 292-306

Fitzgerald, J. D. (1972). The role of beta-adrenergic blockade in acute myocardial ischaemia. In *Effect of Acute Ischaemia on Myocardial Function* (ed. M. F. Oliver, D. G. Julian and K. W. Donald), Churchill Livingstone, Edinburgh, pp. 321-51

Gillis, R. A. (1971). Role of the nervous system in the arrhythmias produced by coronary occlusion in the cat. *Am. Heart J.*, **81**, 677-84

Hampton, J. R. (1981). Presentation and analysis of the result of clinical trials in cardiovascular disease. *Br. med. J.*, **282**, 1371-73

Harris, A. S., Bochae, F. J. and Otero, H. (1975). Role of sympathetic excitation in generating arrhythmias in early and late phases of ectopic responses after coronary artery occlusion in dog heart. In *Recent Advances in Studies on Cardiac Structure and Metabolism*, Vol. V (ed. A. Fleckenstein and N. S. Dhalla), University Park Press, Baltimore, pp. 315-21

Higginson, L., Ross, J., Franklin, D. and McKown, D. (1977). Reduction of myocardial infarct size by propranolol and morphine following coronary occlusion in dogs. *Circulation*, **55/56**, Suppl. III, 111-49

Hoffman, B. F. and Singer, D. H. (1967). Appraisal of the effects of catecholamines on cardiac electrical activity. *Ann. N.Y. Acad. Sci.*, **139**, 914-39

Hope, R. R., Williams, D. O., El-Sheriff, N., Lazzara, R. and Scherlag, P. J. (1974). The efficacy of anti-arrhythmic agents during acute myocardial ischemia and the role of heart rate. *Circulation*, **50**, 507-14

Jurgensen, H. J., Frederiksen, J., Hansen, D. A. and Padersen-Bjergaard, O. (1981). Limitation of myocardial infarct size in patients less than 66 years treated with alprenolol. *Br. Heart J.*, **45**, 583-8

Kane, K. A., McDonald, F. M. and Parratt, J. R. (1979). Coronary artery ligation in anaesthetised rats as a model for the assessment of antidysrhythmic activity; the effects of lignocaine, propranolol and Org. 6001. *Br. J. Pharmac.*, **66**, 463-4P

Kaumann, A. J. and Aramendia, P. (1968). Prevention of ventricular fibrillation induced by coronary ligation. *J. Pharmac. exp. Ther.*, **164**, 326-32

Kelliher, G. J., Widmar, C. and Roberts, J. (1975). Influence of adrenal medulla on cardiac rhythm disturbances following acute coronary artery occlusion. In *Recent Advances in Studies on Cardiac Structure and Metabolism*, Vol. 11 (ed. P. E. Roy and E. Rona), University Park Press, Baltimore, pp. 387-400

Kenedi, I. and Losonci, A. (1973). Effect of beta adrenergic blockade on the arrhythmias following coronary artery ligation in the rat. *Acta physiol. hung.*, **44**, 247-57

Khan, M. I., Hamilton, J. T. and Manning, G. W. (1972). Protective effect of beta adrenoceptor blockade in experimental coronary occlusion in conscious dogs. *Am. J. Cardiol.*, **30**, 832-7

Kupersmith, J., Schiang, H., Litwak, R. S. and Herman, M. V. (1976). Electrophysiological and anti-arrhythmic effects of propranolol in canine acute myocardial ischaemia. *Circulation Res.*, **38**, 302-7

Lancet (1981). Beta blockers after myocardial infarction. *Lancet*, *i*, 873-4

Lown, B. and Wolf, M. (1971). Approaches to sudden death from coronary heart disease. *Circulation*, **44**, 130-42

Lown, B., Verrier, R. L. and Rabinowitz, S. H. (1977). Neural and psychological mechanisms and the problem of sudden death. *Am. J. Cardiol.*, **39**, 890-902

Lubbe, W. F., Podzuweit, T., Daries, P. S. and Opie, L. H. (1978). The role of cyclic adenosine monophosphate in adrenergic effects on ventricular vulnerability to fibrillation in the isolated perfused rat heart. *J. clin. Invest.*, **58**, 1260-9

Maling, H. M. and Moran, N. C. (1957). Ventricular arrhythmias induced by sympathomimetic amines in anaesthetised dogs following coronary artery occlusion. *Circulation Res.*, **5**, 409-13

Matta, R. J., Lawler, J. E. and Lown, B. (1976). Ventricular electrical instability in the conscious dog. Effects of psychological stress and beta adrenergic blockade. *Am. J. Cardiol.*, **38**, 594-8

Menken, U., Wiegard, V., Bucher, P. and Meesmann, W. (1979). Prophylaxis of ventricular fibrillation after experimental coronary occlusion by chronic beta-adrenoceptor blockade. *Cardiovasc. Res.*, **13**, 588-94

Mitchell, J. R. A. (1981). Timolol after myocardial infarction: an answer or a new set of questions? *Br. med. J.*, **282**, 1566-70

Morris, J. J., Wohlegmuth, S., Jackson, D., Whalen, R. E. and McIntosh, H. D. (1967). Quinidine, propranolol and polarising solution in the treatment of experimental myocardial infarction. *Clin. Res.*, **15**, 57

Muller, C. A. and Opie, L. H. (1980). Cardio-selective versus non-selective beta-adrenoceptor antagonism and the incidence of arrhythmias in experimental myocardial infarction. *J. molec. cell. Cardiol.*, **12**, Suppl. 1, 1

Multicentre International Study (1977). Supplementary report: reduction in mortality after myocardial infarction with long-term beta-adrenoceptor blockade. *Br. med. J.*, *ii*, 419-21

Norwegian Multicenter Study Group (1981). Timolol induced reduction in mortality and reinfarction in patients surviving acute myocardial infarction. *New Engl. J. Med.*, **304**, 801-7

Parratt, J. R., Campbell, C. and Fagbemi, O. (1981). Catecholamines and early post-infarction arrhythmias: the effects of α and β-adrenoceptor blockade. In *Catecholamines and the Heart*, Springer Verlag, Heidelberg, pp. 269-84

Pearle, D. L., Williford, D. and Gillis, R. A. (1978). Superiority of practolol versus propranolol in protection against ventricular fibrillation induced by coronary occlusion. *Am. J. Cardiol.*, **42**, 960-4

Pentecost, B. L. and Austen, W. O. (1966). Beta adrenergic blockade in experimental myocardial infarction. *Am. Heart J.*, **72**, 790-6

Peter, T., Heng, M. K., Singh, B. N., Ambler, P., Nisbet, H., Elliot, R. and Norris, R. M. (1978). Failure of high doses of propranolol to reduce experimental and myocardial ischemic damage. *Circulation*, **57**, 534-40

Proger, S. and Naimi, L. (1966). Propranolol in myocardial infarction. *Lancet*, *ii*, 1465-6

Reynolds, R. D., Calzadilla, S. V. and Lee, R. J. (1978). Spontaneous heart rate, propranolol and ischaemia induced ventricular fibrillation in the dog. *Cardiovasc. Res.*, **12**, 653-8

Reimer, K. A., Rasmussen, N. M. and Jennings, R. B. (1973). Reduction by propranolol of myocardial necrosis following temporary coronary artery occlusion in dogs. *Circulation Res.*, **33**, 653-8

Richardson, J. A. (1963). Circulating levels of catecholamines in acute myocardial infarction and angina pectoris. *Progr. cardiovasc. Dis.*, **6**, 56-62

Rosenfeld, J., Rosen, M. R. and Hoffman, B. F. (1978). Pharmacologic and behavioural effects on arrhythmias that immediately follow abrupt coronary occlusion: a canine model of sudden death. *Am. J. Cardiol.*, **41**, 1075-82

Rossi, P. R. F., Yus, S., Ramsdale, D., Peto, R., Furze, L., Bennet, D., Bray, C. and

Sleight, P. (1982). Early intravenous beta blockade decreases ventricular arrhythmias in acute myocardial infarction. In press

Schwartz, P. J., Snebold, N. G. and Brown, A. M. (1976). Effects of unilateral cardiac sympathetic denervation on the ventricular fibrillation threshold. *Am. J. Cardiol.*, **37**, 1034-40

Sethi, V., Haider, B., Ahmed, S. S., Oldewurtel, H. A. and Regan, T. J. (1973). Influence of beta blockade and chemical sympathectomy on myocardial function and arrhythmias in acute ischaemia. *Cardiovasc. Res.*, **7**, 740-7

Sheridan, D. J., Penkoske, P. A., Sobel, B. E. and Corr, P. D. (1980). Alpha adrenergic contributions to dysrhythmia during myocardial ischaemia and reperfusion in cats. *J. clin. Invest.*, **65**, 161-71

Shuster, D. P., Lucchesi, B. R., Nobel, N. L., Mimnaugh, N. M., Counsell, R. E. and Kniffen, F. J. (1973). The anti-arrhythmic properties of UM-272, the dimethyl quaternary derivative of propranolol. *J. Pharmac. exp. Ther.*, **184**, 213-27

Siegmund, W., Leprán, I. and Szekeres, L. (1979). Effect of prolonged beta blocking treatment alone and in combination with parasympatholytic on early arrhythmias arising from sudden coronary occlusion in conscious rats. *Acta physiol. hung.*, **53**, 209

Skinner, J. E., Lie, J. T. and Entman, M. L. (1975). Modification of ventricular fibrillation latency following coronary artery occlusion in the conscious pig: the effects of psychological stress and beta adrenergic blockade. *Circulation*, **51**, 656-67

Snow, P. J. D. (1965). The effect of propranolol in myocardial infarction. *Lancet*, *ii*, 551-3

Sommers, H. L. (1966). The effect of reserpine and propranolol on spontaneous ventricular fibrillation and myocardial necrosis following transient coronary artery occlusion. *Fedn Proc. Fedn Am. Socs exp. Biol.*, **25**, 666

Staszewska-Barczak, J. and Ceremuzynski, L. (1968). The continuous estimation of catecholamine release in the early stages of myocardial infarction in the dog. *Clin. Sci.*, **34**, 531-9

Stephen, K. and Meesmann, W. (1974). Beenflusseung der frühen Arrhythmien nach akuten Koronarverschluss durch Beta-Blockade mit Practolol. *Z. Kardiol.*, **7**, 603-11

Szekeres, L. (1978). Theoretical considerations concerning drug treatment of dysrhythmias due to coronary insufficiency. *Adv. Pharmac. Ther.*, **6**, 257-69

Vatner, S. F., Baig, H., Manders, W. R., Ochs, H. and Pagini, M. (1977). Effects of propranolol on regional myocardial function, electrograms and blood flow in conscious dogs with myocardial ischaemia. *J. clin. Invest.*, **60**, 353-60

Verrier, R. L., Calvert, A. and Lown, B. (1975). Effect of posterior hypothalmic stimulation on ventricular fibrillation threshold. *Am. J. Physiol.*, **228**, 923-7

Vedin, J. A. and Wilhelmsson, C. C. (1979). A review of current beta blocker trials in the world. *Heart Bull.*, **10**, 180-2

Wilcox, R. G., Roland, J. M., Banks, D. C., Hampton, J. R. and Mitchell, J. R. A. (1980). Randomised trial comparing propranolol with atenolol in immediate treatment of suspected myocardial infarction. *Br. med. J.*, **280**, 885-8

Wilhelmsson, C. C., Vedin, J. A., Wilhelmsen, L., Tibblin, G. and Werko, L. (1974). Reduction of sudden deaths after myocardial infarction by treatment with alprenolol. *Lancet*, *ii*, 1158–60

ADDENDUM

Since this review was completed in June 1981, the results of two trials with the β-blocking drugs metoprolol and propranolol in acute myocardial infarction have been published. Both trials show an improved survival rate in drug-treated patients in comparison with placebo. In the metoprolol study (Hjalmarson *et al.*, 1981), 1395 patients from an eligible population of 2619 patients with acute myocardial infarction were allocated to placebo or metoprolol. Treatment was started on arrival and comprised metoprolol 15 mg i.v. followed by 50 mg orally 15 min later. Subsequently, metoprolol 50 mg was given 6 hourly for 48 h followed by 100 mg twice daily for a total period of 3 months. Treatment was commenced within 6 h in 43 per cent of patients. There were 62 deaths in the placebo group (697 patients) and 40 deaths in the metoprolol group (698 patients), giving cumulative mortality rates of 8.9 per cent and 5.7 per cent respectively. These differences in total mortality rates between two comparable groups are statistically significant ($P = 0.025$, Mantel–Haenszel test). This is the first study which shows that β-blocking drugs given early in acute myocardial infarction can improve survival.

The second trial, carried out in the USA, compares the effects of placebo or propranolol given over 30 months to 3837 patients with acute myocardial infarction (Co-operative Trial, 1981). Therapy commenced in hospital on average 13.8 days after the onset of myocardial infarction. The initial dose of propranolol was 40 mg t.d.s., and this dose was increased to 60 or 80 mg t.d.s. 4 weeks later according to the plasma propranolol levels. Thirty-one clinical centres were enrolled between June 1978 and October 1980, and the trial was curtailed in October 1981 as a result of the review of the data by the Policy Board (October 1981). The brief summarising report shows that there was a 9.5 per cent mortality rate in the placebo group (183 deaths in 1921 patients), and a 7.0 per cent mortality rate in the propranolol group (135 deaths in 1916 patients). These differences in mortality rates are statistically significant ($P = 0.005$). The comparability of the groups was satisfactory, and the results confirmed the findings of the metoprolol and timolol trials that treatment of survivors of acute myocardial infarction with β-adrenoceptor blocking drugs improves survival rate, particularly in the first year after the infarction.

A smaller study in high risk patients has recently been reported (Hansteen *et al.*, 1982). Patients with myocardial infarction were selected for study from 12 Norwegian hospitals having a catchment of 1.2 million people. The trial took place between December 1977 and July 1980 and involved patients with an increased risk of death from infarction. In Group 1 the patients had been treated for asystole, *ventricular fibrillation* or prolonged *ventricular tachycardia*. The Group 2 patients had other types of significant arrhythmias or modest heart failure. Patients in shock or pulmonary oedema at the time of trial randomisation were excluded. A total of 560 patients were studied, 49 in Group 1 and 511 in Group 2. They received either placebo or *propranolol*, 40 mg four times daily. Therapy commenced 4–6 days after hospitalisation and lasted for 12 months. The total number of deaths in the treated group was 25 in comparison with 37 in the control group, whilst the total cardiac deaths were 20 and 24 respectively. Neither of these differences were statistically significant but there was a significant reduction in the total number of *sudden deaths*, which were 11 in the treated group and 23 in the placebo group ($P = 0.038$). When sudden deaths on treatment or within 1 month of stopping treatment are considered, the ratio of deaths is 10:19 ($P = 0.097$). The stringent criteria defined for such studies were met in this trial, and it is concluded that propranolol caused a significant reduction in *sudden death* in high risk patients surviving the immediate phase of *myocardial infarction.*

In a recent review (Hampton, 1981) it is suggested that several trials showing a consistent trend are more convincing than a single trial with a dramatic result. The results of the timolol, metoprolol and propranolol studies suggest that β-adrenoceptor blocking drugs are of benefit if given within the first year after infarction, and the results of the other trials (that is, oxprenolol, sotalol, pindolol and metoprolol) are awaited with great interest.

ADDENDUM REFERENCES

Co-operative Trial (1981). The beta blocker heart attack trial. *J. Am. med. Assoc.*, **246**, 2073-4

Hampton, J. R. (1981). The use of beta blockers for the reduction of mortality after myocardial infarction. *Eur. Heart J.*, 2, 259–68

Hansteen, V., Moinichen, E., Lorensten, E., Andersen, A., Strom, O., Soiland, K., Dyrbekk, D., Refsum, A.-M., Tromsdal, A., Knudsen, K., Eika, C., Bakken, J., Smith, P. and Hoff, P. I. (1982). One year's treatment with propranolol after myocardial infarction: preliminary report of Norwegian multicentre trial. *Br. med. J.*, **284**, 155-60

Hjalmarson, A., Herlitz, J., Malek, I., Ryden, L., Vedin, A., Waldenstrom, A., Wedel, H., Elmfeldt, D., Holmberg, S., Nyberg, G., Swedberg, K., Waagstein, F., Waldenstrom, J., Wilhelmsen, L. and Wilhelmsson, C. (1981). Effect on mortality of metoprolol in acute myocardial infarction. *Lancet*, *ii*, 823-7

17

Myocardial α-Adrenoceptors and Arrhythmias Induced by Myocardial Ischaemia

Desmond J. Sheridan

17.1 INTRODUCTION

Although myocardial ischaemia is by far the most frequent cause of ventricular fibrillation, the precise mechanisms which immediately induce this arrhythmia are unclear. Complete coronary occlusion is frequently absent in victims of sudden death (Basche *et al.*, 1975) and experimental studies indicate that both coronary occlusion and reperfusion are associated with ventricular fibrillation (Penkoske *et al.*, 1978). The picture is further complicated by the fact that clinical and experimental arrhythmias are both most intense soon after the onset of myocardial ischaemia, at a time when several pathophysiological processes are occurring simultaneously. Many studies have been carried out in an attempt to distinguish which of these are arrhythmogenic. The present chapter is concerned with the possibility that α-adrenoceptor activity may contribute to the development of ventricular fibrillation during myocardial ischaemia. Interest in this possibility arose out of studies with the α-blocking drug phentolamine, which was found to prevent ventricular arrhythmias induced by a variety of techniques. Thus Leimdorfer (1953) reported that intravenous administration of phentolamine prevented arrhythmias due to nicotine or adrenaline and converted methacholine-induced atrial fibrillation in dogs. Others (Vargaftig and Coignet, 1969) reported that phentolamine prevented arrhythmias induced by aconitine or by inhalation of chloroform. Phentolamine has also been reported to be effective in the treatment of digitalis-induced arrhythmias in experimental animals (Ettinger *et al.*, 1969) and also in man (Gould *et al.*, 1969) and in suppressing ventricular ectopic beats in patients with various forms of heart disease (Gould *et al.*, 1971). More particularly, phentolamine has been shown successfully to suppress ventricular arrhythmias in patients following myocardial infarction (Gould *et al.*, 1975). Recently phentolamine has been shown to suppress ventricular fibrillation in cats during coronary occlusion and reperfusion (Sheridan *et al.*, 1980), and in dogs during coronary reperfusion (Stewart *et al.*, 1980). The question which concerns us is whether these effects of phentolamine result from a direct effect of the drug on the myocardium or whether they are related to α-adrenoceptor blocking properties. There is evidence that phentolamine does have a direct electrophysiological effect on Purkinje fibres similar to those observed with antiarrhythmic agents such as lignocaine (Rosen *et al.*, 1971). These effects, however, are observed at high concentrations of the drug and, as we shall see, phentolamine is effective in preventing ventricular arrhythmias in circumstances where other antiarrhythmic agents are ineffective (Naito *et al.*, 1981).

17.2 EFFECTS MEDIATED BY MYOCARDIAL α-ADRENOCEPTORS

Following the introduction of the α- and β-adrenoceptor concept by Ahlquist in 1948, it was generally believed that the actions of catecholamines on the myocardium are mediated through β-receptors. In 1966, however, Govier *et al.* reported α-adrenoceptor-mediated prolongation of effective refractory period in guinea-pig atria. This effect was confirmed by the demonstration that action potential duration is prolonged in response to α-receptor stimulation in guinea-pig atria (Pappano, 1971) and in sheep Purkinje fibres (Giotti *et al.*, 1973). Stimulation of α-adrenoceptors also has a positive inotropic effect in guinea-pig and rat atria (Govier, 1968; Wagner and Brodde, 1978) and in guinea-pig, cat and rabbit ventricular muscle (Wenzel and Su, 1971; Wagner *et al.*, 1974; Rabinowitz *et al.*, 1975; Schumann *et al.*, 1975; Wagner and Brodde, 1978). The chronotropic response to α-adrenoceptor stimulation is less clear. In studies using canine Purkinje fibres and human atrial tissue (Rosen *et al.*, 1971; Mary-Rabine *et al.*, 1978), apparent α-adrenoceptor-mediated negative chronotropic effects were observed. Other workers have failed to demonstrate any significant chronotropic effect at all (Wagner and Reinhardt, 1974; Wagner and Brodde, 1978). It is of particular interest that although α-adrenoceptor stimulation of atria obtained from normal rats had no chronotropic effect, a positive chronotropic response was obtained (Wagner and Reinhardt, 1974; Wagner and Brodde, 1978) in atria obtained from rats rendered hypothyroid by pretreatment with propylthiouracil, a procedure which is known to increase α-adrenoceptor sensitivity (Nakashima *et al.*, 1973).

Unlike β-adrenoceptor stimulation, the effects of which are mediated through activation of adenylate cyclase, the mechanism of action of myocardial α-adrenoceptor stimulation remains unclear. Stimulation of α-adrenoceptors in isolated myocardial cells of the rat has been claimed to cause a reduction in cyclic AMP (Watanabe *et al.*, 1978). However, in studies using isolated rabbit myocardium there were no changes in the myocardial levels of either cyclic AMP or cyclic GMP during the development of α-adrenoceptor-mediated positive inotropism (Brodde *et al.*, 1978). Using isolated rabbit papillary muscles, partially depolarised by high extracellular potassium, Miura *et al.* (1978) observed that α-receptor stimulation had a positive inotropic effect and restored the action potential. Both of these effects were highly sensitive to the level of extracellular calcium, suggesting that α-receptor stimulation might act by increasing calcium influx during the plateau phase of the action potential.

17.3 SYMPATHETIC ACTIVATION DURING CORONARY ARTERY OCCLUSION AND REPERFUSION

The suggestion that α-adrenoceptor blocking agents might have a role in the treatment of ventricular arrhythmias of course presupposes that α-adrenoceptor stimulation is involved in their genesis. There is considerable evidence in favour of enhanced sympathetic activation during myocardial ischaemia (reviewed in chapters 8–10) and also during reperfusion. For example, plasma and urinary catecholamines are elevated following myocardial infarction and the finding of rapid noradrenaline release from isolated hearts following hypoxia and reperfusion (Wollenberger and Shahab, 1965; Gauduel *et al.*, 1979) suggests that a local effect of ischaemia is probably involved (see, for example, Nazum and Bischoff, 1953; Gazes *et al.*, 1959; Staszewska-Barczak and Ceremuzynski, 1971). This is supported by the fact that myocardial catecholamine depletion is greater in ischaemic than in non-ischaemic regions following coronary occlusion in dogs (Mathes and Gudbjarnason, 1971). The precise mechanisms which cause this neuronal noradrenaline release are not understood, but one possibility is that it may result from the rapid accumulation of extracellular potassium.

Several studies have been carried out to assess the role of sympathetic stimulation during myocardial ischaemia and reperfusion. Surgical denervation of the heart significantly reduces the incidence of ventricular fibrillation following coronary occlusion provided that it is carried out long enough prior to the occlusion to allow depletion of myocardial catecholamines to occur (Ebert *et al.*, 1970). This suggests that sympathetic stimulation is an important contributing factor to the genesis of ventricular fibrillation during coronary artery occlusion and that the critical factor is the concentration of myocardial catecholamines. Further evidence in support of this is provided by cardiac chemical denervation studies with 6-hydroxydopamine. This results in an almost complete abolition of ventricular fibrillation during both coronary occlusion and reperfusion (Sethi *et al.*, 1973; Sheridan *et al.*, 1980). Depletion of myocardial catecholamines with reserpine also reduces the incidence of ventricular fibrillation associated with coronary reperfusion (Sommers and Jennings, 1972), although, paradoxically, this treatment either has no effect on, or may even exacerbate, arrhythmias associated with coronary occlusion itself (Maling *et al.*, 1959; Melville and Varma, 1962). This apparent discrepancy may result from post-synaptic supersensitivity. Further evidence that myocardial catecholamines have a deleterious effect on the myocardium during ischaemia and reperfusion is suggested by studies, in isolated rat hearts, in which enzyme release was used as a marker of damage induced by hypoxia and re-oxygenation (Gauduel *et al.*, 1979). These studies showed that depletion of myocardial catecholamines significantly reduced enzyme release during both hypoxia and re-oxygenation. In addition, the onset of arrhythmias following coronary occlusion in the pig has been shown to be temporarily associated with enhanced coronary arteriovenous noradrenaline differences (Hirche *et al.*, 1980).

17.4 THE ROLE OF MYOCARDIAL α_1-ADRENOCEPTORS IN POST-ISCHAEMIA AND REPERFUSION ARRHYTHMIAS

To what extent α_1-adrenoceptor-mediated effects are responsible for ventricular arrhythmias has only recently been studied. DiMicco *et al.* in 1977 showed that the intracerebral injection of picrotoxin in cats consistently induced ventricular arrhythmias which could be prevented by α-adrenoceptor blockade but not by β-adrenoceptor blockade or by a variety of other antiarrhythmic drugs. In addition, while arrhythmias induced by coronary reperfusion respond dramatically to α-blocking drugs (Sheridan *et al.*, 1980; Stewart *et al.*, 1980) these arrhythmias are generally unresponsive to standard antiarrhythmic drugs (Naito *et al.*, 1981). In a recent study, a chloralose-anaesthetised cat model of coronary occlusion and reperfusion was used to examine the relative importance of α- and β-adrenoceptor stimulation in arrhythmias associated with myocardial ischaemia (Sheridan *et al.*, 1980). The results are summarised in figure 17.1 and show that either α-adrenoceptor blockade with phentolamine, or myocardial catecholamine depletion with 6-hydroxydopamine, significantly reduced the incidence of ventricular fibrillation during occlusion and reperfusion. In contrast, while β-adrenoceptor blockade with propranolol significantly decreased the number of ectopics during occlusion, it failed to reduce the incidence of ventricular fibrillation during either occlusion or reperfusion. Since phentolamine is known to have class 1 antiarrhythmic effects on isolated Purkinje fibres (Rosen *et al.*, 1971), and because it enhances the effect of noradrenaline on isolated atria (Benfey and Greeff, 1961), a second α-adrenoceptor blocking drug (prazosin) was also studied. There was again a significant reduction in ventricular fibrillation during occlusion and reperfusion (Sheridan *et al.*, 1980). Since prazosin does not have direct electrophysiological properties and is largely without presynaptic (α_2) activity, these findings strongly suggest that the protective effect of phentolamine results from its α_1 blocking properties. This is also supported by the finding that myocardial catecholamine depletion prevented ventricular fibrillation whereas β-receptor blockade did not. In order to establish whether the protective effects of phentolamine and prazosin were due to actions on the coronary vasculature, myocardial blood flow was measured in control and treated animals during both occlusion and reperfusion. The results obtained confirmed the marked reduction in flow in the ischaemic zone during occlusion and the transient hyperaemic response during reperfusion; however, flows in control and phentolamine-treated animals did not differ. Neither could the protective effects of α-receptor blockade be attributed to systemic haemodynamic effects. Thus, although both phentolamine and prazosin lowered blood pressure

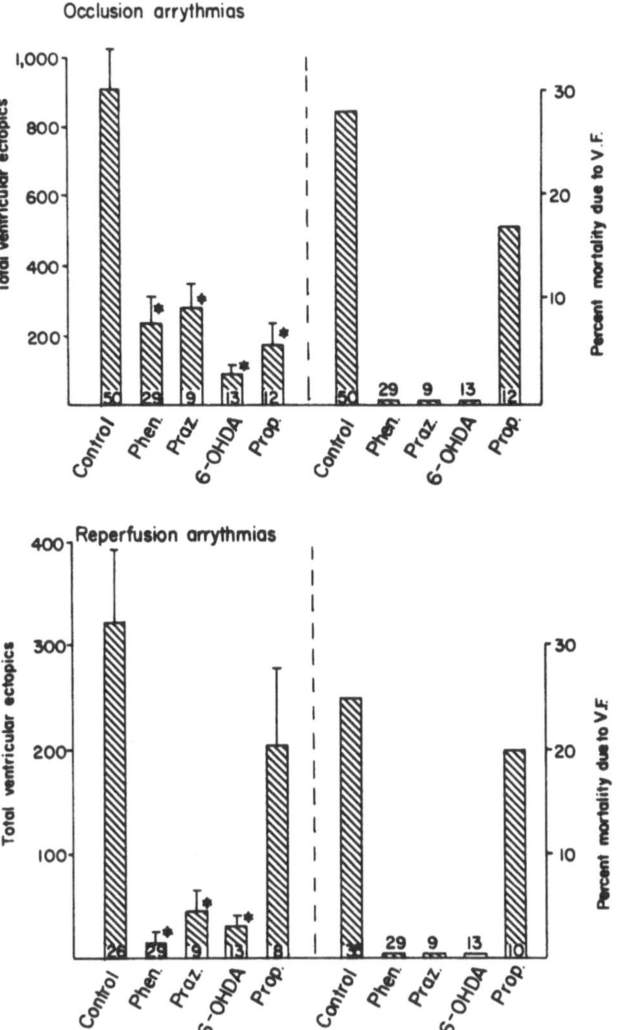

Figure 17.1 The number of premature ventricular contractions (left) and incidence of ventricular fibrillation (right) in open-chest, chloralose-anaesthetised cats subjected to occlusion (upper panel) and reperfusion (lower panel) of the LAD coronary artery in control animals, and animals treated with phentolamine, prazosin, 6-hydroxydopamine or propranolol. Vertical bars represent the S.E.M. and the numbers of animals in each group are also given. $*P < 0.05$ in comparison with controls. (After Sheridan *et al.* (1980).)

compared to control animals, propranolol did so to a similar extent but failed to prevent ventricular fibrillation. A slight reduction in left ventricular end-diastolic pressure (LVEDP) was observed in prazosin and phentolamine-treated animals; however, a similar reduction of LVEDP in control animals by nitroprusside had no antiarrhythmic effect. In addition, maintenance of LVEDP at control levels in phentolamine-treated animals by infusion of dextran did not modify the anti-arrhythmic effect of this drug. Thus, sympathetic stimulation is clearly a factor in the genesis of early arrhythmias during myocardial ischaemia and a major part of the effects involved appear to be mediated through α-receptor stimulation.

The mechanism of this protection effect is unclear; α-receptor stimulation causes a prolongation of action potentive duration (Pappano, 1971; Giotti *et al.*, 1973) and, at least in human atrial tissue, a negative chronotropic effect (Mary-Rabine *et al.*, 1978). That such changes should be compatible with an arrhythmogenic effect is perhaps surprising. However, it must be emphasised that the studies involved were all carried out on normal tissue. In the past decade it has become clear that adrenoceptor numbers may vary according to the physiological environment (Williams *et al.*, 1977; Sharma and Banerjee, 1978). It is also apparent that a change in receptor number is compatible with a change in end-organ responsiveness (Wagner and Reinhardt, 1974; Wagner and Brodde, 1978). Thus, whilst α-receptor stimulation has no clear chronotropic effect on ventricular tissue obtained from normal animals, it produces a distinct positive chronotropic effect when α-receptor sensitivity is increased by rendering animals hypothyroid. This raises the possibility that α-receptor responsiveness may be altered in the presence of myocardial ischaemia (see, for example, Moore and Parratt, 1973). Indeed, recent preliminary evidence suggests that the number of α-adrenoceptors is increased in the early phase of coronary reperfusion (Shayman *et al.*, 1980). More importantly there is evidence of enhanced α-receptor responsiveness soon after commencing reperfusion (Sheridan *et al.*, 1980). Thus, in the chloralose-anaesthetised cat, transient bilateral vagal nerve stimulation induces an intense sinus bradycardia allowing an idioventricular pacemaker to escape. The results of experiments in which this model has been used to measure idioventricular rate during occlusion and reperfusion are shown in figure 17.2. Prior to the onset of occlusion an idioventricular rate of about 65 beats min^{-1} was observed and no significant change occurred during occlusion. However, during early reperfusion a marked acceleration of idioventricular rate was observed which was unaffected by propranolol but completely abolished by α-receptor blockade or by catecholamine depletion. These results suggest that α-adrenoceptors mediate positive chronotropic effect in ventricular tissue during coronary reperfusion.

In order to ascertain whether these effects observed during reperfusion represented enhanced α-receptor responsiveness, a separate group of experiments was carried out in catecholamine-depleted animals to measure the effect of α-adrenoceptor stimulation on idioventricular rate both under normal circumstances and during coronary reperfusion. The results are illustrated in figure 17.3. Prior to coronary occlusion, an infusion of the α-adrenoceptor agonist methoxamine directly into the left anterior descending coronary artery in chloralose-anaesthetised cats had no significant effect on idioventricular rate. However, during early reperfusion methoxamine more than doubled the idioventricular rate, suggesting that the chronotropic effect of α-receptor stimulation is markedly enhanced at this time. This enhanced receptor sensitivity during reperfusion corresponded with the onset and duration of reperfusion arrhythmias.

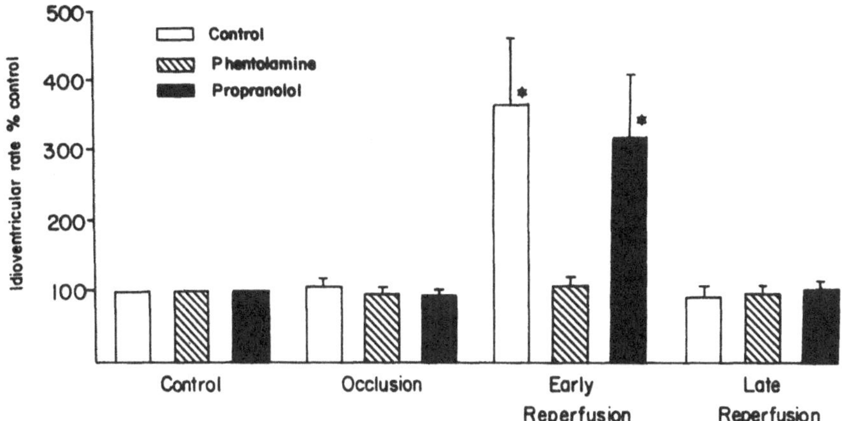

Figure 17.2 Idioventricular rate (expressed as a percentage of the value in controls) measured during efferent vagal nerve stimulation prior to occlusion, during occlusion and during early and late reperfusion in chloralose-anaesthetised control cats (n = 10) and in cats treated with either phentolamine (n = 8) or propranolol (n = 6). Idioventricular rate was unchanged during occlusion but was significantly increased in control and β-blocked animals during early reperfusion; this effect was blocked by phentolamine. (After Sheridan *et al.* (1980).)

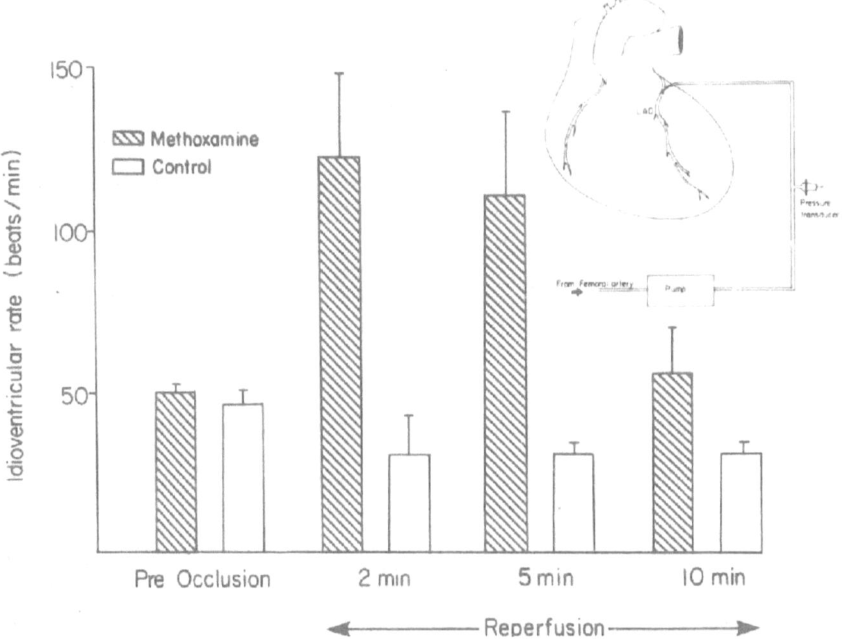

Figure 17.3 Influence of regional (LAD) infusion of methoxamine (0.1 μM) on idioventricular rate in catecholamine-depleted animals. Prior to coronary occlusion methoxamine had no significant effect on idioventricular rate, but this was significantly increased during early reperfusion. The time course corresponded with that of reperfusion arrhythmias. (After Sheridan *et al.* (1980).)

Further evidence in support of the concept of enhanced α-receptor sensitivity during early reperfusion is provided by experiments in which the effects of left stellate nerve stimulation on idioventricular rate were studied. Results from these experiments are illustrated in figure 17.4 and show that left stellate nerve stimulation increased idioventricular rate under normal circumstances. This effect was blocked by propranolol but not by phentolamine; similar findings were obtained during coronary occlusion. However, in propranolol-treated animals, idioventricular rate was accelerated during early reperfusion and increased still further with left stellate nerve stimulation; phentolamine blocked all these increases in idioventricular rate. Fifteen minutes after the onset of reperfusion, adrenoceptor-mediated responses had returned to control values. These findings indicate that myocardial sensitivity to sympathetic nerve stimulation is markedly enhanced during early reperfusion and that these effects are mediated almost entirely through α-receptors. Since the time course of these events corresponds with the onset and duration of

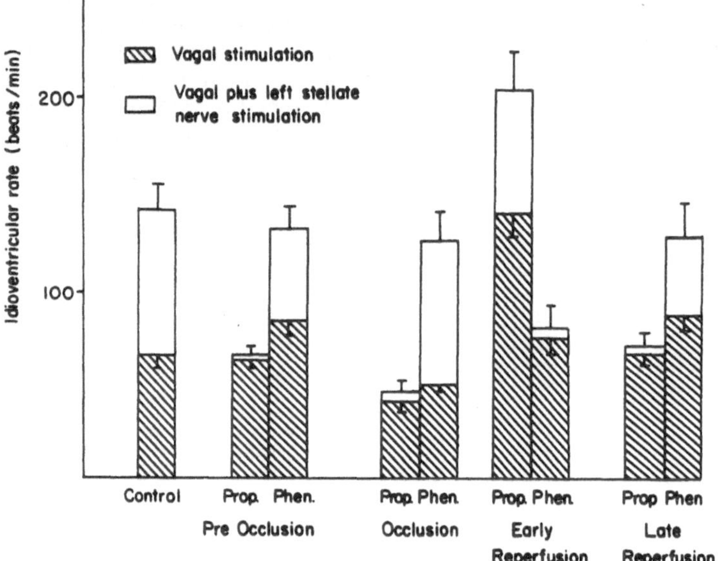

Figure 17.4 The influence of left stellate nerve stimulation on idioventricular rate induced by vagal nerve stimulation in chloralose-anaesthetised cats. The hatched columns indicate the idioventricular rate during vagal nerve stimulation and the open columns the increase observed with stellate nerve stimulation. Results are shown for control animals and for animals treated with phentolamine or propranolol prior to occlusion, during occlusion and during reperfusion. Prior to occlusion propranolol blocked the increase in idioventricular rate observed with stellate nerve stimulation whereas phentolamine did not, a response pattern which was unchanged during occlusion. During early reperfusion, however, propranolol failed to block either the increase in idioventricular rate induced by reperfusion, or the further increase observed with stellate nerve stimulation. In contrast, phentolamine prevented any increase in idioventricular rate at this time. Later during reperfusion (15 min) responses returned to the pre-occlusion pattern. (After Sheridan *et al.* (1980).)

arrhythmias during re-perfusion, and since α-receptor blockade reduces the incidence of ventricular fibrillation, it is difficult to escape the conclusion that α-receptor stimulation is involved in the genesis of these arrhythmias.

Almost all of the experiments which have been described were carried out in order to investigate mechanisms responsible for arrhythmias during myocardial ischaemia rather than to establish therapeutic interventions directly. The doses of adrenoceptor blocking drugs used were chosen in order to establish complete blockade and were therefore higher than would be appropriate for clinical use. Further work is therefore needed to establish whether or not doses which can be safely applied clinically provide a useful antiarrhythmic effect in patients with myocardial infarction. In addition, examination of the cellular electrophysiological changes associated with the antiarrhythmic effects described may provide new insights into possible mechanisms of arrhythmia prevention.

REFERENCES

Basche, W. J., Baba, N., Keller, M. D., Geer, J. C. and Anthony, J. R. (1975). Pathology of atherosclerotic heart disease in sudden death. II. The significance of myocardial infarction. *Circulation*, **52**, Suppl. III, 63-9

Benfey, B. G. and Greeff, K. (1961). Interactions of sympathomimetic drugs and their antagonists on the isolated atrium. *Br. J. Pharmac.*, **17**, 232-5

Brodde, O.-E., Motomura, S., Endoh, M. and Schumann, H. J. (1978). Lack of correlation between the positive inotropic effect evoked by α-adrenoreceptor stimulation and the levels of cyclic AMP and/or cyclic GMP in the isolated ventricle striae of the rabbit. *J. molec. cell. Cardiol.*, **10**, 207-19

Di Micco, J. A., Prestel, T., Pearle, D. L. and Gillis, R. A. (1977). Mechanisms of cardiovascular changes produced in cats by activation of the central nervous system with picrotoxin. *Circulation Res.*, **41**, 446-51

Ebert, P. A., Vanderbeck, R. B., Allgood, R. J. and Sabiston, D. C. (1970). Effect of chronic cardiac denervation on arrhythmias after coronary artery ligation. *Cardiovasc. Res.*, **4**, 141-7

Ettinger, S., Gould, L., Carmichael, J. A. and Tashjian, R. J. (1969). Phentolamine: use in digitalis-induced arrhythmias. *Am. Heart J.*, **77**, 636-40

Gauduel, Y., Karagueuzian, H. S. and De Leiris, J. (1979). Deleterious effects of endogenous catecholamines on hypoxic myocardial cells following reoyxgenation. *J. molec. cell. Cardiol.*, **11**, 717-31

Gazes, P. C., Richardson, J. A. and Woods, E. F. (1959). Plasma catecholamine concentrations in myocardial infarction and angina pectoris. *Circulation*, **19**, 657-61

Giotti, A., Ledda, F. and Mannaioni, P. F. (1973). Effects of noradrenaline and isoprenaline, in combination with α and β receptor blocking substances, on the action potential of cardiac Purkinje fibres. *J. Physiol., Lond.*, **229**, 99-113

Gould, L., Zahir, M., Sharriff, M. and Giuliani, M. G. (1969). Treatment of cardiac arrhythmias with phentolamine. *Am. Heart J.*, **78**, 189-93

Gould, L., Gomprecht, R. F. and Zahir, M. (1971). Oral phentolamine for treatment of ventricular premature contractions. *Br. Heart J.*, **33**, 101-4

Gould, L., Reddy, C. V. R., Weinstein, T. and Gomprecht, R. F. (1975). Anti-arrhythmic prophylaxis with phentolamine in acute myocardial infarction. *J. clin. Pharmac.*, **15**, 191-7

Govier, W. C. (1968). Myocardial alpha adrenergic receptors and their role in the production of a positive inotropic effect by sympathomimetic agents. *J. Pharmac. exp. Ther.*, **159**, 82-90

Govier, W. C., Mosel, N. C., Whittington, P. and Broom, A. H. (1966). Myocardial alpha and beta adrenergic receptors as demonstrated by atrial functional refractory period changes. *J. Pharmac. exp. Ther.*, **154**, 255-63

Hirche, Hj., Franz, C., Bos, L., Bissig, R., Lang, R. and Schramm, M. (1980). Myocardial extracellular K^+ and H^+ increase and noradrenaline release as a possible cause of early arrhythmias following acute coronary occlusion in pigs. *J. molec. cell. Cardiol.*, **12**, 579-93

Leimdorfer, A. (1953). Abolition of cardiac arrhythmias by regitine (parasympatholytic effects of regitine). *Archs int. Pharmacodyn. Thér.*, **94**, 119 and 249

Maling, H. M., Cohn, V. H. and Highman, B. (1959). The effects of coronary occlusion in dogs treated with reserpine and in dogs treated with phenoxybenzamine. *J. Pharmac. exp. Ther.*, **127**, 229-35

Mary-Rabine, L., Hordef, A. J., Bowman, F. O., Malm, J. R. and Rosen, M. R. (1978). Alpha and beta adrenergic effects on human atrial specialized conducting fibers. *Circulation*, **57**, 84-90

Mathes, P. and Gudbjarnason, S. (1971). Changes in norepinephrine stores in the canine heart following experimental myocardial infarction. *Am. Heart J.*, **81**, 211-9

Melville, K. I. and Varma, D. R. (1962). The combined effects of reserpine and various coronary dilator drugs: an experimental study. *Can. med. Assoc. J.*, **86**, 1014-9

Miura, Y., Inui, J. and Imamura, H. (1978). Alpha-adrenoreceptor mediated restoration of calcium-dependent potential in the partially depolarised rabbit papillary muscle. *Naunyn Schmiedebergs Arch. Pharmac.*, **301**, 201-5

Moore, G. and Parratt, J. R. (1973). Effects of noradrenaline and isoprenaline on blood flow in the ischaemic myocardium. *Cardiovasc. Res.*, **7**, 446-57

Naito, M., Michelson, E. L., Kmetzo, J. J., Kaplinsky, E. and Dreifus, L. S. (1981). Failure of antiarrhythmic drugs to prevent experimental reperfusion ventricular fibrillation. *Circulation*, **63**, 70-9

Nakashima, M., Tsuru, H. and Shigei, T. (1973). Stimulant action of methoxamine in the isolated atria of normal and 6-propyl-2-thiouracil fed rats. *Jap. J. Pharmac.*, **23**, 307-12

Nazum, F. R. and Bischoff, F. (1953). The urinary output of catechol derivates including adrenaline in normal individuals in essential hypertension and in myocardial infarction. *Circulation*, **7**, 96-101

Pappano, A. J. (1971). Propranolol-insensitive effects of epinephrine on action potential repolarisation in electrically driven atria of the guinea pig. *J. Pharmac. exp. Ther.*, **177**, 85-95

Penkoske, P. A., Sobel, B. E. and Corr, P. B. (1978). Disparate electrophysiological alterations accompanying dysrhythmia due to coronary occlusion and reperfusion in the cat. *Circulation*, **58**, 1023-35

Rabinowitz, B., Chuck, L., Kligerman, M. and Parmley, W. W. (1975). Positive inotropic effects of methoxamine: evidence for alpha-adrenergic receptors in ventricular myocardium. *Am. J. Physiol.*, **229**, 582-5

Rosen, M. R., Gelband, H. and Hoffman, B. F. (1971). Effects of phentolamine on electrophysiologic properties of isolated canine Purkinje fibers. *J. Pharmac. exp. Ther.*, **179**, 586-93

Rosen, M. R., Hordof, A. J., Ilvento, J. P. and Danilo, P. (1977). Effects of adrenergic amines on electrophysiologic properties and automaticity of neonatal and adult canine Purkinje fibres. *Circulation Res.*, **40**, 390-400

Schumann, H. J., Endoh, M. and Brodde, O.-E. (1975). Positive inotropic effects of phenylephrine in isolated rabbit papillary muscle mediated both by α and β adrenoreceptors. *Naunyn Schmiedebergs Arch. Pharmac.*, **284**, 133-48

Sethi, V., Haider, B., Ahmed, S., Oldewurtel, H. A. and Regan, T. J. (1973). Influence of β blockade and chemical sympathectomy on myocardial function and arrhythmias in acute ischaemia. *Cardiovasc. Res.*, **7**, 740-7

Sharma, V. K. and Banerjee, S. P. (1978). Alpha adrenergic receptor in rat heart. Effects of thyroidectomy. *J. biol. Chem.*, **235**, 5277-9

Shayman, J. A., Kramer, J. B. and Corr, P. B. (1980). Increased α-adrenergic receptors in ischaemic myocardium. *Circulation*, **62**, Suppl. III, 149 (abstract)

Sheridan, D. J., Penkoske, P. A., Sobel, B. E. and Corr, P. B. (1980). Alpha adrenergic contributions to dysrhythmia during myocardial ischaemia and reperfusion in cats. *J. clin. Invest.*, **65**, 161-71

Sommers, H. M. and Jennings, R. B. (1972). Ventricular fibrillation and myocardial necrosis after transient ischaemia: effect of treatment with oxygen, procainamide, reserpine and propranolol. *Archs int. Med.*, **129**, 780-9

Staszewska-Barczak, J. and Ceremuzynski, L. (1971). The reflex stimulation of catecholamine secretion during the acute stage of myocardial infarction in the dog. *Clin. Sci.*, **41**, 419-39

Stewart, J. R., Burmeister, W. E., Burmeister, J. and Lucchesi, B. R. (1980). Electrophysiologic and antiarrhythmic effects of phentolamine in experimental coronary occlusion and reperfusion in the dog. *J. cardiovasc. Pharmac.*, **2**, 77-91

Vargaftig, B. and Coignet, J. L. (1969). A critical evaluation of three methods for the study of adrenergic beta-blocking and antiarrhythmic agents. *Eur. J. Pharmac.*, **6**, 49-55

Wagner, J. and Brodde, O.-E. (1978). On the presence and distribution of α adrenoceptors in the heart of various mammalian species. *Naunyn Schmiedebergs Arch. Pharmac.*, **302**, 239-54

Wagner, J. and Reinhardt, D. (1974). Characterisation of the adrenoceptors mediating the positive ino- and chronotropic effect of phenylephrine on isolated atria from guinea pigs and rabbits by means of adrenolytic drugs. *Naunyn Schmiedebergs Arch. Pharmac.*, **282**, 295-306

Wagner, J., Endoh, M. and Reinhardt, D. (1974). Stimulation by phenylephrine of adrenergic alpha and beta-receptors in the isolated perfused rabbit heart. *Naunyn Schmiedebergs Arch. Pharmac.*, **282**, 307-10

Watanabe, A. M., Besch, H. R., Hathaway, D. R., Harris, R. A. and Farmer, B. B. (1978). Alpha-adrenergic reduction of cyclic adenosine monophosphate levels in rat ventricular myocardial cells. In *Recent Advances in Studies on Cardiac Structure and Metabolism*, Vol. 11 (ed. T. Kobayashi, T. Sano, and N. S. Dhalla), University Park Press, Baltimore, pp. 431-6

Wenzel, D. G. and Su, J. L. (1971). Interaction between sympathomimetic amines and blocking agents on the rat ventricle strip. *Archs int. Pharmacodyn. Thér.*, **160**, 379-89

Williams, L. T., Lefkowitz, R. J., Watanabe, A. M., Hathaway, D. R. and Besch, H. R. (1977). Thyroid hormone regulation of α-adrenergic receptor numbers. *J. biol. Chem.*, **252**, 2787-9

Wollenberger, A. and Shahab, L. (1965). Anoxia-induced release of noradrenaline from the isolated perfused heart. *Nature, Lond.*, **207**, 88-9

18

Inhibitors of the Slow Calcium Current and Early Ventricular Arrhythmias

James R. Parratt

18.1 INTRODUCTION

The effects of 'calcium antagonist' drugs on cardiac muscle are due to interference with those 'slow channels' in the cell membrane through which Ca^{2+} ions enter the cell (for example, during the plateau phase of the action potential in normal ventricular and Purkinje fibres). Calcium ions are also at least partly responsible for so called 'slow potentials' which occur in normal sinus and atrioventricular nodal cells and under conditions, for example during myocardial ischaemia, in which cells are partially depolarised, thereby inactivating Na^{+}-mediated 'fast responses'. The most obvious effects of cardiac cellular 'Ca^{2+} deprivation' are as follows:

(1) Impairment of excitation-contraction coupling, leading to a decline in myocardial contractile force but with no initial alteration in the cardiac muscle action potential.

(2) Depression of pacemaker activity, leading to a decrease in spontaneous (phase 4) depolarisation at the SA and AV nodes and to slowing of AV conduction. These are precisely the effects of inorganic ions such as CO^{2+}, Ni^{2+} and La^{3+} or of specific 'calcium antagonist' drugs which powerfully and selectively inhibit Ca^{2+} flux across the sarcolemma through specific channels. This chapter is concerned particularly with synthetic drugs that inhibit the slow channel transport of calcium.

18.2 CALCIUM INVOLVEMENT IN ARRHYTHMIAS

It has been known since the beginning of the present century that calcium is capable of inducing ventricular arrhythmias, including fibrillation, in isolated

Langendorff-perfused hearts and also following the intravenous administration of large doses (120-200 mg kg^{-1}) in anaesthetised animals. This latter effect was initially ascribed to the central activation of sympathetic nerves but it is also clear that a high extracellular calcium concentration hastens repolarisation in atrial and papillary muscle and, by increasing the permeability to Na^+, hastens depolarisation. The intravenous administration of calcium chloride in rats has been used as a method for evaluating potential antiarrhythmic drugs (Szekeres and Papp, 1971); for example, Campbell, in my own laboratory (unpublished), has shown that there is a 100 per cent incidence of ventricular fibrillation (and over 83 per cent mortality) following the intravenous administration of 100 mg kg^{-1} doses of calcium chloride to pentobarbitone-anaesthetised rats.

It is also well established, in experimental animals and in the clinical situation, that calcium antagonists (slow channel blocking agents) are potentially antiarrhythmic and, on the basis of intracellular recordings of cardiac muscle action potentials, Singh and Vaughan Williams (1972) postulated that they form a distinct (fourth) class of antiarrhythmic drug. The first indication that specific calcium antagonist drugs were antidysrhythmic arose from the early studies of Melville and Benfey in 1965. They found that verapamil protected against ventricular fibrillation induced by either chloroform-adrenaline or ouabain in anaesthetised cats. Subsequent studies have demonstrated that various calcium antagonists prevent arrhythmias induced by calcium chloride *in vitro* (rat atria; Refsum, 1975; Refsum *et al.*, 1979) and *in vivo* (following intravenous administration in anaesthetised rats and dogs; Lynch *et al.*, 1981), by digitalis glycosides (Rodrigues-Pereira and Viana, 1968; Chiou *et al.*, 1976; Piascik *et al.*, 1979; Bergey *et al.*, 1981) and by aconitine (Rodrigues-Pereira and Viana, 1968; Bergey *et al.*, 1981). This review, however, concentrates on the evidence that calcium antagonists prevent, or reverse, ventricular arrhythmias resulting from acute myocardial ischaemia.

18.3 DIFFERENT TYPES OF ARRHYTHMIAS IN THE ISCHAEMIC HEART

It is important to distinguish between ventricular arrhythmias arising at different times after an acute reduction of blood flow to the mammalian myocardium (table 18.1). Ventricular arrhythmias occur soon after the onset of an acute and severe reduction in coronary blood flow. These *early life-threatening* arrhythmias, which are the subject of this book, occur within minutes of coronary artery obstruction, frequently lead to fatal ventricular fibrillation, and are probably responsible for sudden (usually pre-hospital) cardiac death. These arrhythmias almost certainly have a different origin (that is, re-entry as opposed to increased automaticity) to those occurring hours after the onset of infarction. The *late arrhythmias* (4-24 h after infarction in larger experimental animals and in man) are those seen in the coronary care unit. Not only do these arrhythmias have a different mechanism,

Table 18.1 Types of post-infarction ventricular arrhythmias

Early	That is, within minutes. Life-threatening and responsible for sudden cardiac death. Evidence for two distinct phases (1a or 'immediate'; 1b or 'delayed').
Late	That is 4–24 h after the onset of infarction (exact timing very species dependent).
Reperfusion	For instance, following release of a thrombus (not necessarily in a major vessel) or following relief of coronary vasospasm. Also evidence for at least two distinct populations of arrhythmias.

they also have a different sensitivity to drugs. For example, lignocaine is highly effective against those ventricular arrhythmias occurring 12–24 h after two-stage coronary artery ligation in dogs; it is relatively ineffective against early ventricular fibrillation in this species (chapter 15).

There is a third type of ventricular arrhythmia which is relevant to the ischaemic heart. Figure 18.1 makes clear that ventricular arrhythmias occur not only when a

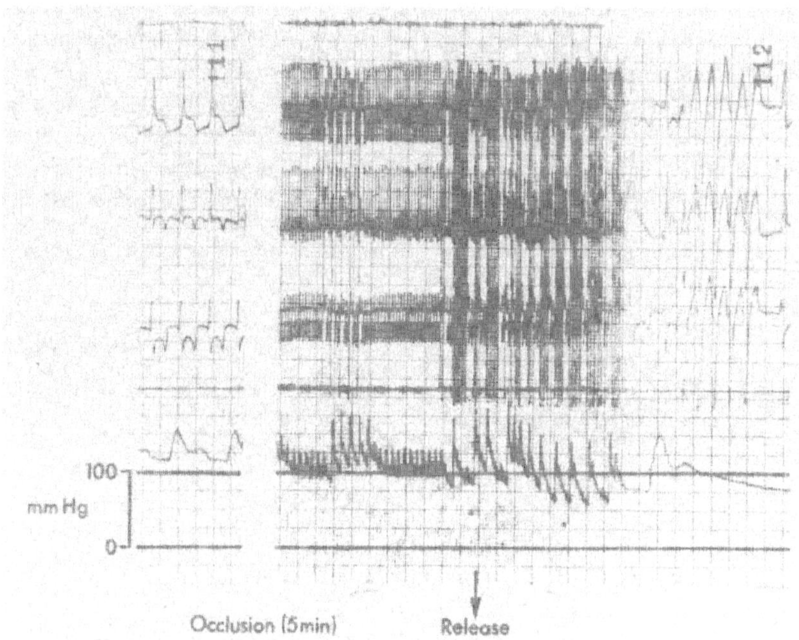

Figure 18.1 The effect of occluding the anterior descending branch of the left coronary artery for 5 min, with subsequent release of the occlusion, in a greyhound anaesthetised with chloralose. The record shows three epicardial leads together with (at the bottom) systemic arterial blood pressure. Notice the occurrence of ventricular ectopic beats during the occlusion but even more pronounced ectopic activity when the occlusion is released ('reperfusion' arrhythmias). (From R. J. Marshall and J. R. Parratt (unpublished).)

branch of a major coronary artery is obstructed, but that they also occur immediately following *reperfusion*. The severity depends upon the time after obstruction that reperfusion occurs; in anaesthetised greyhounds, for example, they are rare after the release of a 3 min coronary artery occlusion, fairly common after the release of a 5 min occlusion and always present after the release of a 30 min occlusion, when the result is invariably ventricular fibrillation (R. J. Marshall and J. R. Parratt, unpublished). It is conceivable that reperfusion-induced ventricular fibrillation (for example, following the release of an occluding thrombus or the sudden relaxation of a coronary artery spasm) is responsible for some cases of sudden cardiac death. Post-mortem examination of such coronary arteries would detect no permanent obstruction. There is again no reason for assuming that reperfusion arrhythmias would be sensitive to the same antiarrhythmic drugs as those which suppress early (or late) post-infarction arrhythmias.

Even the distinction of post-infarction arrhythmias into early, late and reperfusion (table 18.1) is an over-simplification. For example, there is good evidence, reviewed by Meesmann in chapter 6 of this book, that there are two distinct populations of ventricular arrhythmias in the acute, early phase, that is, in the first 30 min of coronary artery obstruction. This has been particularly well documented in the dog (chapter 6) but two distinct early populations of ventricular ectopic beats can also be demonstrated in anaesthetised pigs (Frank *et al.*, 1978) and in the anaesthetised rat model described by Kane, McDonald and Parratt (Kane *et al.*, 1979; Clarke *et al.*, 1980), illustrated in figure 18.2. It is clear from this figure that there is one population of ectopic beats between 4 and 7 min of occlusion and another between 9 and 12 min. The occurrence of ventricular fibrillation, which in the rat often reverts spontaneously, follows a similar biphasic distribution with the first period

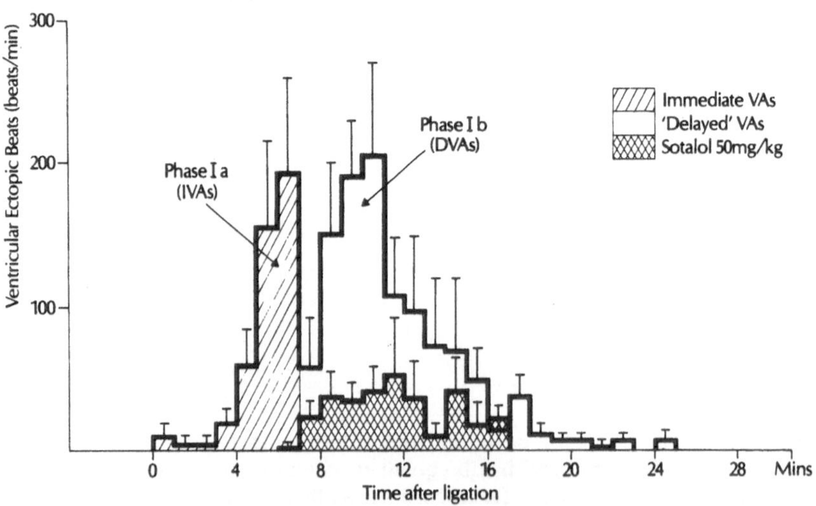

Figure 18.2 The evidence for two periods of early ventricular arrhythmias in the rat infarct model and the effect of β-adrenoceptor blockade with sotalol. (From F. M. McDonald (unpublished).)

of fibrillation occurring between 5 and 8 min. It is possible, as Meesmann believes, that these two phases have a different electrophysiological origin and that they may therefore be sensitive to different drugs, phase 1a being particularly sensitive to β-adrenoceptor blocking drugs (figure 18.2 and chapter 9). As we shall see, the phase 1b arrhythmias are particularly sensitive to calcium antagonists.

18.4 EFFECTIVENESS OF CALCIUM ANTAGONIST DRUGS AGAINST EARLY ARRHYTHMIAS RESULTING FROM EXPERIMENTAL MYOCARDIAL ISCHAEMIA

Verapamil

An early study (Kaumann and Aramendia, 1968) demonstrated clearly that the drug, when given (in a dose of 0.79 mg kg^{-1}) 10 min before coronary artery ligation in pentobarbitone-anaesthetised mongrel dogs, reduced the incidence of early ventricular fibrillation from 10 cases out of 11 (in the controls) to one case out of 10. Similar protection was observed with the β-adrenoceptor blocking drug sotalol. However, the sotalol-treated dogs died later (within 24 h) whereas the verapamil-treated dogs were in apparent good health 10 months after the onset of infarction. Similar results have been obtained by Elharrar *et al.* (1977). In this study pretreatment with a lower dose of verapamil (0.2 mg kg^{-1}) reduced the incidence of ventricular tachycardia or fibrillation induced by pacing during brief (6 min) occlusions of the left anterior descending coronary artery (LAD) from three cases in eight to none in seven and *reduced* the conduction delay occurring within the ischaemic segment. It did not, however, reduce the incidence of VEBs when given 15 min *after* occlusion (Kupersmith *et al.*, 1976). Verapamil also significantly reduced the ventricular fibrillation (VF) which occurred during coronary artery occlusion in the 'occlusion reperfusion' model of Lown (Brooks *et al.*, 1980). During 10 min occlusion of the left anterior descending coronary artery (LAD) the incidence of VF was reduced by verapamil infusion (0.1 mg kg^{-1} min^{-1}) from 23 to 0 per cent. VF during left circumflex occlusion was reduced from 90 to 9 per cent. Verapamil also markedly reduced the incidence of VF during release-reperfusion in those animals subjected to LAD occlusion from 70 per cent in the control to 8 per cent and afforded significant protection against the reduction in the ventricular fibrillation threshold (VFT) which occurred during occlusion and during reperfusion (Brooks *et al.*, 1980).

In contrast to these findings in dogs, studies in the anaesthetised rat model (Kane *et al.*, 1979; Clarke *et al.*, 1980) demonstrated that verapamil, in doses of 0.1 and 0.5 mg kg^{-1} administered intravenously 15 min before ligation, *increased* mortality, although the number of VEBs occurring during the immediate 30 min post-occlusion period was reduced. The incidence of VF was slightly increased by this pretreatment (Kane *et al.*, 1981; McDonald, 1980) and the increased mortality was ascribed partly to AV conduction block, profound systemic hypotension and asystole but mainly to the fact that VF, when it occurred, was invariably terminal. In control rats VF usually reverted spontaneously to sinus rhythm.

Nifedipine and related compounds

It has been stated that nifedipine has no antiarrhythmic activity (Henry, 1980) partly on the basis of its lack of effects on AV conduction. This unique feature of the drug, demonstrated in experimental (Taira and Narimatsu, 1975) and clinical studies (Rowlands *et al.*, 1979), is in marked contrast to other calcium antagonists, especially verapamil and diltiazem (reviewed by Henry, 1980; Ellrodt *et al.*, 1980) and explains the lack of effect of nifedipine on supraventricular arrhythmias.

There is in fact now good evidence that nifedipine, and its related derivatives nisoldipine and niludipine, is extremely effective in reducing serious ventricular arrhythmias that occur soon after experimental myocardial ischaemia. This has been particularly examined in the anaesthetised rat coronary artery ligation model. For example, by intravenous injection, doses as low as 5 μg kg^{-1} completely suppress VF induced by coronary artery ligation (figure 18.3); rather larger doses are required to reduce significantly the number of VEBs (table 18.2; Fagbemi and Parratt, 1981a). Niludipine and nisoldipine are also highly effective in this model, particularly in suppressing VF; the order of potency is niludipine > nifedipine > nisoldipine (Fagbemi and Parratt, 1981a). There was some evidence from these studies that it was the VEBs occurring 16–25 min after ligation, and perhaps equivalent to the phase 1b arrhythmias described by Meesmann (chapter 6 and see also figure 18.1), that were particularly sensitive to the calcium slow channel

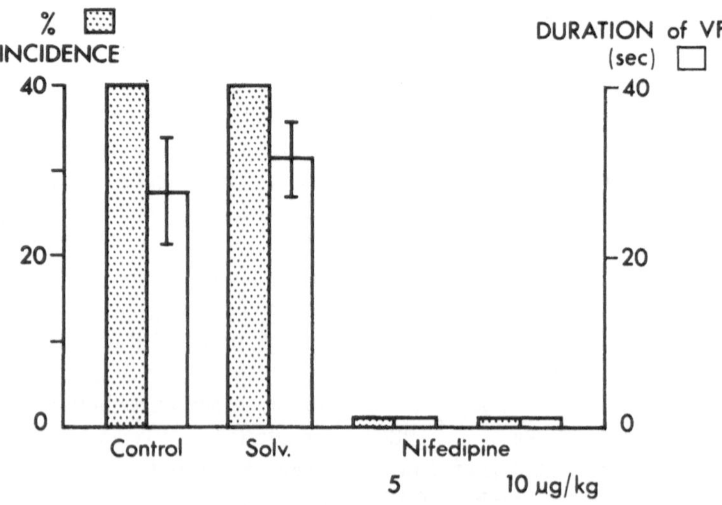

Figure 18.3 The effect of nifedipine (5 or 10 μg kg^{-1}, intravenously) on the incidence and duration of ventricular fibrillation following acute coronary artery ligation in anaesthetised rats.

Table 18.2 The effect of intravenous nifedipine on early post-infarction arrhythmias in anaesthetised rats. Values are means ± S.E.M., $n = 10$

Group	Total number of ectopic beats	Duration of VT (s)	Duration of VF (s)	Incidence of VF (and mortality) (per cent)
Saline controls	1045 ± 206	72 ± 20	28 ± 6	40 (10)
Solvent controls	954 ± 196	69 ± 3	32 ± 4	40 (0)
Nifedipine, 5 μg kg^{-1}	1129 ± 214	67 ± 4	0*	0* (0)
Nifedipine, 10 μg kg^{-1}	558 ± 79*	27 ± 5	0*	0* (0)
Nifedipine, 50 μg kg^{-1}	250 ± 72*	12 ± 4*	0*	0* (0)

From Fagbemi and Parratt (1981a)
$*P < 0.05$.

blockers. This is in contrast to the β-adrenoceptor blocking drugs and, as emphasised by Meesmann, suggests different genesis for these arrhythmias.

Nisoldipine, nifedipine and niludipine are also effective in suppressing VF 1-1.25 h before coronary artery ligation when given by the oral route (Fagbemi and Parratt, 1981b). Again the order of potency was similar to that observed when the drugs were given intravenously. Although the number of VEBs was not markedly reduced by this oral treatment, and the incidence of VF was not markedly affected, the time spent in VF was extremely short and spontaneous reversal to sinus rhythm was made easier (figure 18.4). No animal given these compounds died as a result of

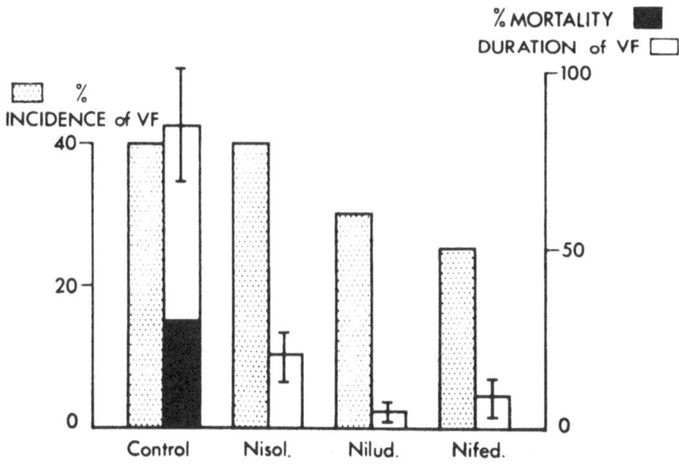

Figure 18.4 The effect of orally administered nisoldipine (Nisol.), niludipine (Nilud.) and nifedipine (Nifed.), each in a dose of 3 mg kg^{-1}, on the incidence and duration (in seconds) of ventricular fibrillation and on mortality in rats anaesthetised with pentobarbitone. (Data from Fagbemi and Parratt (1981b).)

coronary artery ligation, compared to a 40 per cent mortality in the controls (Fagbemi and Parratt, 1981b).

Nifedipine is also effective in suppressing ventricular arrhythmias resulting from coronary artery (LAD) ligation in anaesthetised greyhound dogs (S. J. Coker and J. R. Parratt, unpublished). This is a severe arrhythmia model which results in a 25–30 per cent incidence of VF and (with chloralose anaesthesia) 300–400 VEBs during the initial 30 min post-ligation period (Marshall and Parratt, 1980). Nifedipine (5 μg kg^{-1} bolus injection and a continuous intravenous infusion of 40 μg kg^{-1} h^{-1}) prevented VF and reduced the number of VEBs to less than 20 over the entire 30 min post-ligation period (compare more than 300 in the controls; S. J. Coker and J. R. Parratt, unpublished).

Bepridil

Bepridil (1-[3-isobutoxy-2-(benzylphenyl)amino] propylpyrrolidine hydrochloride) is a recently introduced antianginal drug which increases coronary blood flow, decreases heart rate, has a negative inotropic action and antagonises (although not competitively) the cardiac actions of isoprenaline, theophyline and glucagon (Cosnier *et al.*, 1977; Michelin *et al.*, 1977).

Bepridil has a number of effects on the cardiac muscle action potential. Like the classical calcium antagonists, it reduces or abolishes cardiac contractions in concentrations (10^{-6} M) that have little effect on the upstroke velocity ($+\dot{V}_{max}$) or overshoot of the normal ventricular action potential (Vogel *et al.*, 1979). It thus leads to excitation–contraction uncoupling. Only in concentrations considerably higher than those required to uncouple excitation from contraction in ventricular muscle (that is, 10^{-5} M) are effects seen on $+\dot{V}_{max}$ or on the action potential duration. In contrast, in Purkinje fibres $+\dot{V}_{max}$ is reduced by this concentration of bepridil and the action potential duration is decreased (Kane and Winslow, 1980). In ventricular muscle bepridil depresses the amplitude '$+\dot{V}_{max}$' and duration of slow action potentials generated by isoprenaline, caffeine or tetraethylammonium ions in fibres in which the fast Na^+ current has been voltage-inactivated by partial depolarisation with K^+; these slow action potentials are carried by Ca^{2+} and by Na^+ ions. Since this bepridil-induced depression of the slow channels is reversed by elevating the extracellular Ca^{2+}, and since the negative inotropic action of bepridil is diminished in the presence of agents that enhance the inward Ca^{2+} current, Vogel *et al.* (1979) conclude that bepridil closely resembles the slow channel blockers such as verapamil.

Two recent studies clearly demonstrate that bepridil reduces the early ventricular arrhythmias that result from acute coronary artery ligation in rats (Kane and Winslow, 1980) and dogs (Marshall and Muir, 1981). In the rat study bepridil (2 mg kg^{-1} intravenously) markedly reduced the number of VEBs and abolished fibrillation, an effect equivalent to that of 10 mg kg^{-1} of disopyramide. This dose of bepridil markedly reduced systemic arterial pressure and heart rate. Using chloralose-anaesthetised greyhounds, Marshall and Muir (1981) showed that in an intravenous dose (5 mg kg^{-1}) that caused immediate but transient hypotension and a more prolonged reduction in heart rate and myocardial oxygen consumption, bepridil prevented the VF and VT which invariably result from LAD occlusion in this model (Marshall and Parratt, 1980) and also reduced the number of VEBs occurring in the crucial 10-20 min post-occlusion period. Bepridil is considerably less active than lignocaine, disopyramide or amiodarone in reversing disturbances of ventricular rhythm in conscious dogs 18 h after two-stage LAD ligation (Labrid *et al.*, 1981).

Other calcium antagonists

The Hoffman-La Roche calcium antagonist No. 11-1781 (a substituted homoveratrylamine) is apparently ineffective in preventing VT or VF which result from LAD occlusion in anaesthetised pigs (Frank *et al.*, 1978). The β-adrenoceptor blocking drug pindolol was also ineffective in this severe arrhythmia model. In contrast the coronary vasodilator *lidoflazine*, which has been claimed to possess 'calcium antagonistic properties', reduces early post-occlusion arrhythmias in anaesthetised rats (table 18.3; S. J. Coker, O. Fagbemi and J. R. Parratt, unpublished) and, following acute intravenous administration (2 mg kg^{-1}), in anaesthetised greyhounds (S. J. Coker, O. Fagbemi and J. R. Parratt, unpublished).

A rather similar result in dogs was reported as long ago as 1966 by Schaper *et al.* In this study prolonged (28 day) oral treatment with lidoflazine reduced the incidence of VF (resulting from the abrupt occlusion of the LCFX coronary artery) from 16 cases out of 20 in the controls to only two cases out of 10 in the treated group. It has been suggested (Carmeliet and Xhonneux, 1971) that this protection might be due to a drug-induced increase in the development of coronary collaterals. This, from Meesmann's studies reviewed in chapter 6, might be expected to reduce the severity of early post-ischaemia ventricular arrhythmias. However, this could not explain the effectiveness of the compound after *single* dose administration (S. J. Coker, O. Fagbemi and J. R. Parratt, unpublished). Lidoflazine is apparently not effective against late (24 h) post-infarction arrhythmias (Carmeliet and Xhonneux, 1971).

18.5 POSSIBLE MECHANISMS OF THE ANTIARRHYTHMIC ACTIONS OF CALCIUM ANTAGONISTS

The blocking effect of these drugs on the slow inward current is presumably largely responsible for the antiarrhythmic effects of calcium antagonists in the early stages of acute myocardial ischaemia. It must, however, not be forgotten that these drugs have other and pronounced effects on the ischaemic myocardium that could contribute to their marked ability to suppress the early and serious ventricular arrhythmias resulting from myocardial ischaemia.

Table 18.3 The effect of lidoflazine on early post-infarction ventricular arrhythmias in anaesthetized rats

Group	Duration of		Incidence of VF (per cent)	Mortality (per cent)	Blood pressure (mmHg)	Heart rate (per cent decrease)
	Ventricular tachycardia (s)	Ventricular fibrillation (s)				
Control	68.8 ± 12.6	28.4 ± 2.7	50	30	123 ± 4/103 ± 4	–
Solvent	64.3 ± 6.7	25.7 ± 4.2	40	30	–	–
Lidoflazine, 5 μg kg^{-1}	62.7 ± 16.3	23.5 ± 3.6	40	10	–	–
Lidoflazine, 50 μg kg^{-1}	42.4 ± 14.6	0*	0*	0*	97 ± 4/84 ± 5*	–
Lidoflazine, 2 mg kg^{-1}	18.5 ± 5.1*	0*	0*	0*	85 ± 7*/69 ± 7*	–16.3

Lidoflazine was given intravenously 15 min before coronary artery ligation. There were 10 animals in each group.
*$P < 0.05$.

Blockade of slow calcium channels in the ischaemic myocardium

A strong case can be made for abnormal excitation of myocardial cells early in ischaemia as being due to re-entry mechanisms. Such a circus movement of excitation is favoured by slowly conducting action potentials because 'it permits an impulse to be delayed in the circuitous pathways pending repolarisation of the rest of the heart' (Cranefield, 1980). This means that the delayed (slow impulse) action potential would find excitable tissue when it returned to its origin. The conditions favouring development of slow response potentials are found in the myocardium very soon after the onset of acute myocardial ischaemia. Thus ventricular and Purkinje fibres are exposed to a high concentration of K^+ (chapter 7) and, probably, to locally released noradrenaline (chapters 8–10). The high concentration of K^+ could partially depolarise the cells and, if the membrane potential reaches –50 mV, thus inactivate the fast Na^+ current. High local concentrations of noradrenaline (and also perhaps cyclic AMP or histamine) might then stimulate the slow channels thus resulting in slow response action potentials. The question as to whether these slow responses are mediated early in ischaemia by, for example, calcium is still under discussion. There is little doubt that slow channels are permeable to calcium but, certainly in some types of cardiac cell, the slow channel is also permeable to sodium (Cranefield, 1975), and in fact the current involved might be more nearly a sodium current because there is far more sodium that calcium in the extracellular fluid.

If slow response action potentials are indeed predominantly due to calcium influx through slow channels, then one might expect them to be sensitive to the drugs under discussion in this chapter. There is some evidence that this is indeed so. For example, verapamil increases effective and functional refractory periods of Purkinje cells obtained from the infarcted canine myocardium 24 h after the onset of ischaemia (Dersham and Han, 1981). There is also a decrease in action potential amplitude and a decrease in $\dot{V}_{max}$ only in Purkinje fibres obtained from the infarcted zone (for example, from 48 ± 8 to 22 ± 5 V s^{-1}, a reduction of 52 per cent, with a concentration of 1 μM); these are slow responses. In contrast, $\dot{V}_{max}$ is not altered by verapamil in Purkinje fibres from the uninfarcted zone, a fast response carried predominantly by sodium ions (for example, 253 ± 15 to 266 ± 26 V s^{-1}; n.s.). These results, although obtained in tissue 24 h after coronary artery occlusion, indicate that verapamil preferentially alters slow responses in infarcted tissue, thereby reducing a source of re-entrant-associated arrhythmias. There is other evidence too that verapamil blocks the slow action potentials and the contractions that accompany it (Kohlhardt *et al.*, 1967; Shigenobu *et al.*, 1974; Schneider and Sperelakis, 1975). In contrast, with normal, fast (sodium-mediated) action potentials the same dose of verapamil reduces the muscle contraction to a very low level without altering the shape of the action potential. This incidentally implies that a potassium conductance mechanism is largely responsible for the plateau.

Nifedipine acts mainly to modify the plateau phase of ventricular and Purkinje fibre transmembrane action potentials (Bayer *et al.*, 1977; Dangman and Hoffman,

1980) without depressing phase 4 depolarisation in normal Purkinje fibres (Dangman and Hoffman, 1980). In addition, it depresses spontaneous impulse generation in Purkinje fibres obtained from infarcted tissue 24 h after coronary artery occlusion and also the abnormal automaticity that can be induced in normal Purkinje fibres exposed to low concentrations of barium ions. Both are effects attributable to an action of nifedipine on the slow inward current. Although there are no comparable studies of the effects of calcium antagonists structurally related to nifedipine on ischaemic myocardial cells, there is evidence, from studies on sinus node cells and atrial muscle fibres, that niludipine (table 18.2) also reduces the slow inward current through the myocardial cell membrane.

Improvement of conduction within the ischaemic region

Shortly after coronary artery occlusion, electrograms recorded from the ischaemic region show a decrease in amplitude, an increase in duration and a delayed activation. The resultant slow conduction is associated with electrical inhomogeneity and this favours circus movements by allowing the impulse to be delayed in a circuitous pathway pending repolarisation of the rest of the myocardium. This delayed contraction appears to play an essential role in generating continuous re-entry circuits and recent attempts have been made to correlate the extent of this conduction delay with the incidence of ventricular tachyarrhythmias.

There have been a number of recent canine studies in which the effects of drugs have been examined on early ischaemia-induced conduction delay. Drugs like lignocaine (Kupersmith *et al.*, 1975; Lazzara *et al.*, 1978; Nakaya *et al.*, 1980), diphenylhydantoin (El-Sherif and Lazzara, 1978), tetrodotoxin (El-Sherif and Lazzara, 1979) and aprindine (Elharrar *et al.*, 1977). For example, in the last-mentioned study, aprindine caused a threefold increase in conduction delay in the acutely ischaemic region and increased the incidence of VT and VF from one dog in 11 to eight dogs in 11. In contrast to what one might expect from the electrophysiological effects of calcium slow channel blocking drugs on slow responses, several of these drugs have been shown not to depress still further poor membrane responses of ischaemic cells, but rather to improve conduction. This improvement in conduction is observed not only within the first few minutes of the onset of acute ischaemia (Elharrar *et al.*, 1977; Nakaya *et al.*, 1980), a time corresponding to the onset of early ventricular arrhythmias, but also 3-7 days after LAD ligation (El-Sherif and Lazzara, 1979). Verapamil (Elharrar *et al.*, 1977; Fondacara *et al.*, 1978; El-Sherif and Lazzara, 1979; Nakaya *et al.*, 1980, 1981), D-600 (El-Sherif and Lazzara, 1979) and diltiazem (Nakaya *et al.*, 1980, 1981) are all effective; in contrast, very high doses of nifedipine are required to improve conduction delay even slightly (Nakaya *et al.*, 1981).

The reasons for these effects on ischaemia-induced conduction delay are unknown but there are at least three possibilities.

Increase in blood flow within the ischaemic region

There is good evidence that calcium antagonists increase blood flow in the acutely ischaemic myocardium (see, for example, Henry *et al.*, 1978; Jolly *et al.*, 1981, using nifedipine), although this may depend on the severity of the flow obstruction (Weintraub *et al.*, 1981). Since conduction delay in the ischaemic myocardium has been stated to be critically dependent upon flow (Yamaguchi *et al.*, 1977, but contrast Ruffy *et al.*, 1979), it is conceivable that an increase in blood flow through pre-existing coronary collateral vessels could improve delayed conduction. This would also explain the early observation that the chronic administration of lidoflazine (which has some slow channel blocking activity) reduces the incidence of VF after coronary artery occlusion (Schaper *et al.*, 1966). This possibility has been investigated recently by Nakaya *et al.* (1981). They compared the effects of three calcium antagonists (verapamil, diltiazem and nifedipine) and of the coronary vasodilator dipyridamole (an 'adenosine sparing' agent), as well as a combination of nitroglycerin and phenylephrine, on ischaemia-induced conduction delay and on regional myocardial blood flow. The difficulty of the protocol used in this study was that regional blood flow (using hydrogen clearance) was not measured *during* the short coronary occlusions. This means that flow in the ischaemic myocardium (that is, the area where conduction was delayed) was not assessed; it is well known (reviewed by Parratt *et al.*, 1980) that the effects of coronary vasodilator drugs (for example, dipyridamole, dilazep) on blood flow in the ischaemic myocardium can be quite different to their effects on adjacent, normal regions of the left ventricular wall. For example, such drugs may reduce blood flow in the ischaemic zone through a coronary steal phenomenon. The conclusion, therefore, that a coronary vasodilator action of calcium antagonists is unlikely to play an essential role in reducing conduction delay (Nakaya *et al.*, 1981) may not be valid. It would indeed be technically difficult to measure blood flow in discrete areas of delayed conduction.

Reduction in the degree of myocardial ischaemic damage

Calcium antagonists 'protect' the ischaemic myocardium (limiting infarct size), assessed from changes in epicardial ST-segment mapping (Smith *et al.*, 1975; Wende *et al.*, 1975), from the extent of creatine kinase depletion, from morphometric estimates of necrosis and of ultrastructural damage (Reimer *et al.*, 1977; Henry *et al.*, 1978; Nayler, 1980a), from an ability to protect against depletion of tissue ATP stores (Nayler, 1980a) and from assessments of local mechanical function (Pérez *et al.*, 1980; Sherman *et al.*, 1981). This protection would result partly from increases in blood flow within the ischaemic region and/or from reduced myocardial oxygen demands, for example as a consequence of bradycardia or the effects of reduced after-load or depressed myocardial contractile function (Smith *et al.*, 1975). This beneficial effect on the balance between myocardial oxygen supply and demand might lead to an improvement of ischaemia-induced conduction delay.

Prevention of the damaging effects of Ca^{2+} influx, especially during reperfusion

An increased level of free Ca^{2+} ions in the ischaemic myocardial cells (calcium overload), which occurs especially during reperfusion following prolonged periods of ischaemia or following massive local catecholamine release, leads to cellular damage and to increases in the electrical resistance of cell to cell junctions. These effects are much reduced by pretreatment with calcium slow channel inhibitors such as verapamil and nifedipine (Reimer *et al.*, 1977; Nayler, 1980a,b). In this respect it is of interest that in a number of studies this group of drugs has been shown to protect against the serious ventricular arrhythmias which result from reperfusion (Brooks *et al.*, 1980; Sugiyama *et al.*, 1980; Weishaar and Bing, 1980; but contrast Naito *et al.*, 1981) and to reduce the further lowering of the ventricular fibrillation threshold that results from reperfusion (Brooks *et al.*, 1980; Sugiyama *et al.*, 1980).

REFERENCES

Bayer, R., Rodenkirchen, R., Kaufman, R., Lee, J. H. and Hennekes, R. (1977). The effects of nifedipine on contraction and monophasic action potential of isolated cat myocardium. *Naunyn-Schmiedebergs Arch. Pharmac.*, **301**, 29-37

Bergey J. L., McCallum, J. D. and Nocella, K. (1981). Antiarrhythmic evaluation of verapamil, nifedipine, perhexiline and SKF 525-A in four canine models of cardiac arrhythmias. *Eur. J. Pharmac.*, **70**, 331-43

Brooks, W. W., Verrier, R. L. and Lown, B. (1980). Protective effect of verapamil on vulnerability to ventricular fibrillation during myocardial ischaemia and reperfusion. *Cardiovasc. Res.*, **14**, 295-302

Carmeliet, E. and Xhonneux, R. (1971). Influence of lidoflazine on cardiac transmembrane potentials and experimental arrhythmias. *Naunyn-Schmiedebergs Arch. Pharmac.*, **268**, 210-28

Chiou, C. Y., Malagodi, M. H., Sastry, B. V. R. and Posner, P. (1976). Effects of calcium antagonist, 6-(*N,N*-diethylamino)hexyl-3,4,5-trimethoxybenzoate, on digitalis-induced arrhythmias and cardiac contractions. *J. Pharmac. exp. Ther.*, **198**, 444-9

Clarke, C., Foreman, M. I., Kane, K. A., McDonald, F. M. and Parratt, J. R. (1980). Coronary artery ligation in anaesthetized rats as a method for the production of experimental dysrhythmias and for the determination of infarct size. *J. pharmac. Meth.*, **3**, 357-68

Cosnier, D., Duchene-Marullaz, P., Rispat, E. and Streichenberger, G. (1977). Cardiovascular pharmacology of bepridil (1-[3-isobutoxy-2-(benzylphenyl)-amino] propylpyrrolidine hydrochloride) a new potential anti-anginal compound. *Arch. int. Pharmacodyn. Thér.*, **225**, 133-51

Cranefield, P. F. (1975). *The Conduction of the Cardiac Impulse. The Slow Response and Cardiac Arrhythmias*, Futura, Mount Kisco, N.Y.

Cranefield, P. F. (1980). The slow inward current and the generation of cardiac arrhythmias. In *Ca^{++} Antagonism; Cardiac Arrhythmias and the Slow Ca^{++} Current* (ed. R. G. Richardson), Abbott Laboratories, London, pp. 15-21

Dangman, K. H. and Hoffman, B. F. (1980). Effects of nifedipine on electrical activity of cardiac cells. *Am. J. Cardiol.*, **46**, 1059-67

Dersham, G. H. and Han, J. (1981). Actions of verapamil on Purkinje fibres from normal and infarcted heart tissues. *J. Pharmac. exp. Ther.*, **216**, 261-4

Elharrar, V., Gaum, W. E. and Zipes, D. P. (1977). Effect of drugs on conduction delay and incidence of ventricular arrhythmias induced by acute coronary occlusion in dogs. *Am. J. Cardiol.*, **39**, 544-9

Ellrodt, G., Chew, C. Y. C. and Singh, B. N. (1980). Therapeutic implications of slow-channel blockade in cardiocirculatory disorders. *Circulation*, **62**, 669-79

El-Sherif, N. and Lazzara, R. (1978). Reentrant ventricular arrhythmias in the late myocardial infarction period. 5. Mechanisms of action of diphenylhydantoin. *Circulation*, **57**, 405-11

El-Sherif, N. and Lazzara, R. (1979). Reentrant ventricular arrhythmias in the late myocardial infarction period. 7. Effect of verapamil and D-600 and the role of the 'slow channel'. *Circulation*, **60**, 605-15

Fagbemi, O. and Parratt, J. R. (1981a). Calcium antagonists prevent early post-infarction ventricular fibrillation. *Eur. J. Pharmac.*, **75**, 179-85

Fagbemi, O. and Parratt, J. R. (1981b). Suppression by orally-administered nifedipine, nisoldipine and niludipine of early life-threatening ventricular arrhythmias resulting from acute myocardial ischaemia. *Br. J. Pharmac.*, **74**, 12-14

Fondacaro, J. D., Han, J. and Yoon, M. S. (1978). Effects of verapamil on ventricular rhythm during acute coronary occlusion. *Am. Heart J.*, **96**, 81-6

Frank, J., Dolder, M., Gertsch, M., Althaus, U. and Gurtner, H. P. (1978). Ventriculäre Rhythmusstörungen im akuten Stadium des experimentellen Myokardinfarktes beim Schwein; einfluss des β-Blockers Pindolol und des Calcium-Antagonisten Ro 11-1781. *Schweiz. med. Wschr.*, **108**, 1740-3

Henry, P. D. (1980). Comparative pharmacology of calcium antagonists: nifedipine, verapamil and diltiazem. *Am. J. Cardiol.*, **46**, 1047-58

Henry, P. D., Shuchleib, R., Borda, L. J., Roberts, R., Williamson, J. R. and Sobel, B. E. (1978). Effects of nifedipine on myocardial perfusion and ischemic injury in dogs. *Circulation Res.*, **43**, 372-80

Jolly, S. R., Hardman, H. F. and Gross, G. J. (1981). Comparison of two dihydropyridine calcium antagonists on coronary collateral blood flow in acute myocardial ischemia. *J. Pharmac. exp. Ther.*, **217**, 20-5

Kane, K. A. and Winslow, E. (1980). Antidysrhythmic and electrophysiological effects of a new antianginal agent, bepridil. *J. cardiovasc. Pharmac.*, 2, 193-203

Kane, K. A., McDonald, F. M. and Parratt, J. R. (1979). Coronary artery ligation in anaesthetised rats as a model for the assessment of antidysrhythmic activity. *Br. J. Pharmac.*, **66**, 436P

Kane, K. A., McDonald, F. M. and Parratt, J. R. (1981). What pharmacological properties are necessary for the prevention of early post-infarction arrhythmias? *Br. J. Pharmac.*, 72, 512-3P

Kaplinsky, E., Ogawa, S., Michelson, E. L. and Dreifus, L. S. (1981). Instantaneous and delayed ventricular arrhythmias after reperfusion of acutely ischemic myocardium: evidence for multiple mechanisms. *Circulation*, **63**, 333–40

Kaumann, A. J. and Aramendia, P. (1968). Prevention of ventricular fibrillation induced by coronary ligation. *J. Pharmac. exp. Ther.*, **164**, 326-32

Kohlhardt, M., Happ, K. and Figulla, H. R. (1967). Influence of low extracellular pH upon the Ca inward current and isometric contractile force in mammalian ventricular myocardium. *Pflügers Arch. ges. Physiol.*, **366**, 31-8

Kupersmith, J., Antman, E. M. and Hoffman, B. F. (1975). *In vitro* electrophysiological effects of lidocaine in canine acute myocardial infarction. *Circulation Res.*, **36**, 84-91

Kupersmith, J., Shiang, H. and Litwak, R. S. (1976). Electrophysiological effects of verapamil in canine myocardial ischemia. *Am. J. Cardiol.*, **37**, 149

Labrid, C., Leindt, M., Beaughard, M., Basiez, M. and Duchene-Marullaz, P. (1981). Comparative antidysrhythmic profiles of bepridil, amiodarone and disopyramide in the guinea-pig and dog. *Arch. int. Pharmacodyn. Thér.*, **249**, 87-97

Lazzara, R., El-Sherif, N., Hope, R. R. and Scherlag, B. J. (1978). Ventricular arrhythmias and electrophysiological consequences of myocardial ischemia and infarction. *Circulation Res.*, **42**, 740-9

Lynch, J. J., Rahwan, R. E. and Witiak, D. T. (1981). Effect of 2-substituted 3-dimethylamino-5,6-methylenedioxyindenes on calcium-induced arrhythmias. *J. cardiovasc. Pharmac.*, **3**, 49-60

McDonald, F. M. (1980). Experimental models for the production of cardiac dysrhythmias and for the assessment of activity of antidysrhythmic drugs. PhD thesis, University of Strathclyde

Marshall, R. J. and Muir, A. W. (1981). The beneficial actions of bepridil in acute myocardial infarction in anaesthetized dogs. *Br. J. Pharmac.*, **73**, 471-9

Marshall, R. J. and Parratt, J. R. (1980). The early consequences of myocardial ischaemia and their modification. *J. Physiol., Paris*, **76**, 699-715

Melville, K. I. and Benfey, B. C. (1965). Coronary vasodilatory and cardiac adrenergic blocking effects of iproveratril. *Can. J. Physiol. Pharmac.*, **43**, 339-42

Michelin, M. T., Cheucle, M. and Duchene-Marrulaz, P. (1977). Influence comparée sur l'activité cardiaque et le debit veineux coronaire du bépridil, du dipyridamole et du propranolol chez le chien narcosé. *Thérapie*, **32**, 485-99

Naito, M., Michelson, E. L., Kmetzo, J. J., Kaplinsky, E. and Dreifus, L. S. (1981). Failure of antiarrhythmic drugs to prevent experimental reperfusion ventricular fibrillation. *Circulation*, **63**, 70-9

Nakaya, H., Hattori, Y. and Kanno, M. (1980). Effects of calcium antagonists and lidocaine on conduction delay induced by acute myocardial ischemia in dogs. *Jap. J. Pharmac.*, **30**, 587-97

Nakaya, H., Hattori, Y., Sakuma, I. and Kanno, M. (1981). Effects of calcium antagonists on coronary circulation and conduction delay induced by myocardial ischemia in dogs: a comparative study with other coronary vasodilators. *Eur. J. Pharmac.*, **73**, 273-81

Nayler, W. E. (1980a). The pharmacological protection of the ischaemic heart: the use of calcium and beta-adrenoceptor antagonists. *Eur. Heart J.*, **1**, Suppl. B., 5-13

Nayler, W. G. (1980b). Cardioprotective effects of calcium ion antagonists in myocardial ischemia. *Clin. Invest. Med.*, **3**, 91-9

Parratt, J. R., Marshall, R. J. and Ledingham, I. McA. (1980). Interventions for improving blood flow, oxygen availability and the balance between oxygen supply and demand in the acutely ischaemic myocardium. *J. Physiol., Paris*, **76**, 791-803

Pérez, J. E., Sobel, B. E. and Henry, P. D́. (1980). Improved performance of ischemic canine myocardium in response to nifedipine and diltiazem. *Am. J. Physiol.*, **239**, H658-63

Piascik, M. F., Piascik, M. T., Witiak, D. T. and Rahwan, R. E. (1979). Pharmacological evaluation of new calcium antagonists: 2-substituted 3-dimethylamino-5, 6-methylenedioxyindenes. Antiarrhythmic effects. *Can. J. Physiol. Pharmac.*, **57**, 1350-8

Refsum, H. (1975). Calcium-antagonistic and anti-arrhythmic effects of nifedipine on the isolated rat atrium. *Acta pharmac. toxicol.*, **37**, 377-86

Refsum, H., Landmark, K. and Bjerve, K. S. (1979). Calcium, nifedipine and arrhythmias in isolated rat atrium. *Acta pharmac. toxicol.*, **44**, 71-4

Reimer, K. A., Lowe, J. E. and Jennings, R. B. (1977). Effects of the calcium antagonist verapamil on necrosis following temporary coronary artery occlusion in dogs. *Circulation*, **55**, 581-7

Rodrigues-Pereira, E. and Viana, A. P. (1968). The actions of verapamil on experimental arrhythmias. *Arzneimittel-Forsch.*, **18**, 175-9

Rowland, E., Evans, T. and Krikler, D. (1979). Effect of nifedipine on atrioventricular conduction as compared with verapamil. Intracardiac electrophysiological study. *Br. Heart J.*, **42**, 124-7

Ruffy, R., Lovelace, D. E., Mueller, T. M., Knoebel, S. B. and Zipes, D. P. (1979). Relationship between changes in left ventricular bipolar electrograms and regional myocardial blood flow during acute coronary occlusion in the dog. *Circulation Res.*, **45**, 764-70

Schaper, W. K. A., Xhonneux, R., Jageneau, A. H. M. and Janssen, P. A. J. (1966). The cardiovascular pharmacology of lidoflazine, a long-acting coronary vasodilator. *J. Pharmac. exp. Ther.*, **152**, 265-74

Schneider, J. A. and Sperelakis, N. (1975). Slow Ca^{++} and Na^{+} responses induced by isoproterenol and methylxanthines in isolated perfused guinea pig hearts exposed to elevated K^{+}. *J. molec. cell. Cardiol.*, **7**, 249-73

Sherman, L. E., Liane, C.-S., Boden, W. E. and Hood, W. B. (1981). The effect of verapamil on mechanical performance of acutely ischemic and reperfused myocardium in the conscious dog. *Circulation Res.*, **48**, 224-32

Shigenobu, K., Schneider, J. A. and Sperelakis, N. (1974). Verapamil blockade of slow Na^{+} and Ca^{++} responses in myocardial cells. *J. Pharmac. exp. Ther.*, **190**, 280-8

Singh, B. N. and Vaughan Williams, E. M. (1972). A fourth class of antidysrhythmic action? Effect of verapamil on ouabain toxicity, on atrial and ventricular intracellular potentials, and on other features of cardiac function. *Cardiovasc. Res.*, **6**, 109-19

Smith, H. J., Singh, B. N., Nisbet, H. D. and Norris, R. M. (1975). Effects of verapamil on infarct size following experimental coronary occlusion. *Cardiovasc. Res.*, **9**, 569-78

Sugiyama, S., Ozawa, T., Suzuki, S. and Kato, T. (1980). Effects of verapamil and propranolol on ventricular vulnerability after coronary reperfusion. *J. Electrocardiol.*, **13**, 49-54

Szekeres, L. and Papp, Gy. J. (1971). *Experimental Cardiac Arrhythmias and Antiarrhythmic Drugs*, Akademiai Kiado, Budapest

Taira, N. and Narimatsu, A. (1975). Effects of nifedipine, a potent calcium antagonistic coronary vasodilator, on atrioventricular conduction and blood flow in the isolated atrioventricular node preparation of the dog. *Naunyn Schmiedebergs Arch. Pharmac.*, **290**, 107-112

Vogel, S., Crampton, R. and Sperelakis, N. (1979). Blockade of myocardial slow channels by bepridil (CERM-1978). *J. Pharmac. exp. Ther.*, **210**, 378-85

Weintraub, W. S., Hattori, S., Agarwal, J., Bodenheimer, M. M., Banka, V. S. and Helfant, R. H. (1981). Variable effect of nifedipine on myocardial blood flow at three grades of coronary occlusion in the dog. *Circulation Res.*, **48**, 937-42

Weishaar, R. E. and Bing, R. J. (1980). The beneficial effect of a calcium channel blocker, diltiazem, on the ischemic-reperfused heart. *J. molec. cell. Cardiol.*, **12**, 993-1009

Wende, W., Bleifeld, W., Meyer, J. and Stühlen, H. W. (1975). Reduction of the size of acute, experimental myocardial infarction by verapamil. *Basic Res. Cardiol.*, **70**, 198-208

Yamaguchi, Z., McCullen, A. and Mandel, W. J. (1977). The electrophysiological time course after graded reduction in coronary flow and reperfusion. *Am. J. Cardiol.*, **39**, 312

19

Sulphinpyrazone and Early Post-infarction Arrhythmias

R. C. Browning

19.1 INTRODUCTION

The pyrazolidine derivative sulphinpyrazone has been in clinical use for over 20 years because of its potent uricosuric properties (Burns *et al*., 1957). In 1962 a study of arteriosclerotic patients by Murphy and Mustard revealed, by chance, that those taking sulphinpyrazone had prolonged platelet survival and reduced platelet turnover; this effect was confirmed by Smythe *et al*. (1965), who noted also reduced platelet adhesiveness. These findings were demonstrated later to be independent of reductions in uric acid (Mustard *et al*., 1967). These facts, somewhat expanded, formed the basis for an opportunity directly to affect platelets, pathological processes associated with them and resulting clinical manifestations.

The results of subsequent clinical studies in conditions where platelet economy is known to be disturbed were confirmatory. Patients with prosthetic mitral valves and a reduced platelet survival time had this parameter corrected to normal by sulphinpyrazone whilst platelet adhesiveness was also reduced (Weily and Genton, 1970). Sulphinpyrazone was also demonstrated to prolong the pathologically shortened platelet survival found in patients with coronary artery disease (Steele, *et al*., 1975).

As a result of these findings and the role which platelets were known to play in the initiation and growth of thrombi, therapeutic trials into diseases associated with thrombosis were undertaken. In patients with *amaurosis fugax* sulphinpyrazone was effective in the short term reduction of symptoms (Evans and Gent, 1972) and the drug significantly reduced the incidence of recurrent attacks of clinically detectable venous thrombosis in patients with that disorder. Kaegi *et al*. (1974) also demonstrated that in patients with arteriovenous shunts, sulphinpyrazone markedly reduced the incidence of documented thrombosis and prolonged shunt survival.

In 1975, Blakely and Gent reported a study which showed in a geriatric population that sulphinpyrazone prevented vascular-related death in patients who had suffered a previous myocardial infarction either alone or in combination with stroke.

An extensive multicentre study set up in the light of previous knowledge to look at the effect of sulphinpyrazone versus those of placebo on cardiac mortality following an acute myocardial infarction was reported from North America (Anturane Reinfarction Trial Research Group. 1980). The results showed an apparent reduction in cardiac mortality over the whole 24 month trial period. Looking at the cause of cardiac mortality in more detail revealed that there was no difference in mortality due to re-infarction but a reduction in the incidence of sudden cardiac death over this same time. Furthermore, it was in the first 6 months of treatment that sulphinpyrazone was having its greatest effect. What mechanism of action is responsible for the preventative effect of sulphinpyrazone on sudden death is not yet clear, and a multiplicity of theories have been proposed.

No single rationale is currently held to explain sudden death, although the final event is almost certainly ventricular fibrillation. Since sulphinpyrazone is effective in reducing this in the early post-infarction period, it may be that the drug in man supresses fatal arrhythmias (Margulies *et al.*, 1980). The evidence which supports this possibility will first be considered.

19.2 EVIDENCE FOR THE ANTIARRHYTHMIC ACTIVITY OF SULPHINPYRAZONE

A summary of the evidence for an antiarrhythmic effect of sulphinpyrazone is shown in table 19.1. Holter 24 hour monitorings were made on patients in one of the ART participating centres during the study and deferred for report until the end of the trial (Cuddy, 1980). Qualitative analysis according to a modified Lown classification revealed a significantly different distribution of arrhythmias between the two patient groups. Classified according to the most abnormal rhythm detected, classes I-III were found in 67.5 per cent of sulphinpyrazone patients and 40.5 per cent of those on placebo. Classes IV and V occurred in 32.5 per cent of sulphinpyrazone patients and 59.5 per cent of those on placebo. Comparison of characteristics known to increase the likelihood of ventricular arrhythmias showed no difference between the two groups sufficient to explain this finding. Conversely, in a recent study of cardiac rhythm on the first day and 5-8 days after acute myocardial infarction (Wilcox *et al.*, 1980), the investigators reported that sulphinpyrazone, given as soon as possible after the acute event, caused no significant reduction in serious arrhythmias.

The data available from animal arrhythmia models is less contradictory. Thus, Kelliher *et al.* (1980) pretreated cats with sulphinpyrazone (100 mg kg^{-1} intravenously) or an appropriate volume of vehicle. In one group of animals the vagus nerve was sectioned whilst in another it was left intact. After 1 h the left anterior descending coronary artery was ligated in all animals. In the intact vagus group sulphinpyrazone significantly reduced the incidence and duration of ventricular tachycardia and the number of premature ventricular complexes. In the vagotomised

Table 19.1 A summary of the evidence for the antiarrhythmic activity of sulphinpyrazone

Arrhythmia model	Sulphinpyrazone dose	Effect reported	Reference
Man	200 mg q.d.s., oral	Lown class IV + V arrhythmias	Cuddy (1980)
Cat	100 mg kg^{-1}, i.v.	VT, PVCs, VF onset	Kelliher *et al.* (1980)
Dog	30 mg kg^{-1} day^{-1}, oral	VF mortality	Povalski *et al.* (1980)
Dog	300 mg day^{-1}, oral	VF mortality	Moschos *et al.* (1980)
Rat	30 mg kg^{-1}, s.c.	Mortality	Brunner *et al.* (1980)
Rat	100 mg kg^{-1} day^{-1}, oral	Arrhythmias	Leprán *et al.* (1981) and chapter 14
Rabbit	100 mg kg^{-1} day^{-1}, oral	VE	Rabkin and Ohmae (1980)
Rabbit (isolated heart)	Infusion	VF	Shragge *et al.* (1980)

cats the usual abbreviation of the time to the onset of ventricular arrhythmias was prevented by sulphinpyrazone and the normally increased incidence of ventricular fibrillation was reduced.

An effect on ventricular arrhythmias and in particular fibrillation has also been reported by other authors. Thus, in the dog, Povalski and his colleagues (Povalski *et al.*, 1980) demonstrated that occlusion and reperfusion of the left anterior descending coronary artery caused appreciably less ventricular fibrillation (17 per cent) and a lower mortality (50 per cent) in animals pretreated for 7 days with sulphinpyrazone (30 mg kg^{-1} day^{-1}) compared with those receiving placebo (58 per cent and 75 per cent respectively). The same authors found that the incidence of abnormal or ectopic beats after complete left circumflex coronary artery occlusion was lower in dogs pretreated for 4 days with sulphinpyrazone (30 mg kg^{-1} day^{-1}). Again, a study by Moschos *et al.* (1980) showed in dogs that after totally occluding the LAD coronary artery by means of a balloon catheter there was a decreased mortality (and no ventricular fibrillation) in those animals which had been given sulphinpyrazone (300 mg daily for 7 days previously).

A model of coronary ischaemia utilising ligation of the LAD coronary artery in rats has been used to study the effects of sulphinpyrazone. Brunner *et al.* (1980) pretreated animals for 2 days either with sulphinpyrazone (30 mg kg^{-1} subcutaneously twice daily) or saline. During the first 30 min after ligation, 14 per cent of the control group and 3.3 per cent of the treated animals died; up to the sixth day after ligation (5 days after the last sulphinpyrazone dose) less deaths occurred in the treatment group. Thereafter both groups had the same mortality up to 21 days. The same experimental model, but in conscious animals, was used by Leprán *et al.* (1981) (see also chapter 14). These workers pretreated one group with sulphinpyrazone (50 mg kg^{-1} orally only 60 min before ligation) and showed that the number of animals showing no arrhythmias after ligation increased from 0 per cent in the controls to 20 per cent on treatment. The duration of arrhythmias was reduced by one-third and the time taken for arrhythmias to appear was increased. There was a marked and significant increase in survival (33 per cent in the controls and 65–80 per cent in animals pretreated with sulphinpyrazone, 50 and 10 mg kg^{-1}).

Adriamycin-induced cardiotoxicity in the rabbit was studied by Rabkin and Ohmae (1980), who claim that the kind of arrhythmias produced in this model are simlar to those associated with sudden death in man. Pretreatment with sulphinpyrazone (100 and 200 mg kg^{-1} daily) was associated with a dose-dependent reduction in the time of appearance and the frequency of ventricular ectopics. Rabbit hearts perfused with an asanguinous solution containing sulphinpyrazone had a lower incidence (10 per cent) of ventricular fibrillation on reperfusion compared to control isolated hearts (72 per cent).

The results of these studies are supportive evidence for an antiarrhythmic effect of sulphinpyrazone. This effect is manifest in the ischaemic myocardium of the rat, cat, dog and rabbit. The situation in man is less clear, although in the study by Wilcox *et al.* (1980), by its very nature, sulphinpyrazone could not be given until after vascular occlusion; in all the animal studies it was given prior to the acute event.

Table 19.2 Possible mechanisms for antiarrhythmic effect of sulphinpyrazone for which there is supportive evidence

Primary antiarrhythmic effect

Electrophysiological stabilisation of ischaemic cells

Secondary antiarrhythmic effect

Primary effect on myocardial ischaemia:

(a) Haemodynamic alterations
(b) Enhancement of the coronary circulation
(c) Reduction of thrombosis and embolism

Platelet adhesion
Platelet aggregation
Platelet release reaction
Endothelial protection
Uricosuric effect

(d) Effects on prostaglandin synthesis

It is not a simple task to elucidate from the available evidence by what mechanism sulphinpyrazone affects arrhythmias (table 19.2). One possibility is that the drug has a direct antiarrhythmic action. However, re-entrant arrhythmias arise from ventricular muscle and are frequently the result of myocardial ischaemia. It may be that it is by influencing events giving rise to ischaemia that sulphinpyrazone has a (secondary) antiarrhythmic effect.

19.3 ELECTROPHYSIOLOGICAL EVIDENCE FOR A PRIMARY ANTIARRHYTHMIC EFFECT OF SULPHINPYRAZONE

The evidence available to date is not conclusive. Roos and Dunning (1980) studied the effects of sulphinpyrazone in 20 patients, 17 of whom had abnormal electrocardiograms. They found that sulphinpyrazone had no effect on sinus rate, sinuatrial conduction time, sinus node recovery time or refractory periods in the atrium, AV node, His–Purkinje system or right ventricle. A study of the drug on isolated superfused canine Purkinje fibres using micro-electrode recording techniques (Benditt *et al.*, 1980) also showed that sulphinpyrazone does not have direct electrophysiological actions comparable to those of conventional antiarrhythmic drugs.

Biochemical changes within the ischaemic area (for example, acidosis) predispose to re-entry phenomena. On examination of the effect of sulphinpyrazone on tissues exposed to such an environment, Iansmith *et al.* (1979) showed that the drug protected cells against acidosis, prolonging survival time to the onset of uncontrollable automaticity in isolated canine Purkinje fibres from 15 to 60 min.

To date, therefore, it would not seem that available evidence has shown sulphinpyrazone to exert a recognised direct antiarrhythmic effect on the heart.

19.4 EVIDENCE FOR SECONDARY ANTIARRHYTHMIC MECHANISMS

Reduction in myocardial oxygen demands

Heart rate and blood pressure are both major determinants of myocardial oxygen consumption. Recently Forfar *et al.* (1980) studied the effect of sulphinpyrazone in human volunteers and found that 2 h after a 200 mg oral dose there was a significant fall in the product of heart rate and blood pressure during exercise and for 2 min after recovery from exercise. This resulted mainly from a reduced rise in systolic blood pressure. Animal studies have also shown that sulphinpyrazone reduces absolute levels of blood pressure in dogs (Moschos *et al.*, 1980) and decreases heart rate during myocardial ischaemia in the cat (Kelliher *et al.*, 1980) and dog (Folts and Beck, 1980; Forfar *et al.*, 1981). A reduction in the rate-pressure product during exercise by sulphinpyrazone would reduce myocardial oxygen demand and so thereby lessen the extent and duration of myocardial ischaemia which might predispose toward arrhythmias.

Effects on coronary blood flow

Thomas *et al.* (1980) showed in dogs that the intracoronary administration of large doses of sulphinpyrazone (50 mg) led to an increase in blood flow of up to 500 per cent; this persisted for periods in excess of 20 min. A possibly related effect was reported by Davenport *et al.* (1979), who demonstrated that in dogs, using labelled microspheres, sulphinpyrazone caused an increase in collateral blood flow to the epicardium and also, to a lesser extent, to the endocardium of the ischaemic region. This increase in tissue oxygenation resulting from an augmented blood flow to the ischaemic zone would be likely to reduce the severity of myocardial ischaemia and the likelihood of electrical instability. However, the mechanisms involved cannot be elucidated from this data, although the increase in blood flow in the Davenport study was still observable after the plasma drug levels had disappeared.

Effect on prostaglandin synthesis

It has been shown by Needleman *et al.* (1977) that thromboxane A_2 causes profound constriction of coronary arteries and the resultant reduction in blood flow might predispose to electrical instability. It has also been demonstrated conclusively that sulphinpyrazone inhibits thromboxane formation (Cerskus *et al.*, 1980).

Ali and McDonald (1977) have demonstrated, in human platelet lysates incubated with arachidonic acid, that sulphinpyrazone was an inhibitor of platelet prostaglandin synthesis. Inhibition was competitive with respect to substrate and 50 per cent inhibition occurred at arachidonic acid concentrations of 2.5 μmol and sulphinpyrazone at 50 μmol. The production of thromboxane B_2 and PGD_2 in rabbits in response to infusions of arachidonic acid (Cerskus *et al.*, 1978) was eliminated by pretreatment with sulphinpyrazone.

It has been proposed that a balance between the production of thromboxane A_2 by the platelets and the production of prostacyclin by the vessel wall (Moncada *et al.*, 1977) is important as a vascular protective mechanism. In human platelets sulphinpyrazone has been demonstrated to inhibit equally the formation of PGD_2 and thromboxane A_2 (measured by thromboxane B_2), indicating that the drug inhibits cyclo-oxygenase. However, in rats, Livio *et al.* (1980) reported that, whilst production of thromboxane A_2 (as measured by malondialdehyde production) was progressively inhibited during the first 3 h after sulphinpyrazone administration, prostacyclin activity was not inhibited at any time. Although some of the more detailed evidence is conflicting, it would seem conclusive that sulphinpyrazone does indeed affect prostaglandin synthesis. Apart from being important on its own as a mechanism (see chapter 13), the generation of prostaglandins has a part to play in the pathways through which several other mechanisms interact.

Effect on arterial thrombosis and embolism

Arterial thrombi are not stable structures. They tend to grow and fragment as parts are shed off, pass downstream as platelet-fibrin emboli and reform. Emboli showering into the myocardial circulation may cause transient ischaemia and fatal arrhythmia (Mustard and Packham, 1975). This is supported by the work of Robbins *et al.* (1969), demonstrating that temporary obstruction of small coronary vessels in the pig by platelet aggregates can produce fatal arrhythmias.

Sulphinpyrazone inhibits platelet aggregation induced by collagen and arachidonic acid (Butler *et al.*, 1979b; Butler and White, 1980) and also reduces the formation of experimentally induced thrombi *in vivo*. This has been demonstrated by Lewis and Westwick (1977), who stimulated the hamster cheek pouch electrically and showed that pretreatment with sulphinpyrazone reduced thrombus formation in a dose-dependent fashion. Butler and White (1980) also showed that sulphinpyrazone inhibited the sequestration of platelet aggregates in the lungs which results from the Forssman reaction in guinea-pigs. Further, these workers demonstrated in the same species inhibition by sulphinpyrazone of the thrombocytopaenia associated with induction of the Arthus reaction. Whilst the drug doses used were rather high it should be emphasised that sulphinpyrazone is metabolised extremely rapidly in this species and that plasma levels measured 1 h after such intravenous doses are similar to those found in man after therapeutic doses of the drug (Butler and White, 1980). The formation of white bodies in physically damaged cerebral arteries of rabbits is also prevented by sulphinpyrazone (Adams and Mitchell, 1979).

It has been proposed that platelet aggregation frequently results from catecholamines released as a result of stress (Haft and Fani, 1973) and that the resulting platelet plugging may generate arrhythmias. In this respect, Folts and Beck (1980) demonstrated, in a dog model with a fixed stenosis of a coronary artery, that platelet plugs actively form and produce cyclical reductions in blood flow. Sulphinpyrazone given after the stress was produced abolished these reductions in flow. These investigators also demonstrated that infusions of adrenaline caused cyclical flow reductions, which were abolished by sulphinpyrazone (Folts and Rowe, 1979).

Important in the generation of platelet thrombi and possibly also in the genesis of atherosclerosis is endothelial damage. Sulphinpyrazone has been shown by Harker and Ross (1978) to reduce endothelial damage resulting from the infusion of homocysteine in baboons; aortic damage (measured by endothelial cell desquamation) decreased from 9.6 per cent to 0.4 per cent on treatment.

The ability of sulphinpyrazone to interfere with the renal tubular transport of uric acid and thereby promote uricosuria led to its description as a uricosuric agent (Burns *et al.*, 1957). Newland (1979) has proposed that, since ADP is a mediator of platelet aggregation and since ADP is degraded enzymatically to the final metabolite uric acid, high levels of blood uric acid may inhibit the rate of ADP degradation and thereby increase the stability of platelet aggregates. Patients with high uric acid could therefore have more stable platelet aggregates and an increase in thrombosis; conversely, treatment with sulphinpyrazone would reduce the levels of uric acid and the incidence of resulting thrombosis.

It would seem, therefore, that there are many mechanisms by which sulphinpyrazone can exert an effect of arterial thrombosis and embolism and thereby reduce the incidence of coronary ischaemia, leading to arrhythmias and sudden death.

ACKNOWLEDGEMENTS

The author would like to thank Dr I. M. Jackson and Dr R. B. Wallis for their advice in the preparation of this manuscript.

REFERENCES

Adams, J. H. and Mitchell, J. R. A. (1979). The effect of agents which modify platelet behaviour and magnesium ions on thrombus formation *in vivo*. *Thrombosis Haemostasis*, **42**, 603–10

Ali, M. and McDonald, J. W. D. (1977). Effects of sulfinpyrazone on platelet prostaglandin synthesis and platelet release of serotonin. *J. Lab. clin. Med.*, **89**, 868–75

Anturane Reinfarction Trial Research Group (1980). Sulfinpyrazone in the prevention of sudden death after myocardial infarction. *New Engl. J. Med.*, **302**, 250–6

Benditt, D. G., Grant, A. O., Hutchinson, A. B. S. and Schauss, H. C. (1980). Electrophysiological effects of sulfinpyrazone on canine cardiac Purkinje fibres. *Can. J. Physiol. Pharmac.*, **58**, 738-42

Blakely, J. A. and Gent, M. (1975). Platelets, drugs and longevity in a geriatric population. In *Platelets, Drugs and Thrombosis* (ed. J. Hirsch), Karger, Basle, pp. 284-91

Brunner, L., Stepanek, J. and Brunner, H. (1980). Reduction of mortality by sulphinpyrazone after experimental myocardial infarction in the rat. *J. Pharm. Pharmac.*, **32**, 714-5

Burns, J. J., Yu, T. F., Ritterband, A., Perel, J. M., Gutman, A. B. and Brodie, B. B. (1957). A potent new uricosuric agent, the sulfoxide metabolite of the phenybutazone analogue G-25671. *J. Pharmac. exp. Ther.*, **119**, 418-26

Butler, K. D. and White, A. M. (1980). Inhibition of platelet involvement in the sublethal Forssman reaction by sulfinpyrazone. In *Cardiovascular Actions of Sulphinpyrazone: Basic and Clinical Research* (ed. M. McGregor, J. F. Mustard, M. F. Oliver and S. Sherry), Symposia Specialists Inc., Miami, pp. 3-17

Butler, K. D., Wallis, R. B. and White, A. M. (1979a). A study of the relationship between *ex vivo* and *in vivo* effects of sulphinpyrazone in the guinea pig. *Haemostasis*, **8**, 353-60

Butler, K. D., Pay, G. F., Roberts, I. M. and White, A. M. (1979b). The effect of sulphinpyrazone and other drugs on the platelet response during the acute phase of active Arthus reaction in guinea pigs. *Thombosis Res.*, **15**, 319-40

Butler, K. D., Dieterle, W., Maguire, E. D., Pay, G. F., Wallis, R. B. and White, A. M. (1980). Sustained effects of sulphinpyrazone. In *Cardiovascular Actions of Sulphinpyrazone: Basic and Clinical Research* (ed. M. McGregor, J. F. Mustard, M. F. Oliver and S. Sherry), Symposia Specialists Inc., Miami, pp. 19-35

Cerskus, A. L., Ali, M., Zamecnik, J. and McDonald, J. W. D. (1978). Effects of indomethacin and sulfinpyrazone on *in vivo* formation of thromboxane B_2 and prostaglandin D_2 during arachidonate infusion in rabbits. *Thrombosis Res.*, **12**, 549-53

Cerskus, A. L., Ali, M. and McDonald, J. W. D. (1980). Thromboxane B_2 and 6-keto-prostaglandin $F_{1\alpha}$ synthesis during infusion of collagen and arachidonic acid in rabbits: inhibition by aspirin and sulphinpyrazone. *Thrombosis Res.*, **18**, 693-705

Cuddy, T. E. (1980). Sulphinpyrazone and ventricular arrhythmias after acute myocardial infarction. In *The Clinical Impact of Beta-Adrenoceptor Blockade* (ed. D. M. Burley and G. F. B. Birdwood), Ciba Laboratories, Horsham, Surrey, pp. 31-2

Davenport, N., Goldstein, R. E., Capurro, N. L., Shulman, N. R. and Epstein, S. E. (1979). Sulfinpyrazone increases collateral blood flow following acute coronary occlusion. *Am. J. Cardiol.*, **43**, 396

Evans, G. and Gent, M. (1980). Effect of platelet suppressive drugs on arterial and venous thromboembolism. In *Platelets, Drugs and Thrombosis* (ed. J. Hirsch), Karger, Basle, pp. 258-62

Folts, J. D. and Beck, R. A. (1980). Inhibition of platelet plugging in stenosed dog coronary arteries with sulfinpyrazone. In *Cardiovascular Actions of Sulphin-*

pyrazone: Basic and Clinical Research (ed. M. McGregor, J. F. Mustard, M. F. Oliver and S. Sherry), Symposia Specialists Inc., Miami, pp. 211-28

Folts, J. D. and Rowe, G. G. (1979). Inhibition of platelet plugging in stenosed dog coronary arteries with sulfinpyrazone. *Clin. Res.*, **27**, 612A

Forfar, J. C., Russell, D. C. and Oliver, M. F. (1980). Haemodynamic effects of sulphinpyrazone on exercise responses in normal subjects. *Lancet*, *ii*, 718-20

Forfar, J. C., Russell, D. C. and Oliver, M. F. (1981). Haemodynamic effects of sulphinpyrazone: clinical and experimental studies. *Br. Heart J.*, **45**, 350-1

Haft, J. I. and Fani, K. (1973). Intravascular platelet aggregation in the heart induced by stress. *Circulation*, **47**, 353-8

Harker, L. A. and Ross, R. (1979). Prevention of homocysteine-induced arteriosclerosis: sulphinpyrazone endothelial protection. In *A New Approach to Reduction of Cardiac Death* (ed. T. Abe and S. Sherry), Huber, Basle, pp. 59-71

Iansmith, D. H. S., Riddle, J. R. and Bandura, J. P. (1979). Protection against acid-induced changes in canine cardiac microelectrophysiology by sulfinpyrazone. *Circulation*, **60**, Suppl. II, 209 (abstr. 815)

Kaegi, A., Pineo, G. F., Shimizu, A., Trivedi, H., Hirsh, J. and Gent, M. (1974). Arteriovenous-shunt thrombosis. Prevention by sulfinpyrazone. *New Engl. J. Med.*, **290**, 304-6

Kelliher, G. J., Dix, R. K., Jurkiewicz, N. and Lawrence, T. L. (1980). Effects of sulfinpyrazone on arrhythmia and death following coronary occlusion in cats. In *Cardiovascular Actions of Sulfinpyrazone: Basic and Clinical Research* (ed. M. McGregor, J. F. Mustard, M. F. Oliver and S. Sherry), Symposia Specialists Inc., Miami, pp. 193-209

Leprán, I., Koltai, M. and Szekeres, L. (1981). Effect of non-steroid anti-inflammatory drugs in experimental myocardial infarction in rats. *Eur. J. Pharmac.*, **69**, 235-8

Lewis, G. P. and Westwick, J. (1977). An *in vivo* model for studying arterial thrombosis. In *Thromboembolism – A New Approach to Therapy* (ed. J. R. A. Mitchell and J. G. Domenet), Academic Press, London. pp. 40-54

Livio, M., Villa, S. and Gaetano, G. de (1980). Long-lasting inhibition of platelet prostaglandin but normal vascular prostacyclin generation following sulphinpurazone administration to rats. *J. Pharm. Pharmac.*, **32**, 718-9

Margulies, E. H., White, A. M. and Sherry, S. (1980). Sulfinpyrazone: a review of its pharmacological properties and therapeutic use. *Drugs*, **20**, 179-97

Moncada, S., Higgs, E. A. and Vane, J. R. (1977). Human arterial and venous tissues generate prostacyclin (prostaglandin X), a potent inhibitor of platelet aggregation. *Lancet*, *i*, 18-21

Moschos, C. B., Escobinas, A. J. and Jorgensen, O. B. (1980). Effects of sulfinpyrazone on ischaemic myocardium. In *Cardiovascular Actions of Sulphinpyrazone: Basic and Clinical Research* (ed. M. McGregor, J. F. Mustard, M. F. Oliver and S. Sherry), Symposia Specialists Inc., Miami, pp. 175-91

Murphy, E. A. and Mustard, J. F. (1962). Coagulation tests and platelet economy in atherosclerotic and control subjects. *Circulation*, **25**, 114-25

Mustard, J. F. and Packham, M. A. (1975). Platelets, thrombosis and drugs. *Drugs*, **9**, 19-76

Mustard, J. F., Rowsell, H. C., Smythe, H. A., Senyi, A. and Murphy, E. A. (1967). The effect of sulphinpyrazone on platelet economy and thrombus function in rabbits. *Blood*, **29**, 859-66

Needleman, P., Kulkarni, P. S. and Raz, A. (1977). Coronary tone modulation: formulation and actions of prostaglandins, endoperoxides and thromboxanes. *Science, N. Y.*, **195**, 409-12

Newland, H. (1979). Hyperuricemia in coronary, cerebral and peripheral arterial disease: an explanation. *Med. Hypoth.*, **1**, 152-5

Povalski, H. J., Olson, R., Kopia, S. and Furness, P. (1980). Comparative effects of sulfinpyrazone and aspirin in the coronary occlusion-reperfusion dog model. In *Cardiovascular Actions of Sulphinpyrazone: Basic and Clinical Research* (ed. M. McGregor, J. F. Mustard, M. F. Oliver and S. Sherry), Symposia Specialists Inc., Miami, pp. 153-73

Rabkin, S. W. and Ohmae, M. (1980). Effect of sulfinpyrazone on adriamycin-induced acute cardiotoxic arrhythmias in rabbits. *Pharmac. Res. Commun.*, **12**, 195-204

Robbins, S. L., Berger, R. L., Suda, Y. and Ryan, T. J. (1969). Myocardial infarction produced by temporary microcoronary occlusion. *Circulation*, **40**, Suppl. III, 171

Roos, J. C. and Dunning, A. J. (1980). Clinical electrophysiological effects of sulfinpyrazone. *Circulation*, **62**, Suppl. III, 83 (abstr. 302)

Shragge, B. W., Robertson, M. A., Nolan, W. T., Buchanan, M. R. and Hirsh, J. (1980). The antiarrhythmic properties of sulfinpyrazone in the isolated rabbit heart. *Circulation*, **62**, Suppl. III, 83 (abstr. 301)

Smythe, H. A., Ogryzlo, M. A., Murphy, E. A. and Mustard, J. F. (1965). The effect of sulfinpyrazone (Anturan) on platelet economy and blood coagulation in man. *Can. med. Assoc. J.*, **92**, 818-21

Steele, P., Battock, D. and Genton, E. (1975). Effects of clofibrate and sulfinpyrazone on platelet survival time in coronary artery disease. *Circulation*, **52**, 473-6

Thomas, M., Gabe, I. T. and Mills, C. J. (1980). Vasodilator effects of sulfinpyrazone in dogs. *J. cardiovasc. Pharmac.*, **2**, 771-6

Weily, H. S. and Genton, E. (1970). Altered platelet function in patients with prosthetic mitral valves. Effects of sulfinpyrazone therapy. *Circulation*, **42**, 967-72

Wilcox, R. G., Richardson, D., Hampton, J. R., Mitchell, J. R. A. and Banks, D. C. (1980). Sulphinpyrazone in acute myocardial infarction: studies on cardiac rhythm and renal function. *Br. med. J.*, **281**, 531-3

20

Treatment of Arrhythmias in the Early Stages of Clinical Acute Myocardial Infarction

R. G. Shanks

20.1 THE NATURE OF THE PROBLEM

Ventricular fibrillation is the commonest cause of death in the early stages of acute myocardial infarction. Prompt correction of this arrhythmia by external cardiac massage and direct current countershock may prevent death. Coronary care units were established in the belief that in many cases ventricular fibrillation was preceded by warning arrhythmias and that these could be suppressed by drug treatment (Lown and Vassaux, 1968). Even though these statements were made over 13 years ago, there is still no agreement on the relationship between the occurrence of the so-called warning arrhythmias and the appearance of ventricular fibrillation. Although these arrhythmias may precede ventricular fibrillation, this fatal arrhythmia may occur without warning arrhythmias (*Lancet*, 1979). On the basis that warning arrhythmias did precede ventricular fibrillation, drug treatment regimes were developed to try and prevent or abolish these arrhythmias.

In 1968, Lown stated,

> 'Since the occurrence of catastrophic arrhythmias appears to be most common at the very inception of a coronary attack, this is the very time to institute prophylactic treatment. Lidocaine (lignocaine) should, therefore, be one of the earliest measures employed as soon as the diagnosis is made.'

Surprisingly, 13 years later, there appears to be little information available to either support or refute this recommendation. After reviewing the available literature Harrison (1978) concluded that,

> 'the routine administration of lidocaine to all patients in the coronary care unit (c.c.u.) seems indicated. . . . The rationale for these recommendations are: (1) routine prophylaxis prevents primary ventricular fibrillation; (2)

warning arrhythmias are absent or are missed in a high percentage of patients in the coronary care unit; and (3) rational programmes for administration minimise the likelihood of toxicity.'

In contrast, an editorial in *The Lancet* (1979) on the same subject concluded that

'prophylactic lignocaine in the c.c.u. is unnecessary, since V.F. can be so readily treated, whereas its administration to patients before they have access to monitors and defibrillators might save lives. Unhappily, there are no adequate controlled trials to show whether this is so (Lovell, 1978).'

As these two opposing conclusions were reached after consideration of much the same material, it would appear that there is considerable confusion about the effectiveness of antiarrhythmic drugs in treating ventricular arrhythmias. There are a number of areas in which there is disagreement, confusion and an absence of hard information. These include the value of warning arrhythmias in predicting ventricular fibrillation; the effect of antiarrhythmic drugs in preventing and in abolishing these arrhythmias; the effect of these drugs on mortality.

Antiarrhythmic drugs can be used in several different ways in patients with acute myocardial infarction. They may be given to treat an established arrhythmia or to prevent an arrhythmia occurring and leading to ventricular fibrillation and death.

Many studies have confirmed the effectiveness of drugs in the treatment of arrhythmias in the later stages of acute myocardial infarction, but there are few studies in the very early stages of infarction. This paper is confined to a survey of the effects of antiarrhythmic drugs on arrhythmias occurring in the very early stages of acute myocardial infarction - defined as the first 2 h after the onset of symptoms. The studies are of two types - those in which the drugs are given as treatment and those in which they are given prophylactically to prevent arrhythmias, ventricular fibrillation and death.

A survey of the literature indicates that there have been very few studies on the efficacy of antiarrhythmic drugs in the treatment of arrhythmias occurring within the first 2 h after acute myocardial infarction. Although several drugs are used to treat arrhythmias occurring in the later stages of acute myocardial infarction, for example, mexiletine, disopyramide, procainamide, phenytoin and quinidine, lignocaine is the most widely used drug; however, recent studies indicate that it may be less effective than mexiletine (Horowitz *et al.*, 1981). For treatment within the first few hours of the onset of acute myocardial infarction, lignocaine is clearly the drug of choice as it is easier to maintain the plasma concentration within the therapeutic range and there is probably a greater ratio between the plasma concentration for a therapeutic effect and for adverse effects than with the other drugs.

There are several reasons for the paucity of investigations on the efficacy of lignocaine in the early stages of infarction, these include the following:

(1) There is a high mortality rate in the first 2 h after the onset of symptoms of infarction with about 50 per cent of patients dying within the first 2 h, and in the majority of these death occurs before it has been possible to institute treatment. In men of middle age or younger, 63 per cent of deaths occur within 1 h of the onset of symptoms (Bainton and Peterson, 1963). The rate of mortality then rapidly declines (Pantridge, 1970). Thus the number of patients available for treatment falls rapidly during the first 2 h.

(2) The onset of symptoms of acute myocardial infarction occur in a large majority of patients when they are removed from medical attention. A study has shown that only 16 per cent of patients reach hospital within 4 h of the onset of symptoms and probably less than 5 per cent in less than 2 h (Pantridge, 1970). Thus the number of patients who reach hospital and are available for study or treatment with antiarrhythmic drugs will be extremely small. Although it may be rewarding to study the effects of treatment in the early stages of infarction, it is difficult because of the rapid increase in mortality and the small number of patients seen at this time. The introduction of mobile coronary care has enabled patients to be seen much earlier after the onset of symptoms of acute infarction (Pantridge and Geddes, 1967). As a result, events occurring in the first few hours after the initial event and the effects of intervention have been able to be monitored.

Before considering the effects of drugs on the arrhythmias occurring in the early stages of infarction, it is necessary to examine their nature and occurrence. The most detailed study was that described by Pantridge and his colleagues (Pantridge *et al.*, 1975). Observations were made in 294 patients seen within 1 h of the onset of symptoms of acute infarction and followed for at least 4 h. The occurrence of ventricular ectopics, ventricular fibrillation and ventricular tachycardia in the first and second hours respectively were 171 (58 per cent) and 80 (27 per cent); 28 (9.5 per cent) and 13 (4.5 per cent); six (2 per cent) and four (1.5 per cent). Thus ventricular ectopic beats occurred in 85 per cent of patients within the first 2 h of the onset of symptoms. There was a higher incidence of all arrhythmias in the first hour than in the second. This study clearly shows a very high incidence of ventricular arrhythmias in patients who have survived an acute infarction and are seen within the first 2 h.

Treatment of ventricular arrhythmias in the early stages may be commenced either in the belief that suppression of such arrhythmias may reduce the chances of ventricular fibrillation occurring, or that their correction may correct any adverse haemodynamic effects that may be present as a result of the arrhythmia.

20.2 LIGNOCAINE IN THE TREATMENT OF EARLY POST-INFARCTION ARRHYTHMIAS

Pantridge (1971) has described the effects of lignocaine on ventricular ectopics occurring within the first 2 h of the onset of symptoms. Lignocaine was given intravenously as a loading dose of 100 mg followed immediately by an infusion of 2 mg min^{-1} to patients in whom ventricular ectopics persisted at a rate greater than 5 min^{-1}, or when ventricular ectopics were frequent in the presence of a heart rate not less than 90 beats min^{-1}. Lignocaine was given to 96 patients seen within 2 h and its effects were determined in 66 of these patients. Lignocaine abolished ventricular ectopics in 33 per cent of patients, reduced them in 38 per cent and had no effect in 29 per cent of patients.

Plasma concentrations of lignocaine were not measured in this study, and it is not clear if the failure to respond to lignocaine resulted from low plasma lignocaine concentrations. It was also not stated whether there were any differences between the patients who responded and those that did not respond, for example, in age, severity of arrhythmia, location of infarct, and haemodynamic status. The outcome of treatment on prevention of ventricular fibrillation or on mortality was not included.

Further observations on the efficacy of lignocaine in the early stages of acute infarction have been reported by Webb and his colleagues in Belfast (Webb, 1974). Patients seen within 4 h of the onset of symptoms of acute myocardial infarction complicated by ventricular ectopics were considered for inclusion in the study. Patients with severe left ventricular failure, cardiogenic shock, AV block, continuous ventricular tachycardia or ventricular fibrillation were excluded. Pain was relieved with diamorphine and cyclizine. Patients were randomly allocated to treatment with lignocaine (100 mg bolus intravenously followed immediately by an infusion at 2 mg min^{-1}) or practolol (10 mg intravenously). The effects of the two drugs was assessed from a continuous recording of the electrocardiogram obtained for 5-10 min before drug administration and for 10 min after treatment. The number of sinus beats and ventricular ectopics was counted in each minute. The number of ventricular ectopics during the control period was compared with the number which occurred during a similar period after drug administration.

One hundred and four patients entered the trial but the effect of the test drug could not be assessed in 57 patients, 30 of whom received lignocaine and 27 practolol. These patients were excluded for the following reasons: infrequent ectopics during the control period (13 and 12); a control period of less than 5 min (seven and nine); acute coronary insufficiency (eight and six) and atrial fibrillation (two and zero). The first of each pair of numbers in brackets is the patients who *would* have received lignocaine and the second patient who *would* have been allocated to practolol.

The final study comprised 47 patients, 23 of whom received lignocaine and 24 practolol. The patients were well matched for sex, age, site of infarction, previous history of infarction and number of patients with heart rate either greater or less than 90 beats min^{-1}. Each treatment group was divided into those patients with heart rates less than 90 and above 90 beats min^{-1}.

The results of treatment are given in tables 20.1 and 20.2. Lignocaine abolished or reduced ventricular ectopics in 67 per cent and had no effect in 33 per cent of patients with an initial heart rate in the range 60-90 beats min^{-1}. The effect of lignocaine was less in the patients whose initial heart rate was greater than 90 beats

Table 20.1 Effect of lignocaine on ventricular ectopics in 23 patients with acute myocardial infarction treated within 4 h of the onset of symptoms (from Webb, 1974)

Heart rate (beats min^{-1})	Number of patients	Effect of lignocaine		
		> 75 per cent reduction	50–75 per cent reduction	No effect or increased
60–90	15	8 (54 per cent)	2 (13 per cent)	5 (33 per cent)
> 90	8	1 (12.5 per cent)	2 (25 per cent)	5 (62.5 per cent)

Table 20.2 Effect of practolol on ventricular ectopics in 24 patients with acute myocardial infarction treated within 4 h of the onset of symptoms (from Webb, 1974)

Heart rate (beats min^{-1})	Number of patients	Effect of practolol		
		> 75 per cent reduction	50–75 per cent reduction	No effect or increased
60–90	11	3 (27.5 per cent)	2 (18 per cent)	6 (54.5 per cent)
> 90	13	3 (23 per cent)	6 (46 per cent)	4 (31 per cent)

min^{-1} as ectopic activity was only reduced or abolished in 37.5 per cent. Practolol reduced or abolished ectopics in 45.5 per cent of patients whose heart rate was less than 90 beats min^{-1} and in 69 per cent of patients with an initial rate over 90 beats min^{-1}.

None of the patients who received lignocaine developed ventricular fibrillation within 10 min of the commencement of lignocaine therapy but it occurred in two patients 2 and 10 min after practolol administration.

This appears to be the only study of the effects of lignocaine on ventricular ectopic beats occurring within 2 h of the onset of symptoms of acute myocardial infarction with random allocation of patients to lignocaine therapy. In retrospect the study may be criticised on a number of grounds. No placebo group was included as it was thought unjustified. This may have been a correct decision at the time but subsequent studies on the prophylactic use of lignocaine have included placebo treatment and with the absence of a placebo group it is more difficult to be certain that the effects observed resulted from drug administration as spontaneous disappearance of ventricular ectopics may occur (Allen, 1972). However, this would not account for the absence of an effect of lignocaine in a high percentage of patients.

The electrocardiogram was only monitored for 10 min after drug administration. While this will show the immediate effects of the drug, it does not indicate whether the drug will continue to have an effect in those patients in whom it was initially effective or would have a delayed onset of action in those patients in whom it was not initially effective. Thus a longer period of monitoring may have provided further important information, but the problems of carrying out such studies outside hospital may be considerable. Further information about any additional treatment given to those patients who did not respond to lignocaine would have been of value. Information on mortality or outcome of treatment is important and was also not provided. The plasma concentrations of the drugs were not measured.

This study provided little explanation for the relative ineffectiveness of lignocaine in abolishing ventricular ectopic beats during the first 2 h after the onset of symptoms of acute infarction. In contrast, several studies have shown that lignocaine is much more effective in abolishing arrhythmias in the later stages (greater than 24 h) after infarction (Ribner *et al.*, 1979). By dividing the patients into two groups with initial heart rates below or above 90 beats min^{-1}, the effects of a high heart rate on the response to lignocaine was isolated. However, in patients with a heart rate below 90 beats min^{-1}, the drug was ineffective in 33 per cent of patients. A number of factors may contribute to this poor response.

It is generally accepted that the plasma concentration of lignocaine required for a therapeutic effect is above 2 $\mu g\ ml^{-1}$ (Winkle *et al.*, 1975). Although the plasma concentrations of lignocaine were not measured in this study, it is most likely that during the 10 min period of observation the plasma concentration will be above this value after a bolus injection of 100 mg and an infusion of 2 mg min^{-1} (Campbell *et al.*, 1978). The plasma concentration is more likely to fall below 2 $\mu g\ ml^{-1}$ 30-60 min after the start of this regime. Thus it is unlikely that the poor response in the patients with heart rates below 90 beats min^{-1} resulted from a low plasma concentration of lignocaine.

During the early stages of acute infarction there may be increased activity of the autonomic nervous system (Pantridge *et al.*, 1975). In this study sympathetic over-activity was assessed by the presence of sinus tachycardia, transient hypertension (blood pressure 160/100 mmHg) or both in patients seen within 30 min of the onset of symptoms of acute infarction. Among 89 patients seen within this time, 35 per cent had evidence of sympathetic over-activity, 25 per cent with a sinus tachycardia. Parasympathetic over-activity (sinus bradycardia, second degree or complete AV block, transient hypotension - systolic pressure less than 100 mmHg) was present in 48 per cent of patients with 40 per cent having bradyarrhythmia. Only 17 per cent had a normal heart rate and blood pressure.

As the study by Webb (1974) showed that lignocaine was less effective in patients with heart rates greater than 90 beats min^{-1} and such patients may be classified as having increased sympathetic activity, it may be that increased sympathetic activity may interfere with the antiarrhythmic action of lignocaine. In patients with normal heart rates and blood pressures the effects of increased sympathetic and parasympathetic activity may nullify each other on these parameters, but the increase in sympathetic activity may still interfere with the antiarrhythmic action of lignocaine. Such a hypothesis requires testing in laboratory animals.

The third possibility is that the mechanism of the arrhythmia in the first 2 h may be different to that in the later stages after infarction. At present there is little evidence from human clinical studies to support this hypothesis, although there is good animal data to support such a concept. However, there is probably inadequate scientific information at present available to conclude that lignocaine is less effective in the early than in the late stages after the onset of symptoms of acute infarction as there are limitations to the studies that have been completed. Furthermore, it is probably not correct to compare the effectiveness of lignocaine given to one group of patients seen within the first 2 h of infarction (and in whom its effect was only followed for 10 min) with the response in other groups seen, not only later after infarction, but in different centres under different conditions. Ideally one would hope to see a comparison of the effects of lignocaine using dosage regimes to maintain the plasma concentration in the therapeutic range both in patients within the first 2 h after the onset of symptoms and at a later stage after infarction. A longer period of monitoring (for example 2-4 h) after drug administration should be utilised and the effects of the drug should be compared on a randomised basis with a properly matched group receiving placebo.

20.3 OTHER ANTIARRHYTHMIC DRUGS IN THE TREATMENT OF EARLY POST-INFARCTION ARRHYTHMIAS

Several other drugs have been used for the treatment of ventricular ectopics including quinidine, procainamide, mexiletine and disopyramide. The latter two drugs have been more recently introduced and appear to have a greater therapeutic ratio than lignocaine. Studies have not yet been described of the effects of these drugs on the arrhythmias in the very early stages of acute infarction; however, as there may be differences in the pharmacological properties of these drugs (Opie, 1980) such studies are indicated, especially as mexiletine and disopyramide appear to be effective in treating ventricular ectopics that are resistant (non-responsive) to lignocaine (Campbell *et al.*, 1977; Sbarbaro *et al.*, 1979).

20.4 PROPHYLACTIC ADMINISTRATION OF DRUGS

Several studies have been carried out to see if the prophylactic administration of lignocaine to patients with acute infarction prevents the development of ventricular arrhythmias and, in particular, ventricular fibrillation and death. These studies can generally be criticised on several grounds, but the majority have had to be excluded from consideration in this paper as patients were often admitted for up to 24 h after the onset of symptoms of acute myocardial infarction.

A comprehensive analysis of these studies has recently been completed by Noneman and Rogers (1978). They document 13 trials of the prophylactic administration of lignocaine in patients with acute myocardial infarction but found that only six were double blind, admission time was not given in two, and in three trials only mean admission time was given; in two studies no loading dose of lignocaine was given and in five studies lignocaine was given by the intramuscular route, which meant that plasma levels were not in the therapeutic range during the first few hours of observation.

Of the trials, Noneman and Rogers (1978) considered that the study by Lie and his associates (Lie *et al.*, 1974) was the best designed for the selection of patients with the administration of adequate doses of lignocaine. In this study all patients started treatment in a coronary care unit within 6 h of the onset of symptoms of acute infarction. Patients received intravenously either lignocaine (100 mg with an infusion of 3 mg min^{-1}), or glucose and water for 48 h. There were 107 patients in the treated group and 105 in the control group. Ventricular fibrillation occurred in nine patients in the control group and in none in the treated group; but only one of the patients with ventricular fibrillation died. The mortality in the two groups was the same, deaths being due to causes other than ventricular fibrillation (cardiac rupture, cardiogenic shock and pulmonary oedema). However, it is important to note that if direct current cardioversion had not been available, the patients with ventricular fibrillation in the control group would have died and lignocaine would have had a beneficial effect on mortality. The dose of lignocaine in this study was probably adequate to maintain therapeutic plasma concentrations, but there may have been a trough in the early part of the study. At 6 h the blood lignocaine levels ranged from 1.5 to 6.4 μg ml^{-1} and side effects attributable to lignocaine occurred in 15 per cent of patients.

During the 48 h period of treatment and observation, ventricular fibrillation occurred in 11 of the control patients and in none of the treated patients; ventricular tachycardia occurred in six controls and in two treated patients and warning arrhythmias occurred in 61 controls and in 34 treated patients. Thus the administration of lignocaine prevented the occurrence of ventricular fibrillation but only produced a modest reduction in the frequency of warning arrhythmias. It is interesting that in this controlled study, where lignocaine in adequate doses was compared with placebo, the drug was not always effective in preventing ventricular arrhythmias. These results would support those of Pantridge and Webb (described earlier) that lignocaine was not effective in all patients after acute infarction.

This study also showed that four of the nine patients with primary ventricular fibrillation did not exhibit warning arrhythmias before the occurrence of ventricular fibrillation and that warning arrhythmias were documented in 59 per cent of the patients in the control group who did not have ventricular fibrillation. This study suggested that the administration of lignocaine to patients with acute myocardial infarction prevented the occurrence of ventricular fibrillation but had little effect on warning arrhythmias and that warning arrhythmias were not necessarily of value in predicting ventricular fibrillation. However, the patients were admitted for up to 6 h after the onset of symptoms of acute myocardial infarction, while this current review is only concerned with the first 2 h after the onset of symptoms. This study by Lie and his colleagues (Lie *et al.*, 1974) clearly indicates that lignocaine may be of considerable value to patients in the early stages of acute infarction but that studies must be carried out in which the drug is given within the first 2 h after infarction and the patients followed for some time. Such studies must reach given standards and be organised to provide information that would be of practical value.

20.5 CONCLUSIONS

Since lignocaine has been widely used to prevent and treat ventricular arrhythmias occurring after acute myocardial infarction for nearly 20 years, it is surprising that little information is available about its effects within the first few hours after the onset of symptoms of acute myocardial infarction. The studies which have been summarised in this paper show that lignocaine was only effective in abolishing ventricular arrhythmias in 33 per cent of patients (Pantridge, 1971). With the development of mobile or pre-hospital coronary care systems, facilities are now being made available for the treatment of patients shortly after the onset of symptoms of infarction. Thus more information must be obtained about the role of drug therapy in abolishing or preventing ventricular ectopics in the early stages of infarction.

Such studies must be organised to eliminate the limitations present in some of the previous studies in this field. Observations must be made in patients within 2 h of the onset of symptoms of acute infarction. This will probably necessitate making observations using mobile coronary care, which will restrict the number of centres in which such observations can be made. Furthermore, it is more difficult to carry out double blind controlled trials under such conditions and to adhere to the critical standards that may require to be followed. Patients for such studies may be selected in two different ways. First, patients who have ventricular ectopics may be selected for inclusion. In this way the effect of an antiarrhythmic drug on an established arrhythmia may be shown. In this case the electrocardiogram would need to be followed before a decision is made about starting treatment. Secondly, or alternatively, patients with symptoms of acute infarction may be accepted for inclusion regardless of the presence or absence of arrhythmias. In this way, not only the effect of a drug in treating an established arrhythmia will be studied but in addition its effectiveness in preventing ventricular ectopics will also be investigated. Information is required in both of these areas. In these studies the patients should be divided into two groups which should be matched to compare the effects of active drug against a placebo. Electrocardiographic monitoring should be carried out in patients before and for at least 2 h after the start of drug administration. This period should be adequate to investigate an effect on ventricular arrhythmias in the short term, but if possible should be longer to see if the response of such arrhythmias varies with time. As there is little information available on the response of ventricular arrhythmias to antiarrhythmic drugs in the early stages of infarction, it is important that the effect of the active drug is compared to that of an inactive placebo, with drug and placebo randomly allocated in a single or double blind fashion. While short time drug administration may be of value in demonstrating an effect on established arrhythmias, longer periods of administration will be required to establish an effect on mortality. It is essential that an adequate dose of drug is administered to maintain the plasma concentration in the therapeutic plasma concentration range from as soon after the commencement of drug administration as possible. This, for lignocaine, will involve a regime other than the standard practice of a bolus of 100 mg and an intravenous infusion of 2 mg min^{-1}; suitable regimes may be those described by Aps *et al.* (1976), who gave a bolus or 100 mg followed by a constant intravenous infusion of 4 mg min^{-1} for 30 min, 2 mg min^{-1} for 2 h and 1 mg min^{-1} thereafter, and by Barber *et al.* (1977), who used a regime combining 100 mg intravenously and 300 mg by intramuscular injection.

Similar studies should be carried out with the newer antiarrhythmic drugs such as mexiletine and disopyramide using adequate doses of drugs to maintain plasma concentrations in the therapeutic range.

ACKNOWLEDGEMENT

Tables 20.1 and 20.2 are published by kind permission of Dr S. W. Webb.

REFERENCES

Allen, J. D. (1972). Studies of the effects of drugs on cardiac arrhythmias. Thesis for the degree of Doctor of Medicine, The Queen's University, Belfast

Aps, C., Bell, J. A., Jenkins, B. S., Poole-Wilson, P. A. and Reynolds, F. (1976). Logical approach to lignocaine therapy. *Br. med. J.*, *i*, 13-15

Bainton, C. R. and Peterson, D. R. (1963). Deaths from coronary heart disease in persons fifty years of age and younger; community-wide study. *New Engl. J. Med.*, **268**, 569-75

Barber, J. M., Boyle, D. McC., Hussani, Z., Kelly, J. G. and McDevitt, D. G. (1977). Simple lignocaine regimen for transit to hospital after myocardial infarction. *Br. Heart J.*, **39**, 1361-3

Campbell, N. P. S., Kelly, J. G., Adgey, A. A. J., McDevitt, D. G. and Pantridge, J. F. (1978). Observations on intravenous administration of lignocaine in patients with myocardial infarction. *Br. Heart J.*, **40**, 1371-5

Campbell, N. P. S., Pantridge, J. F. and Adgey, A. A. J. (1977). Mexiletine in the management of ventricular dysrhythmias. *Eur. J. Cardiol.*, **6**, 245-58

Harrison, D. C. (1978). Should lidocaine be administered routinely to all patients after acute myocardial infarction. *Circulation*, **58**, 581-4

Horowitz, J. D., Anavekar, S. N., Morris, P. M., Goble, A. J., Doyle, A. E. and Louis, W. J. (1981). Comparative trial of mexiletine and lignocaine in the treatment of early ventricular tachyarrhythmias after acute myocardial infarction. *J. cardiovasc. Pharmac.*, **3**, 409-19

Lancet (1979). Antidysrhythmic treatment in acute myocardial infarction. Editorial. *Lancet*, *i*, 193-4

Lie, K. I., Wellens, H. J., van Capelle, F. J. and Durrer, D. (1974). Lidocaine in the prevention of primary ventricular fibrillation. *New Engl. J. Med.*, **291**, 1324-6

Lovell, R. R. H. (1978). Review of the present status of drug treatment for preventing sudden death. *Br. Heart J.*, **40**, Suppl., 94-8

Lown, B. and Vassaux, C. (1968). Lidocaine in acute myocardial infarction. *Am. Heart J.*, **76**, 586-7

Noneman, J. W. and Rogers, J. F. (1978). Lidocaine prophylaxis in acute myocardial infarction. *Medicine*, **57**, 501-15

Opie, L. H. (1980). Drugs and the heart. *Lancet*, *i*, 39-57

Pantridge, J. F. (1970). Mobile coronary care. *Chest*, **58**, 229-34

Pantridge, J. F. (1971). Emergency treatment of cardiac arrhythmias in myocardial infarction. In *Lidocaine in the Treatment of Ventricular Arrhythmias* (ed. D. B. Scott and D. G. Julian), Livingstone, Edinburgh and London, pp. 77-81

Pantridge, J. F. and Geddes, J. S. (1967). A mobile intensive-care unit in the management of myocardial infarction. *Lancet*, *ii*, 271-3

Pantridge, J. F., Adgey, A. A. J., Geddes, J. S. and Webb, S. W. (1975). *The Acute Coronary Attack*, Pitman Medical, Tunbridge Wells, Kent

Ribner, H. S., Isaacs, E. S. and Frishman, W. H. (1979). Lidocaine prophylaxis against ventricular fibrillation. *Progr. cardiovasc. Dis.*, **21**, 287-313

Sbarbaro, J. A., Rawling, D. A. and Fozzard, H. A. (1979). Suppression of ventricular arrhythmias with intravenous disopyramide and lidocaine. Efficacy comparison in a randomized trial. *Am. J. Cardiol.*, **44**, 513-20

Webb, S. W. (1974). The acute phase of myocardial infarction. Thesis for the degree of Doctor of Medicine, The Queen's University, Belfast

Winkle, R. A., Glantz, S. A. and Harrison, D. C. (1975). Pharmacologic therapy of ventricular arrhythmias. *Am. J. Cardiol.*, **36**, 629-50

Index

In this index, chapter numbers are indicated by the use of italic type and page numbers by roman type.